Disability in Medieval Europe

This is the first book that comprehensively describes disability and physical impairment in the Middle Ages. What attitudes did the medieval world have towards disabled people? Was every physical impairment a punishment for sin? And how did impairment affect the normal, everyday life of medieval disabled people? *Disability in Medieval Europe* presents a serious account of these and other aspects of the cultural construction of disability in that period of European history.

This book looks beyond the stereotype of physically impaired people as either beggars or court jesters by drawing upon modern disability studies, ethnology, history, medieval natural philosophy, medical texts and religious discourse. Medieval miracle narratives are examined for the invaluable information they can provide about the lived experience of impaired people, their social, economic and cultural position, right down to descriptions of what mobility aids were used. The book analyses the intellectual frameworks within which physical disability was positioned during the European Middle Ages, investigating medieval notions and constructs of disability. The emerging picture shows the ambivalence and fluidity of medieval attitudes to the physically impaired, revealing it was not necessarily viewed as being primarily caused by sin, as many historians have previously assumed.

Irina Metzler is a Research Fellow in the Department of Theology and Religious Studies, University of Bristol, UK.

Routledge Studies in Medieval Religion and Culture

Edited by George Ferzoco
University of Leicester

Carolyn Muessig
University of Bristol

This series aims to present developments and debates within the field of medieval religion and culture. It will provide a broad range of case studies and theoretical perspectives, covering a variety of topics, theories and issues.

1. **Gender and Holiness**
   Men, women and saints in late Medieval Europe
   Edited by Samantha J. E. Riches and Sarah Salih

2. **The Invention of Saintliness**
   Edited by Anneke B. Mulder-Bakker

3. **Tolkien the Medievalist**
   Edited by Jane Chance

4. **Julian of Norwich**
   Mystic or visionary?
   Kevin J. Magill

5. **Disability in Medieval Europe**
   Thinking about physical impairment during the high Middle Ages, *c.*1100–1400
   Irina Metzler

Disability in Medieval Europe

Thinking about physical impairment during the high Middle Ages, *c.*1100–1400

Irina Metzler

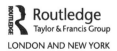
LONDON AND NEW YORK

First published 2006
by Routledge
2 Park Square, Milton Park, Abingdon, Oxon OX14 4RN

Simultaneously published in the USA and Canada
by Routledge
270 Madison Ave, New York, NY 10016

Routledge is an imprint of the Taylor & Francis Group

Transferred to Digital Printing 2010

© 2006 Irina Metzler

Typeset in Baskerville by
Newgen Imaging Systems (P) Ltd, Chennai, India

British Library Cataloguing in Publication Data
A catalogue record for this book is available from the British Library

Library of Congress Cataloging in Publication Data
A catalog record for this book has been requested

ISBN10: 0–415–36503–1 (hbk)
ISBN10: 0–415–58204–0 (pbk)

ISBN13: 978–0–415–36503–1 (hbk)
ISBN13: 978–0–415–58204–9 (pbk)

Contents

Acknowledgements   vii
List of abbreviations   viii

1   Introduction   1
   1.1   Structure, methodology and scope 1
   1.2   Definitions and stereotypes of disability 3

2   The theoretical framework of disability   11
   2.1   A historiography of disability 11
   2.2   Modern theories of disability and disability studies 20
   2.3   Summary 36

3   Medieval theoretical concepts of the (impaired) body   38
   3.1   Thisworldly: notions of health, impairment and sin 38
   3.2   Otherworldly: impairment and corporal resurrection 55
   3.3   Summary 62

4   Impairment in medieval medicine and
    natural philosophy   65
   4.1   Impairment and the medieval 'sciences' 65
   4.2   Aetiologies of impairment 71
   4.3   Preventative medicine 98
   4.4   Social and 'alternative' medicine 115
   4.5   Summary 122

5   Medieval miracles and impairment   126
   5.1   The context of saints, miracles and healing 126
   5.2   Medicine, transgression and miracle 138
   5.3   Narratives of impairment in medieval miracles 153
   5.4   Summary 183

6 Conclusion   186

Appendix: medieval miracle narratives   191

V   *Miracles* in vitae *from St Gall 191*
F   *Miracles of St Foy at Conques 194*
I   *Miracles of St Ithamar at Rochester 205*
W   *Miracles of St William of Norwich 207*
M   *Miracles of the Virgin Mary at Rocamadour 215*
J   *Miracles of the Hand of St James at Reading 224*
G   *Miracles of St Godric of Finchale 227*
E   *Miracles of St Elisabeth at Marburg 235*

Notes and references   260
Select bibliography   332
Index   347

Acknowledgements

To be able to metamorphise a thesis that was originally written for a limited readership consisting of a handful of academic examiners, and perhaps the odd future research student, into a published book, to be read by a wide audience, is perhaps the culmination of years of work, and vindication for those of us who saw beyond the depressed horizons of institutional grant applications. My heartfelt gratitude goes out to all those individuals who supported this project.

In the first instance, I am indebted to the Department of History at the University of Reading for the generous financial support given to me over the years towards my registration fees. I am further most grateful to the Institute of Historical Research at University College London for providing me with a Scouloudi Fellowship, which helped me during a pecuniarily desperate time. The Royal Historical Association assisted me with a travel grant, which enabled me to carry out necessary research at various libraries in London, while a further travel grant from the Wellcome Trust for the History of Medicine permitted me to carry out much-needed research at the Institut für Geschichte der Medizin at the University of Münster, Germany.

My thanks are further owed to my supervisor, Prof. Malcolm Barber, for his constructive criticisms with regards to work in progress, as well as my co-supervisor, Prof. Anne Curry, for her encouragement. While work was in progress on the thesis, Prof. Michael Biddiss and Dr Helen King read parts of my research which were eventually published as a separate, independent article. To turn what started life as a thesis into a proper book would not have been possible without the advice and support of the editors of this series, Dr Carolyn Muessig and Dr George Ferzoco, and the thoughtful critique of the anonymous reviewer for Routledge.

Overall, the completion of years of research and study, resulting in this present volume, would not have been achieved without the support and encouragement of my partner, extended family and friends.

Abbreviations

E   Jürgen Jansen (ed. and transl.), *Medizinische Kasuistik in den »Miracula Sancte Elyzabet«. Medizinhistorische Analyse und Übersetzung der Wunderprotokolle am Grab der Elisabeth von Thüringen (1207–1231)* (Marburger Schriften zur Medizingeschichte Band 15), Frankfurt am Main, Bern and New York: Verlag Peter Lang, 1985

F   Pamela Sheingorn (transl. with an introduction and notes), *The Book of Sainte Foy*, Philadelphia, PA: University of Pennsylvania Press, 1995

G   J. Stevenson (ed.), *Libellus de Vita et Miraculis S. Godrici, Heremitæ de Finchale, auctore Reginaldo Monacho Dunelmensi*, Surtees Society, 20, 1845

I   Denis Bethell (ed.), 'The Miracles of St Ithamar', *Analecta Bollandiana*, 89, 1971, pp. 421–37

J   Brian Kemp (ed. and transl.), 'The Miracles of the Hand of St James', *Berkshire Archaeological Journal*, 65, 1970, pp. 1–19

M   Marcus Bull, *The Miracles of Our Lady of Rocamadour: Analysis and Translation*, Woodbridge: Boydell, 1999

V   J. Duft, *Notker der Arzt. Klostermedizin und Mönchsarzt im frühmittelalterlichen St. Gallen*, St. Gall: Fehr'sche Buchhandlug, 1972

W   A. Jessop and M. R. James (ed. and transl.), *The Life and Miracles of St William of Norwich by Thomas of Monmouth*, Cambridge: Cambridge University Press, 1896

1 Introduction

1.1 Structure, methodology and scope

Disability and impairment have generally been used as quasi-synonymous terms by medical historians as well as by historians of the medieval period. Drawing on theories developed by modern sociology and anthropology, which allow a distinction to be made between the two terms, it is possible to discuss notions of impairment and disability in the Middle Ages as separate concepts. Such an approach provides a more meaningful form of enquiry, since it does not automatically assume that all impaired people were treated as disabled, in the Middle Ages or in other historic societies. It also allows us to treat physical impairment as a separate category from 'illness' in general, so that medieval concepts of impairment will no longer be confused with those relating to diseases such as plague or leprosy, as many medical historians have done. Questions this book addresses with regard to medieval notions of impairment, for example, revolve around ideas concerning the liminality of impairment, the differences between congenital impairment and impairment acquired in later life, and how strong or important the connection between spiritual sin and physical impairment was deemed to be in the Middle Ages. To answer these questions, I have chosen three more or less contingent fields of enquiry: medieval, theological and philosophical notions of the impaired body and how it was seen to differ from the perceived 'normal' body; medieval 'scientific' (medical and natural philosophical) views of impairment relating to causalities and prevention of such conditions; and medieval therapeutic measures in the form of miracle healings of the impaired. These areas can be regarded as contingent due to the nature of the sources which describe, position and explain impairment in the Middle Ages.

The sources I have employed in the main belong to those types of written record that one associates with the product of an intellectual and cultural elite, texts, that is, emanating from the environment of monasteries, cathedral schools and universities and from writers trained at such institutions. Since no unique or identifiable single corpus of medieval sources exists that deals specifically with physical impairment, in contrast to those studies which, for example, have a set of taxation records or manorial accounts to draw upon, my own investigations have had to be far more wide-ranging than is perhaps the norm for a medievalist. To achieve this, I have started with a reading of the secondary literature from various disciplines, including sociology, anthropology, medical history, as well as histories of medieval culture, before working backward, so to speak, to the original medieval material. The advantages of such an approach lie in the broad scope this brings to the subject, which allows one to gain an understanding of medieval impairment which is not restricted to, say, impairment in medical texts alone, but permits the (re)construction of wider cultural attitudes to and theories of impairment.

Chronologically, the book focuses on the period generally referred to as the high Middle Ages, that is the twelfth through to the middle of the fourteenth centuries. In part, this chronological restriction has been imposed by the nature of the sources: the greatest intellectual output, both in the quantity as well as the quality, of medieval writings on theology, (natural) philosophy, medicine and healing miracles falls within this period. Therefore, in effect, I am concentrating on sources influenced by and derived from the culture of Scholasticism. However, since many of the sources themselves (re)used earlier writers, it has been necessary to expand the time-span covered by this book to include references to important texts from ancient, biblical, patristic and early medieval sources.

Geographically, the text concentrates on what can be loosely described as Western Europe, that is those areas now part of modern France, Germany and England. The Mediterranean region is covered to a lesser extent, drawing mainly on examples from what now constitutes modern Italy and Spain. Some cultural cross-references are made to ancient or Islamic cultures, while occasionally the odd non-Occidental example from anthropology is cited to highlight specific cultural constructions of disability.

Because physical impairment in the Middle Ages has (to the best of my knowledge) never been researched before in a monograph as a distinct and identifiable subject, it seemed that the best way to initiate such a study was to focus on the theoretical framework and intellectual context of impairment in that period. This means that many other areas that could have been studied in relation to medieval impairment, such as the iconographic representation of physical impairment, the legal, economic and social situation of impaired people, and the care (or lack of it) provided for the impaired by medieval hospitals, have had to be omitted from this present research. It is anticipated, however, that by providing an outline of medieval cultural attitudes towards physical impairment, as is the aim of this book, future research into medieval impairment can build on the basic structures of a theoretical frame which will permit a qualitatively better interpretation and analysis of these other aspects.

One of the issues central to my research is the question whether we can at all refer to medieval 'disabled' persons, or whether we are dealing historically with medieval 'impaired' persons who might not share much of the 'special needs' status of their modern counterparts. It is therefore preferable to speak of 'impairment' during the medieval period, rather than of 'disability', which implies certain social and cultural connotations that medieval impaired persons may not have shared with modern impaired people. Notions of 'impairment', though attempts can be made to define them physiologically or medically, are never far removed from culturally constructed notions or from sociological notions. Any historical approach to 'impairment' or 'disability' should therefore explore not just past medical or biological theories of impairment, but tie these in with contemporary cultural notions, such as religious and philosophical ideas during the Middle Ages. Hence approaching the topic from an angle which utilises more than just literature relating to the history of medicine.

Throughout I try to differentiate 'impairment' and 'disability' (there may be the occasional lapses where force of habit and linguistic convention take over and 'disability' is used as the main term). The reason for this is that I have taken on board the distinctions posited by disability studies scholars, of impairment being the physical condition and disability the social construction of an impairment. Or, to explain it more precisely, impairment is the 'medically classified condition' whereas disability is the 'generic term used to denote the social disadvantage experienced by people with an accredited impairment'.[1] This terminology, first suggested by the British disabled people's movement, has essentially remained unchanged since 1981.[2] Some terminological tolerance, however, is needed by the modern reader, in that since I am dealing with a historical topic, I perforce have to quote historical words, labels and terms. Hence I will use the now archaic, abusive or politically incorrect terms 'cripple', 'dumb', 'mute' and such like without in future placing them in quotes. Lastly, I will be using the non-gendered term 'they' instead of the clumsy 'he and/or she', and certainly preferable to the biased 'he'.[3]

1.2 Definitions and stereotypes of disability

One should commence this enquiry into historic aspects of disability by asking what is meant by the terms 'disabled' and 'impaired'. Therefore I shall briefly address the problems involved in categorising disability in a modern context, followed by a discussion of what terminology the medieval period employed for disabled or impaired people. On the basis of the resulting findings, I outline what criteria I have followed in delineating certain physiological conditions as 'impairing'. Before embarking on a closer investigation of what 'impairment' and/or 'disability' meant in a medieval context (in the following chapters), I will also allude to modern stereotypes and prejudices concerning disability, as well as examining possible reasons why disability during the Middle Ages has so far not been deemed a suitable area for study.

Impairment is ubiquitous in human society, and as far as we can tell from the archaeological record, has been so in past human societies,[4] even being present in other vertebrate animals.[5] The World Health Organisation suggested that approximately 10 per cent of the world's population is either physically or mentally impaired at any given time,[6] which means that we may assume a similar proportion for past societies, including, the Middle Ages, as well. Impairment therefore is and has been a factor in a large number of people's lives, and it is necessary to study the implications and effects of impairment in past as well as present societies.

There are a number of problems relating to a study of impairment and disability in historic societies. To begin with, there is the wide scope of disability, both as a linguistic term and as a biological condition in the shape of impairment; there are many different kinds of physiologically impairing conditions, and there is also no one singular agreement in modern times on what constitutes 'disabled'. A World Health Organisation list of impairments[7] is the closest thing to this, but not everyone is happy either with these definitions or with using them. Essentially, definitions of disability are arbitrary and entirely subjective. As an example, Reading University has its own categories of disability as found in student registration documents, listing disabilities as follows:

> 1 dyslexia, 2 blind/partially sighted, 3 deaf/hearing impediment, 4 wheelchair user/mobility difficulties, 5 personal care support needed, 6 mental health disabilities, 7 unseen disability e.g. diabetes, epilepsy, asthma, 8 multiple difficulties, 9 a disability not listed above (please specify).[8]

Note the use of the phrase 'unseen disability' as distinct from the other categories. Maybe one way, for some people, to define a disability would be through an index of visibility, that is, the more noticeable an impairment is to others, the more of a disability it becomes.[9] Greater visibility of an impairment would therefore bring with it greater cultural or social consequences for the affected individual. This was also pointed out in a study of the representation of disabled people in cinema, where it was observed that cerebral palsy and epilepsy were the topics of only a minority of Hollywood films out of the many others that dealt with disability of all types.[10] The distinction between visible and invisible disability has important consequences for social expectations, that is, whether a person's disability is visible to others or not makes a profound difference as to how that person is perceived by their society. 'And because invisible disabilities are not readily apparent, their existence in the population tends to get forgotten or dismissed as inconsequential when the subject of disability is raised.'[11] The term 'disabled' in contemporary society stereotypically tends to conjure up the image of the wheelchair user, to the exclusion of people with auditory, visual or other invisible impairments.

The problem of categories of disability is further confounded by the lack of an umbrella term such as 'disability' during the medieval period. Medieval people were less 'politically correct' and more direct in their terminology, so a wide variety of descriptions of physical impairments that we would now reclassify as disabling exists in this period. Some physical impairments were recognised as such by medieval people, in other words the crippled (*contracti, defecti, decrepiti*), blind (*caeci*), mute (*muti*) or deaf (*surdi*) people, epileptics (*epileptici* or people with *morbus caducus*),[12] and children born with congenital deformities. For these afflictions the medieval period did have a specific terminology, albeit one that by modern standards is rather politically incorrect – some terminological tolerance is required of the reader – or deemed too vague by modern medicine. How vague medieval terminology could be is already evident if one looks at just one linguistic example, Middle English. 'Disease' (*disese*) was a general term in Middle English usage for trouble, misfortune or misery, encompassing both a notion of bodily discomfort, suffering or pain, as well as a notion of corporal infirmity or impairment. 'Sickness' (*siknes[se]*) was also a blanket term for an abnormal or special state of health, and could sometimes signify a specific mental or physical disorder.[13] In medieval Latin (which is the language of the vast majority of my sources), *infirmi*, *aegri* and *egroti* were often used as interchangeable terms for 'diseased', 'sick' and 'impaired'. *Infirmi* appears to be another umbrella term, referring to a wide range of afflictions. In hospital charters of the twelfth century, as in the hospital of St John at Jerusalem for example, inmates were nearly always described as *infirmi*, which modern translators usually render simply as 'sick', although strictly speaking that term should be translated in such a way as to convey the implicit meaning of 'chronically ill' or 'impaired', since *aegri* or *egroti* referred to 'sick'.[14]

Besides *infirmus*, there are any number of other vague references to disability as a concept, again mainly in Latin, for example, *deformans*, *malformans*, *decrepitus*, *imbecillis*, *impotens*, *debilitans*, *defectus*. So apart from the direct, precise terms, we can never be too certain that the vaguer terms actually imply the notion of disability, as they would in our parlance. If one accepts the distinction between the two terms 'impairment' and 'disability' as being contrasting notions, one a physical, the other a cultural one, then it is likely that the medieval period had only an awareness of the former but not the latter. The lack of the modern umbrella term 'disability' and the cultural implications it carries with it may also entail during the Middle Ages the lack of the entire notion of an impaired person as being disabled. This would be one of the propositions to examine. The medieval period certainly had a notion of impairment in the physical sense, as can easily be evidenced from medical texts.

For the sake of argument, therefore, I concentrate on somatic and sensory impairments. To establish some criteria as to which of the huge variety of potential impairments will be discussed, I utilised the outline categorisation of impairments worked out by ethnologists Neubert and Cloerkes,[15] as follows:

- extreme deformations or monstrosities, for example, two heads, lack of mouth, twisted head, misplaced eyes, twisted feet;
- impairments which notably restrict normal functions, for example, crippled or missing individual limbs, hunchback, clubfoot, lameness and paralysis, harelip, soft bones, and among sensory impairments: total blindness or deafness;
- little or no restriction of normal function, for example, surplus or deficit of toes or fingers, misshapen mouth, short stature (achondroplasia), partial or minor sight or hearing impairments.

Therefore not all orthopaedic disabilities (regardless of the modern medical aetiology, so including paralysis, amputation and musculo-skeletal deformations) would be equally 'disabling', nor would the visual, oral and auditory disabilities. I exclude deliberately the discussion of leprosy since it falls into a category of its own, with its own symbolism, meaning and aetiology.[16] For related reasons I also exclude mental illnesses, especially since a fair amount of research has already been done in this area.[17] Epilepsy is not discussed either, on the one hand since predominant medieval attitudes tended to regard epilepsy as either a form of mental illness (in the medical discourse) or demonic possession (in the theological discourse), on the other hand since a fairly exhaustive historical study of epilepsy has been conducted already.[18] Old age, however, will feature to some extent in my research. There has been an increasing recognition by theorists of disability of the overlap between disability and chronic illness, an overlap that had previously been downplayed. Most people in old age suffer some kind of chronic illness; hence most people in old age will at some point be disabled.[19] There is no reason to suppose that this situation will have been any different in the Middle Ages; therefore some of the problems of the ageing body will also be looked at.[20]

Before turning to a discussion of impairment in the Middle Ages, an excursion is necessary into modern attitudes, prejudices and assumptions with regard to 'disability'. I deem this necessary because our contemporary, modern attitudes influence how we try to analyse and interpret the past; that is, when faced with an impaired medieval person we would tend to judge their impairment, and how it might be disabling, by our culture's assumptions. Since this book is primarily concerned with medieval theoretical approaches to impairment, or 'attitudes', to put it another way, we have to be aware of our own cultural attitudes towards 'disability' before embarking on a historical study.

Policy makers in twentieth-century Britain, in the health services and government, too often concentrated purely on the material circumstances, that is the economic situation and employment question, of disabled people, to the neglect of factors that can broadly be classed as 'cultural'. The Leonard Cheshire charity, working with disabled people, emphasised this point in their research on the UK government's social exclusion policy: 'By limiting social exclusion to the effects of extreme poverty, the Government ignores a whole area which disabled people – not to mention a whole lot of other groups – know only too well: that of being excluded from society because of the attitudes of others.'[21]

An example of how arbitrary perceptions of disability may be in present culture, and how pervasive certain stereotypes are, is found in the following incident: a disabled airline passenger was asked to fill in a form prior to a flight asking whether the 'patient' was 'in any way offensive to other passengers (smell, appearance, conduct)' and also what arrangements had been made for his 'delivery' and 'collection'.[22] The disabled person here emerges as an 'object', to be handled like a piece of air freight. Additionally, the sensitivities, aesthetic or otherwise, of fellow non-disabled passengers are to be the deciding factors in assessing the level of disability – disability as defined by its visibility to non-disabled people.[23] Another case of the importance of disability being 'visible' to non-disabled people is the controversial use of cosmetic surgery on children with Down's syndrome with the aim of making them look more 'normal' so that they might be better accepted by other people,[24] as is happening in the United Kingdom at present. These examples of 'attitudes' to disabled people in modern

British society emphasise my point that 'disability' is created through more than medical or economic factors, but that cultural factors, the attitudes and reactions of non-disabled people, are just as significant. Hence my exploration of medieval disability will primarily concentrate on those types of sources that allow us to gain a picture of the cultural context of disability in that historic period.

Institutionalisation of impaired people in modern Western societies has had a significant effect on how impaired people viewed themselves, as well as how others viewed them. There is an argument that prior to the institutionalisation which happened in Western society increasingly from the nineteenth century on, the non-segregated presence of impaired people in their home communities, often in small, face-to-face societies, did not lead to the forming of a 'disabled identity' for the individual. How applicable this theory is will be seen in my discussions of modern disability theories (Chapter 2.2). With regard to the medieval period, the question of notions of 'disabled identity' will be addressed in Chapter 3. Nevertheless, the presence in society as a whole of the concept of 'disability' does not automatically lead to individual impaired persons being regarded, or seeing themselves, as 'disabled', as the following example may demonstrate: Snowy Harding, suffering from muscular dystrophy all his life, spent his childhood in the 1930s in London's East End, participating in the activities and play of the other children in his area, albeit having to do everything crawling (as his mother could not afford a wheelchair), which was accepted by the other children.[25] Interviewed, Harding said: '*I didn't know I was disabled* [my emphasis] until during the war, when I was 14 and the other kids were evacuated to families in the country. I was sent to an institution.'[26] Whereas impairment is a non-negotiable reality, disability, in this instance, is very much a matter of perception, both by others and by the individual concerned. A similar discrepancy between self-perception and the gaze of society as a whole was already found in a 1918 US study, the so-called Cleveland Cripple Survey. Among the impaired participants of the survey '[s]ome were amazed that they should be considered cripples, even though they were without an arm or a leg, or perhaps seriously crippled as a result of infantile paralysis. They had never considered themselves handicapped in any sense'.[27]

One crucial aspect of disability revolves around the issue of work. An interesting observation can be made on the relationship between an individual's impairment and the degree to which that individual is deemed incapable of earning their living as an indicator of 'disability' in our society. In some ways this relationship forms *the* main definition of 'disabled' in modern Western society. As Herzlich and Pierret have pointed out in the context of their study of illness and social attitudes:

> In a society in which we define ourselves as producers, illness and inactivity have become equivalents. That is why today we have come to perceive the sick body essentially through its incapacity to 'perform', rather than through the alteration of its appearance.[28]

In a country where work, and the ability to work, held almost religious significance, such as the United States in the nineteenth and early twentieth centuries, disability becomes of prime importance to the aspiring immigrant. Legislation enacted by the US government to exclude unwanted 'aliens' on medical grounds concerned mainly those with contagious diseases, but also covered some disabilities. Such immigrants had been 'regarded as a menace both to the public health and to the public purse'.[29] Prospective immigrants were classed A, B or C according to the perceived danger of their disease, A being the most serious category. The various regulations enforced between 1903 and 1917 stipulated that persons with 'physical defects affecting their ability to earn a living' were excluded as class B diseased aliens; these included hernia, chronic rheumatism, deformities, senility and debility, varicose veins, serious defects in vision (defined as unaided vision of 20/70 or less), also 'poor physique' and pregnancy.[30] If the criteria of ability to work are so important in modern Western society, it is worth enquiring as to their importance during the medieval period, and if there were any cultural or economic circumstances during which the importance shifts or changes, although this is beyond the scope of the present work, but an important area for further study. Some aspects of a medieval person's ability or inability to work are, however, briefly discussed in Chapter 5.3, since occasionally the miracle narratives I have studied mention how physical impairment affected ability to sustain one's livelihood.

One aspect of disability that is very important with regard to the medieval period is the apparent connection between physical disability and sin made in medieval times – 'apparent', since, as will be discussed in Chapters 3.1 and 4.2, such a link between sin and disability (or ill-health in general) is not as straightforward as the secondary literature has tended to assume. As a preamble to my further discussion of sin and disability in the Middle Ages I will here cite one modern, contemporary expression of the idea that sin and disability are connected. In early 1999, England football coach Glen Hoddle remarked that the disabled were paying for the sins of a previous life. Hoddle seemed to mix a quasi-Buddhist idea of reincarnation with Christian prejudicial notions of sin. As will be demonstrated later (in Chapter 4.2 on aetiologies of impairment), the idea that an impairment present from birth is the result of a sinful action by the parents, or that an acquired impairment is punishment for one's own sins (some examples in Chapter 5.3 on narratives of impairment in medieval miracles), is not exactly unheard of in Christian thought. Hoddle was justly criticised, amongst many by Phil Greer in *Disability Times*, who pointed out that his remarks 'pander to the type of prejudices that all those involved in disability issues have striven to eradicate from our society'.[31] In nineteenth-century literature, one finds the example of Samuel Butler's (1835–1902) utopian satire *Erewhon*, where the citizens of the imaginary land Erewhon regard disability and sickness as a crime and punish the 'offence', treating their sick and disabled like criminals while treating their criminals like sick people. How prevailing such attitudes appeared to be in the Middle Ages remains to be considered in this volume.

Having explored some of the more recent prejudices against disabled people I think it is only worth pointing out some of the prejudices against the Middle Ages and that period's perceived conduct towards disability. In other words, why study disability in the Middle Ages, of all historic periods? Popular notions of the medieval period as dark, barbaric and superstitious, to name but a few stereo-types, still abound. In the context of disability, this period is almost invariably held up as *the* worst time in human history to have been a disabled person. Such a popular perception is described, for example, by actor Stacy Keach, himself disabled and chair of the American Cleft Palate Foundation, who, with regard to people with cleft palate, 'counts his blessings': '...Had I been born in the Middle Ages, I would never have lasted. I would have been instantly killed, because children like me would have been considered the instruments of the devil.'[32] In a culture where popular concepts of the Middle Ages[33] are a result of a digestion of a steady diet of the 'fast-food world'[34] of fantasy films and novels, Dungeons and Dragons role playing games or New Age pseudo-philosophies one might expect such attitudes. However, even amongst scholars of the medieval period the subject of disability is treated so ahistorically that similar statements can be made: 'The medievals felt that disfiguration, deformation or any abnormality was a sentence imposed by God. They freely laughed at such people. Throwing stones at cripples, lepers, etc. was considered great fun. So of course the monarch would laugh "at" [the court jester or fool]. That was the whole reason why such people existed.'[35] If the Middle Ages are a neglected area of history, and disability history is also neglected – see Chapter 2.1 on historiography – then disability in the Middle Ages is a doubly neglected field of study.

The aim is not just to catalogue evidence of different impairments or 'disabilities' in the Middle Ages, but to try and explain their meanings within a specific cultural context. Hence the important question: What constitutes a disability, or an ability for that matter, in a given culture? To answer this the crucial point to be borne in mind is that 'disability' is a cultural construction. Disability has no 'inherent meaning'[36] outside of culture; one cannot therefore speak automatically of all impaired persons as disabled at all times, in all places. The main theory to be examined, then, could be that there were no 'disabled' people in the Middle Ages, only impaired people. If the distinction between biological, physical impair-ment on the one hand and cultural, constructed disability on the other is made, then one also has to take issue with the medical model of disability, which does not permit such a distinction. To the medical model, impairment and disability are practically co-terminous. The medical model, moreover, is not appropriate to an investigation of disability in historic terms, in that past societies (or contemporary societies other than our own) have had impairment but may not have had 'disability'. If the medical model is used, then it is at the risk of 'contam-inating the...evidence with modern cultural assumptions'.[37] To an extent, one has to examine whether and how (modern) disability theories, which make the distinction between 'impairment' and 'disability', can be applied to the medieval period, for the simple reason that until now no other theoretical framework for a discussion of disability within a cultural context exists.

As such, my approach to the source material can be described as an emic[38] approach, as opposed to the etic[39] approach so often found in medical histories. I hereby follow on from concepts formulated first by linguists and picked up by ethnological theorists, namely in distinguishing between an emic and an etic perspective. An emic perspective describes the specific world-view of a culture as it is usual within that culture, while an etic perspective is generalising and comparative, and the categories used by the ethnologist are equally utilised for different cultures. One of the most important differences between emic and etic perspectives is that an emic approach treats cultural criteria as related to internal characteristics (i.e. within that culture) while an etic approach treats cultural criteria as absolutes or universals.[40] Hence it is possible to regard 'disability' as an emic condition, in that it is culturally constructed, and therefore culturally specific, and 'impairment' as an etic condition, in that it is biological and (apparently) transcultural.

2 The theoretical framework of disability

2.1 A historiography of disability

Disability *per se* is only recently becoming an area of interest academically, outside the medical disciplines. As Charles T. Wood has pointed out in the context of an historical analysis of menstruation, historians have viewed their discipline as being primarily concerned with the very processes of change, and since 'like the poor, taxes, and death, menstruation has always been with us, *it seemed a subject scarcely in need of historical explanation*'[1] (my emphasis). One could easily add disability to Wood's list. Like other under-studied groups, such as women, the working classes, or ethnic minorities, it is only in recent decades that they have been discovered by academic disciplines, and, in the case of disability, really only within the last decade and a half – they have been marginalised historiographically. Even then (the history of) disability has been one of the more neglected areas. Here most academic pursuits hinge around the history of the development of facilities for the disabled, the 'rehabilitation' of the disabled into society, the impact of the Welfare State, the idea of special needs, and, of course, the politicisation of disability – all of which pertain exclusively to modern history. In general, as far as histories of disability are concerned, I agree with the comments made by one disability studies scholar:

> A key defect of most accounts of handicap is their blind disregard for the accretions of history. Insofar as such elements do enter into accounts of handicap, they generally consist of a ragbag of examples from Leviticus via Richard III to Frankenstein, all serving to indicate the supposed perennial, 'natural' character of discrimination against the handicapped. Such 'histories' serve paradoxically to produce an understanding of handicap which is...an ahistorical one.[2]

Many modern texts on disability from a sociological, psychological or medical perspective regard it almost as a compulsory exercise to present a brief outline of the intercultural or historical reasons behind the social reactions to disability. In such texts, the respective position of the author means that either disability is seen from a progressionist viewpoint, whereby the fate of disabled people has steadily improved over time, or it is treated from a pessimistic viewpoint, stating that humanity as such has 'always' reacted to disability in the same, negative way, and therefore it is inevitable that disabled people would be treated badly.[3] Evolutionistic viewpoints such as the progressionist theory can be refuted easily enough through empirical evidence. To counter the culturally optimistic notion of a steady betterment in the treatment of disabled people from 'primitive' societies onward one need only look at the reaction to disabled people in modern, industrialised Western societies to question such simplistic assumptions: issues revolving around the sterilisation of mentally impaired people, the eugenic approach to pregnancy termination or the isolation of disabled people in institutions are factors that belie the progressionist theory.[4]

Earlier attempts at a history of disability stem mainly from the 1920s and 1930s – this dating is in itself significant – and then tend to focus on orthopaedic impairments. I would venture here that the impact of the First World War, and especially the visible, large numbers of maimed soldiers returning from the front, prompted academic as well as medical interest in disability and 'rehabilitation'. An article by Seth Koven appeared on precisely this historiographical point.[5] These decades between 1914 and 1939 produced a variety of articles, tracts and monographs on disability-related issues, the sheer number of which can be seen in the extensive bibliography to Deborah Cohen's work on disabled war veterans.[6] The most notable attempt at an overall history of disability was a book by Frederick Watson with the title *Civilisation and the Cripple* published in 1930[7] – the juxtaposition of 'civilisation' with 'cripple' says it all, I believe. Medicine is presented in this tome as the great benefactor of humanity, but only from the medicine of the Enlightenment onwards; the medieval period is passed over in one and a half paragraphs;[8] furthermore, in 'primitive' societies all cripples died quickly, which was only logical according to Watson's notions, no doubt based on ideas of 'survival of the fittest'. For Watson, the issue of disability was essentially a social 'problem'[9] that rational, scientific approaches, like medicine and institutionalisation, could resolve. A similar book purporting to write the history of disability was H. W. Haggard's *The Lame, the Halt and the Blind: The Vital Role of Medicine in the History of Civilization* published in 1932.[10] This was a popular-style book not intended for an academic audience, and in that respect was even more damaging in its reinforcement and shaping of popular misconceptions (the collapse of all things civilised during the medieval period) and stereotypes (disabled people are a problem to society). Here again the dominant discourse is progressionist: everything in the past, and of course especially in the medieval 'Dark Ages' of popular imagination, is seen as filthy and generally unhealthy, and only modern science can save people. Haggard went one step farther than Watson, though, in that Haggard did not even pretend any more to actually write about disabled people, as is evident from the title alone, instead seeing disability purely as a medical 'problem' of the past which civilisation has overcome.

This unfortunate expression of the stereotype of the 'Dark Ages' also still crops up in more recent works of medical history, in reference to discussing any period of history prior to the eighteenth century, it seems. In ancient societies, and this by implication includes the Middle Ages, according to one group of authors, people who were impaired were regarded as completely expendable since they failed to contribute to their society (a notion which is more closely linked with the Protestant work ethic than any observable facts about ancient societies); furthermore, mental illness and physical impairment are bundled together, so that the authors can state that '...mental illnesses and physical afflictions were generally viewed as the work of evil mana, or spirits. If, after considerable coaxing, the spirits did not leave a possessed body, this was believed to be indisputable evidence that the individual was being punished. In order to prevent contamination, people possessed with evil spirits were to be either avoided or killed.'[11] For the Middle Ages directly, a standard textbook of (orthopaedic) medical history repeats more such ill-informed stereotypes, asserting that from the fifth to the fifteenth century 'there was a [*sic*] utter lack of any sense of responsibility on the part of society for those who suffered from visible deformities (one supposes the counterpart of the ancient Indian attitude to cripples as evil incarnate). This may be true for Central and Western Europe...it is unfortunate that disease and deformity were considered to be the punishment for sin'.[12] Things are not much better when academics from the field of disability studies turn their attention to historical aspects of disability. Deborah Mark's otherwise excellent analysis of modern disability dismisses the Middle Ages in a few sentences, which are worth citing in full as they exemplify the full range of stereotypes and unsubstantiated assumptions the researcher encounters when reading modern texts.

> ...in the Middle Ages, disabled people were subjected to a host of superstitious ideas, which led to their persecution. Impairment was believed to be the result of divine judgement and therefore a punishment for sin. Abuse of disabled people was sanctioned by the church. ...During the Middle Ages disability was associated with evil and witchcraft.[13]

This belief of modern authors that ancient or medieval societies *invariably* saw a link between sin and illness appears to be the dominant historiographical notion on the subject of disability.

A rather curious book on disability entitled *Zerbrecht die Krücken*[14] (Smash the Crutches) was published in Germany in 1932, written by Hans Würtz, who, as he stated in his introduction, had by then had a quarter of a century's worth of experience working with the 'crippled' in institutions. This book essentially tried to rehabilitate 'crippled' persons as people who were just as capable of great achievements throughout human history and culture as non-disabled people were, an early form of the 'supercrip' notion, by cataloguing famous infirm and disfigured people[15] who had been notable as educators, scientists, religious thinkers, writers, artists, musicians and actors, inventors, sports personalities, politicians, military leaders, courtiers and, here regrettably returning to stereotypes, 'Schaukrüppel' ('cripples' put on display, presumably an allusion to the 'freak shows' popular in the late nineteenth and early twentieth centuries).

The volume represents a phenomenal trawl through world history, also listing representations of disabled people in the arts (painting, sculpture, fictional literature, folklore), though most of Würtz's examples are from the nineteenth century onwards. However, the book is permeated by a benign patronisation of the disabled, something which is all the more obvious when one turns to the introductory chapter on 'the cripple and his problems'[16] and the aphorisms and mottos for disabled people which are appended to the book.[17] Here the emphasis is on overcoming the psychological 'problems' of the physically disabled through instigating in them an 'iron willpower', which will enable them to achieve economic independence through their participation in the labour market. The real person inside the physically disabled can only be healed in their soul and spirit; they are to be 'de-crippled',[18] as Würtz puts it. For him, it appears, disability is all in the mind. Life is about achieving a spiritual and psychological victory over one's disabled body, and Würtz's catalogue of the successful disabled appears to intend a demonstration of that very point.

However, Würtz appears to have been an unusual and rare voice. In contrast, Haggard and Watson were not atypical in their views. The orthodox view of history appears to encompass the notion that all impaired people must always have been either beggars and/or a burden. This view is expressed even as recently as 1970, when it is assumed that disabled people have always been 'problematical for all societies throughout history, since they could not usually perform their social responsibilities satisfactorily and became dependent upon the productive able bodied'.[19] Still more recently, a lot of interest by academics has been in histories of medicine, illness and demography, but such histories often fail to mention disability altogether. This failure by texts on the history of medicine to deal with disability may have something to do with the definition of disability as something separate from disease/illness, and therefore disability may not be seen as a truly appropriate subject for the history of medicine. In some ways, even medieval medical texts, as we shall see in Chapter 4.1, already neglected 'disability', in that untreatable conditions were dealt with rather perfunctorily in such texts. An example of the modern neglect of disability by medical historians is a recent work by G. Melvyn Howe[20] which, in the context of the medieval period, discusses leprosy and the sixth- and seventh-century 'pestilences' (which are possibly associated with the plague striking Justinian's Byzantium in 540), thereafter only dealing with the Black Death of 1348/50 and subsequent plagues, together with a brief mention of the dance epidemics of St Vitus' dance,[21] but has no reference to impaired people whatsoever.

However, some general work on disability in a historical setting has been done in the last two decades. Moving on, historiographically, to the present we have the interest of scholars of classical antiquity in disability and deformity, with publications on this topic in the late 1980s and throughout the 1990s. Works include an article by Luca Giuliani[22] which tries to interpret the Hellenistic stat-uettes of impaired or deformed people partly from an art historical perspective, partly from a cultural history approach. Then there is V. Dasen's study of dwarfs in the ancient world,[23] which tries to discover whether dwarfs were marginalised and feared, or whether they were accorded special powers within a religious setting (note, however, that in either case, dwarfs would be deemed part of the 'Other' – this line of enquiry automatically positions dwarfs within a discourse of difference). A more wide-ranging study by Robert Garland[24] investigated the social symbolism and physical condition of the impaired and deformed in the Graeco-Roman world, concluding that it is 'a perennial problem confronting those afflicted with severe deformity' as to 'how to escape the myths and stereotypes which divest them of a full, complex and rounded humanity'.[25] Garland parallels the antique experience of impairment with that of modern times, in that in both periods, physical difference which did not 'conform to the norms of the dominant group' was treated 'either with suspicion, terror and contempt, or alternatively with an unhealthy blend of amusement, fascination and embarrassment'[26] – the impaired as 'Other' again. In similar vein, a collection of essays edited by Beth Cohen[27] explored the notion of otherness by focusing on deviance from the 'Classical ideal' in Greek art, especially emphasising the depiction as 'ugly' of people with a physical deformity, the aged or people with 'monstrous' behaviour. A study by Daniel Ogden examined orthopaedic impairments in the mythical and legendary kings of ancient Greece.[28] Less fatalist in conclusion was an article by Nicholas Vlahogiannis[29] on disability, the body and cultural attitudes, which firmly placed classical notions of disability into their historical context; similarly an essay on hearing- and speech-impaired people in ancient Greece by M. L. Edwards[30] argued from the point of view of the social construction of disability.

Like earlier general histories of disability, though, earlier studies by classicists looked at disability in antiquity from a purely medical angle. A case in point is an article by M. Michler[31] on the treatment of crippling disorders in the corpus of Hippocratic texts. The author is interested in the two Hippocratic texts he studies from the angle of medical 'advancement'; the importance of the texts lies for him in the fact that they are the first to mention congenital impairments of an orthopaedic kind, also that these texts try to explain 'rationally'[32] how such conditions came about. The social position of disabled people is more of a secondary issue, they are seen as marginal figures who are badly treated by the rest of society,[33] and therefore the Hippocratic texts are 'revolutionary' to Michler because they express concern in helping congenitally impaired people.[34]

Exceptions within studies of disability in antiquity have been the handful of monographs and articles published on disability in the non-Classical world, in other words in a region where the cultural stereotypes of the Western world, both ancient and modern, do not automatically crop up. One would therefore expect these authors to approach the history of impairment in a slightly different vein to those dealing with Classical antiquity, which, because of our modern Classicism, predisposes us to cultural assumptions and stereotypes that might prevent us from asking less biased questions. Unfortunately, one of the first historical studies of disability in a non-Western, non-Classical context, Fareed Haj's *Disability in Antiquity*,[35] is firmly entrenched in the medical dialogue of disability, interested mainly in the advancement of medical knowledge and treatment of impairments, such as those sustained during war, as in the crippling of both Muslims and Christians during the Crusades. However, more recently an article by Johannes Renger[36] questioned the automatic marginalisation of the sick, cripples and mentally impaired in Babylonia or Mesopotamia, concluding that, from a study of cuneiform texts, the picture presented of disability is rather more diffuse and complex, whereby disabled people were not marginalised primarily because of their physical appearance, but because of other factors, such as loss of family and/or income, which then forced them into a marginal position they shared with other, equally marginal, groups of society, basically those socially and economically powerless, such as the aged, widows or the poor. In similar vein, M. Miles's article[37] on disability in an Eastern religious context attempts to approach disability in a non-Western context without the usual Western, Classicist or Christian bias, focusing on popular notions of disabled people in Islam, Buddhism and Hinduism.

One very notable exception to the dearth of modern scholarly texts on the history of disability is a book by a French academic, Henri-Jacques Stiker. Stiker's *History of Disability* was first published in France in 1982 as *Corps infirmes et sociétés*, followed by a second French edition in 1997, before being published in the United States in 1999. He is the only author of either a text of medical history or of disability studies to devote more than a few cursory sentences to medieval disability; indeed he has an entire chapter ('The System(s) of Charity') on the subject. It is therefore important to take a closer look at the main theories Stiker has proposed. Stiker investigates some remarks made by Philippe Ariès on disability; that 'for the Middle Ages as a whole, physical aberrancy like all monstrosities was a "normal anomaly" in the face of which there was neither revulsion, nor terror, nor treatment',[38] but disagrees with this, choosing to use the abundant secondary literature on poverty in the medieval period to address the question of whether the disabled did 'simply melt into the crowd of the poor'.[39] He disagrees with the idea that in France before the seventeenth and early eighteenth centuries there was no specific vision of the disabled, even if he believes that to a great extent the disabled were included among the poor.[40] However, he admits that there is a 'difficulty of knowing just where the disabled were'[41] throughout the entire medieval period, and repeats this view, saying that 'the silence about the disabled is remarkable'.[42] He emphasises the absence of specific documents to do with the disabled, and concentrates instead on understanding and reconstructing the various mentalities,[43] which is in fact exactly what my findings have been and subsequent aims are, too, in the present book.

Following Jean Delumeau's work on fear in the later Middle Ages and the Renaissance, Stiker surmises that this general culture of fear encompassed the disabled and commenced the process of their sequestration and 'back to work' ethics,[44] a process which culminated later in the 'great confinement' famously studied by Michel Foucault. Stiker cites a few secondary sources on poverty and the art of Brueghel to support his views of the 'striking mixture of the poor and the disabled'.[45] Towards the end of his chapter, Stiker takes up the theme of fear again, citing a few secondary sources on the increasingly repressive treatment of marginalised groups (such as the poor, disabled, petty criminals) by the later Middle Ages, that is, from the fourteenth century onwards. Stiker concludes there was an 'essentially ambiguous situation of the disabled that prevailed at the time. Clearly distinguished on the one hand and the object of traditional charity, and almost undistinguished on the other . . . the repression, forced labor, and establishment concern for security that had earlier disregarded the disabled would end up by reaching them.'[46] In particular, the popular preachers of the fourteenth and fifteenth centuries are blamed by Stiker for promulgating attitudes of fear: 'The great dignity of lepers, the disabled, sick, and, in a general way, the poor has been forgotten.'[47]

With regard to the change in perception of the disabled from antiquity, Judaism, or the Old Testament texts to a Christian, New Testament religious world-view, Stiker says that in the earlier period 'religious fear' informed attitudes to the disabled, caused by challenging the order of 'the species and the social unit', whereas from the time of the church fathers onwards this fear becomes purely a 'subjective fear', whereby the disabled may not be 'integrated in the contemporary sense of the term', but are to be recipients of love, help and charity.[48] Stiker concludes that while the disabled had a status 'which was quite clear in the classical world, and in the Jewish world even though often disadvantaged, [it] remained very fluid in the Middle Ages'.[49] According to Stiker, rather simplistically, the charity given to the disabled was provided almost by default since people did not really know what to else do with them. 'The mentality and attitudes were variable and ambiguous at the same time. Never truly excluded, for the disabled were always spiritually integrated; never integrated, for they were always on the social fringes.'[50] Although a very valuable contribution, mainly because it is the only multi-period history of disability to address the Middle Ages in more detail, there are some issues with Stiker's approach and methodology. He has relied almost entirely, it seems, on secondary texts in favour of primary material; hence he has placed too much emphasis on the apparent poverty of the majority of the disabled in the medieval period. Also, leprosy is seen as just another impairment by Stiker, which distorts some of the material he cites with regard to disabled people, since, as I have pointed out above, leprosy was seen as a distinct and specific illness with its own cultural meaning. Most importantly, Stiker has made no distinction between impairment (physiological phenomenon) and disability (cultural construct); hence he is forced to assume a priori the existence of an anachronistic notion of 'disability' in the Middle Ages.

Slightly more work on disability in all historical epochs has been done in the German-speaking academic world. Here such diverse topics have been studied as the healing of the blind as depicted in art,[51] and the physically disabled in myth and art,[52] both from an art historical perspective with less emphasis on social or cultural factors; the social history of the disabled in Germany[53] (or 'cripples, idiots and lunatics', as the subtitle puts it) and the forgotten history of the war-wounded and crippled in European literature;[54] and most interestingly, a study of the cripple from a cultural anthropology and historic perspective (subtitled 'the ethnography of human suffering').[55] Yet none of these studies deals specifically with the medieval period. Once again the Middle Ages are viewed in a decidedly dark fashion, the Dark Ages of popular perception.

Why should it be the case that the medieval period is neglected in historical studies of disability? To sum up the historiographical overview, histories of disability concentrated either on a 'medical advancement' view of disability, or, if they treated specific historical epochs prior to the modern period, have concentrated on the culture of Classical antiquity. To a degree the methodology employed by researchers and/or the questions asked by them elicit certain predetermined answers. In other words, if one subscribes to a view of 'culture' as being essentially Western, Classical or modern, then one is not going to be interested in the Middle Ages. Also, if one's perspective of history is shaped by these Western, modernist tendencies, then one's understanding of 'body' will be similarly biased; that is, the disabled body will be viewed as unchanging throughout history. In a sense this leads to a subscription to the idea that things have 'always been like that', so that it is easy to reach the conclusion that in the Middle Ages all impaired people were either beggars or court jesters, to name but two dominant stereotypes – which even the otherwise exceptional work by Stiker does.[56]

The Middle Ages are out on both counts (medical history and histories of the Classical body) within such a limited discourse: the medieval period has been viewed by the medical historians, until fairly recently at least, as an unwelcome interruption in the glorious advancement of medical science from (Classical) antiquity to the present day, with at best an apparent stagnation, or at worst even collapse of medical knowledge during that time; similarly, cultural and postmodernist historians have concentrated either on the modern, that is post-Enlightenment period, or on Classical antiquity, which was of course the philosophical and intellectual basis for the subsequent 'Enlightenment' (though sometimes a 'Renaissance' is seen to take the position of 'Enlightenment'). In this respect Foucault has a lot to answer for, since his seminal work in the areas of body, sexuality, gender, madness, institutionalisation and so on, which justly forms the intellectual basis for subsequent studies of these fields, does not deal much with culture outside the Classical period or the (early) modern period based on (re)discovery of that Classical culture.[57] Foucault was 'a good philosopher but a bad historian', as it has been put. The postmodern analysis of the body therefore tends to assume a Classical body, the modern body being essentially a Classical body, and has difficulties with paradigms other than that. I would therefore argue that, since most work on the body in recent years has been done by postmodernist scholars (using 'postmodernist' in its widest sense), the medieval period has been neglected because the general culture of the Middle Ages was deemed non-Classical. This is not to disparage postmodern theories on the body, which are very useful to gain an understanding of cultural assumptions surrounding such phenomena. It is, however, more a failing of those scholars practising postmodern history to disregard the medieval period. Notable exceptions, such as the work by Caroline Walker Bynum,[58] are a case in point: her investigation of the boundary crossings[59] between male and female, spiritual and physical, in late medieval religion presents a much more complex picture than a strictly postmodern interpretation of the binaries of Classical and modern culture allow for, and argues for a far more fluid, diverse and shifting paradigm within later medieval culture.

> [T]he very dualisms [male/female, body/soul] modern commentators have emphasized so much were far from absolute in the late Middle Ages. Not only did theology, natural philosophy and folk tradition mingle male and female in their understanding of human character and human physiology; theological and psychological discussion also sometimes mingled body and soul. ... the philosophical, medical and folk understandings of body saw men and women as variations on a single physiological structure. ... theology and natural philosophy saw persons as in some real sense body as well as soul.[60]

The postmodern critique of history has focused the historian's gaze on the world of language and texts, and allowed historians to develop more complex analyses, as well as to take a heightened interest in previously disregarded topics (of which disability is one example). There is a danger, though, that the 'linguistic turn'[61] in the discipline of history may make us ignore the very real facts of illness, poverty, death, and so on, which are not simply reducible to textuality alone. One postmodern author, Elizabeth Deeds Ermarth,[62] has reduced everything to pure text and discourse, thereby eliminating notions of time or society as anything other than linguistic constructs. Criticism has come from historians against the 'postmodernist concentration on words [which] diverts attention away from real suffering and oppression and towards the kinds of secondary intellectual issues that matter in the physically comfortable world of academia'.[63] Postmodernist history therefore has its uses when dealing with topics like 'body' and 'disability', but one must be cautious not to eliminate discursively the very thing one is trying to write about.

A further possibility as to the lack of historiographic writings on the disabled may stem from the medieval period itself. Historiography and the writing of history in the Middle Ages followed certain conventions,[64] of which one was the definition of the topic(s) seen to be appropriate for inclusion in a history. As an example, in the twelfth century Otto of Freising states in the dedication of his encyclopaedic *History of the Two Cities* that what he had intended was that he 'did not merely give events (*gestae*) in their chronological order, but rather wove together, in the manner of a tragedy (*in modum tragoediae*), their sadder aspects, ...'.[65] Therefore history is the proper subject of tragedy, but what then, one may ask, is the proper subject of history? Tragedy, and by implication according to Otto's notion, also history, is dealing with the great, the good (or evil) and the powerful in society. Such a notion can be traced to the influential Isidore of Seville, who defined tragedy as dealing with public matters and the histories of rulers, done in a sorrowful manner, whereas comedy deals with the private affairs of people and is made up of cheerful things.[66] The marginalised in society, that is the lower orders, peasants, the poor and the sick and disabled would then be subjects of comedy rather than tragedy. The *comici*, writers of things comic, that is, would be left to write about the disabled, for example, and since, as one notion of history shows, comedy is not the proper subject of history, the poor, disabled and other powerless groups find no place in history (even if nominally a history such as Otto of Freising's is not about deeds alone). Not so far removed is the definition of 'history' and historiography of the Middle Ages by one modern scholar: 'The historiographer collects knowledge about actions of individuals or groups that are able to act.'[67] Like the poor or peasants, disabled people do not 'act' since in society they are not in a position to act, they are *un*able to act, *dis*-abled, as the very etymology of the word exemplifies (it is another question, one that is beyond the scope of the present work, whether impaired people, as opposed to disabled, are able to act in the Middle Ages) and one could conclude that therefore disabled people do not prove themselves suitable subjects of *historia*.

Against this historiographical background, then, disability in the medieval period has been neglected partly because medical histories had little or no interest in the period, and partly because most work on the body and meanings of bodies has been conducted in the main by scholars more interested in the familiar 'Classical' body than the more complex medieval one, let alone the even more complex disabled body. Perhaps also notions of what is and what is not appropriate to write as 'history' have had an impact on the absence of disability from historiography. As the next stage then it is worth examining how the school of disability studies, coming mainly from a sociological angle, has looked at historical disabilities.

2.2   Modern theories of disability and disability studies

Disability studies emerged as an academic discipline only in the last two decades from the political disability movement of the 1970s and 1980s in Europe, especially in the United Kingdom, and in the United States. Within disability studies there have been a multitude of scholars who have theorised disability from equally diverse perspectives, such as from historical–geographical and materialist angles, from anthropological or comparative cultural angles, and from psychology and sociology. What most disability studies theorists have in common is an emphasis on the distinction between the social construction of disability and the physiological reality of impairment.

As outlined above, I distinguish between 'impairment' (the term preferred in the social model of disability) and 'disability' (the term preferred in the medical model of disability). In the terminology of disability studies, impairment is seen as the biological 'fact', the bodily manifestation, and describes the purely anatomical, so that impairment lacks social connotations. By contrast, 'disability' refers to the social constructedness of the relationship between the impaired body and the culture and society that body's owner inhabits. In Britain, the *Union of the Physically Impaired Against Segregation* suggested the following definition:

> Impairment: Lacking part or all of a limb, or having a defective limb, organ, or mechanism of the body. Disability: The disadvantage or restriction of

activity caused by a contemporary social organisation which takes no or little account of people who have physical impairments and thus excludes them from the mainstream of social activities.[68]

In other words, one may be born impaired but one is made disabled (to paraphrase Simone de Beauvoir's famous dictum on women). The notion of the social construction of disability therefore permits historical investigation and analysis – if disability is a social construct, as times and societies change so should notions of what is and what is not disability. In contrast, the medico-biological model of disability regards impairment and disability as virtually synonymous, and treats disability as a 'natural' occurrence, thereby negating any necessity for a historical explanation: if disability is natural, it is by definition unchanging and not within the realms of human agency, and it would therefore be futile to try and look for change let alone historical processes when discussing disability – possibly one of the reasons why disability has so far been overlooked in historical writing. One of the few historians to acknowledge the paucity of disability as a topic within traditional historical writing has been J. C. Riley[69] in an article which, even then, focuses only on the post-medieval period. Though it is important to distinguish the physical 'reality' of impairment from the social constructedness of disability, it needs to be pointed out that too rigorous a distinction or intellectual gulf between the two brings further problems with it, in that the notion of impairment as physical 'fact' is as ahistorical as the notion of disability as an unchanging constant. That is to say, though factual or real, impairment is just as much a manifestation of time and space as disability: how the same specific physiological phenomenon of impairment is described by the particular science or medicine of the time varies from period to period. As Hughes and Patterson have expressed it:

> The social model [of disability] – in spite of its critique of the medical model – actually concedes the body to medicine and understands impairment in terms of medical discourse. …the social model requires to mount a critique of its own dualistic heritage and establish…that the impaired body is part of the domain of history, culture and meaning, and not – as medicine would have it – an ahistorical, pre-social, purely natural object.[70]

It is therefore possible to analyse impairment in the medieval period, and then within that period across geographical space as well as smaller time-periods, as something distinct from impairment in other eras. Or to put it another way, a 'cripple' in the thirteenth century could share the same physiological condition with a 'cripple' in the later twentieth century, yet the scientific, medical or biological discourse of each time would already describe each body, though outwardly manifesting the same symptoms, in different ways. The theological and philosophical positioning of impairment in the Middle Ages (discussed in Chapter 3) and the medieval 'scientific' notions of impairment (Chapter 4) therefore provide the central evidence which enables us to appreciate the theoretical distinctions between medieval and modern concepts of impairment.

The notion of disabled people as inferior, dependent, and by implication, of little or no value to their society, has been termed 'disablism', that is the -*ism* of disability, as in racism or sexism. Such notions of disabled people are still dominant in modern Western society.[71] The term 'disablism' was coined to describe the socio-political processes which marginalise and oppress disabled people. Mainstream sociological theory is more of a hindrance than a help with regards to theorising disability, as such theory is at present theoretically backward, according to disability studies. This is because the dominant strands of sociological theory individualise the nature and experiences of disability, suggesting it is akin to a medical condition that requires treatment.[72] 'In this way, any negative experiences which disabled people encounter in, for instance, moving around their environments or failing to obtain employment, is conceptualised as linked to individual impairment rather than resulting from forms of social and political discrimination.'[73] Conversely, Ann Shearer[74] starts from the premise that every individual has their personal share of diverse abilities, and that therefore the line drawn between able and disabled is a fluctuating one, a line that can be constantly re-drawn by society. The problems revolving around disability are not personal tragedies that would need overcoming, in her view, but instead they constitute the responses of other people: the problems of prejudice, the attitudes of health professionals working with disabled people, the wider issues of politics and economics. The main problem is formed by the exclusion of the disabled from 'normal' activities. However, in the dominant 'disablist' perspective, disability is seen as a personal stigma which hinders the impaired person from leading a normal life, and is therefore theoretically still stuck in the social psychology theory of some 40 years ago, as is exemplified by Goffman's theories.

Positioning disability within a social context was achieved (to a degree) in a seminal text on stigma by Erving Goffman[75] in the early 1960s, where he looked at issues such as visibility, identity and deviancy. This is the social psychology view, which sees disability as an ideological construct arising out of the negative attitudes of society. The material conditions of life, for example mobility, space, work, are brushed aside in favour of psychological and discursive structures. For Goffman, there were three types of stigma, namely the 'abominations of the body – the various physical deformities', character blemishes, and the 'tribal stigma' of race, ethnicity or religion.[76] A person with a stigma is said to have both a virtual social identity and an actual social identity,[77] where the virtual identity is that inscribed on the stigmatised person by others, and the actual identity describes the character and attributes which that person could actually be proven to possess, if only we could look at them objectively.[78] Furthermore, 'visibility' is very important for Goffman, though he preferred 'perceptibility' as the better term.[79] By this he meant that not all stigmatic manifestations are visible to 'normals' all the time, but that some phenomena are more apparent than others to different groups of people; one could think of the different ways, for example, in which a medical professional and a lay person perceive a stigmatised person such as a wheelchair user. Goffman therefore placed 'visibility' firmly within a cultural context by emphasising that '...the decoding capacity of the audience must be specified before one can speak of degree of visibility.'[80]

More recently, a French structuralist, René Girard, investigating issues of religion, mythology, anthropology and psychology, has reiterated notions of 'stigma', and asserted the cross-cultural universality of such ideas. In his work on the 'scapegoat', Girard discusses the signifiers according to which scapegoat-victims are selected:

> In addition to cultural and religious there are purely *physical* criteria. Sickness, madness, genetic deformities, accidental injuries, and even disabilities in general tend to polarise persecutors. We need only look around or within to understand the universality. Even today people cannot control a momentary recoil from physical abnormality. ...The 'handicapped' are subject to discriminatory measures that make them victims, out of all proportion to the extent to which their presence disturbs the ease of social exchange.[81]

In his language, Girard echoes the sentiments of Goffman, by effectively ascribing a kind of 'stigma' to the victim which, albeit unjustifiably, prompts discriminating reactions among the rest of society. He posits disability among a 'large group of banal signs of a victim' and equates any outsider within a specific group as 'more or less interchangeable with a cripple'.[82] He furthermore distinguishes between 'real' disability, by which he appears to mean physiological impairments, and metaphorical, unreal disabilities: 'If the disability or deformity is real, it tends to polarise 'primitive' people against the afflicted person. Similarly, if a group of people is used to choosing its victims from a certain social, ethnic, or religious category, it tends to attribute to them disabilities or deformities that would reinforce the polarisation against the victim, were they real.'[83] Social abnormalities are included in this definition, as well as physical or mental abnormalities. 'Disabled' can then become a figurative expression for 'victimhood' in Girard's theory, and in this he seems to be thinking along the same lines as Goffman was some decades earlier.

With the politicisation of disability and the finding of a voice by and for disabled people in the last two decades, Goffman's work has been challenged. (Girard would be challenged, too, one presumes, were it not for the possibility that few scholars in the area of disability studies had encountered his theories.) Goffman has been accused of coming from an interactionist perspective.[84] An individual's 'personality' for Goffman is constituted by the social interaction between people – a set of attitudes is therefore formed on the basis of personal attributes, both positive and negative, as they are perceived by others. Disability becomes a stigma which emerges from the ritualistic interactions of actors in a society, and thereby Goffman can posit a 'disabled personality' which is moulded by the stigmatising encounters with others in society. One of the main critics of Goffman in the United Kingdom has been Paul Abberley,[85] but newer approaches to theorising disability have also come from Mike Oliver[86] and Tom Shakespeare, both of whom are themselves impaired. Goffman's theories live on, in a sense, in

Reginald Golledge's work. Golledge has defined disability as 'those situations where an individual is prevented wholly or partially from performing the full range of actions and activities usually performed by members of the society or culture in which the person lives'.[87] However, the prevention of participation for the impaired person is seen to stem from that individual's physical incapability; physiological difference places limitations upon an individual, and physiological impairment automatically leads to social handicap, a view for which Golledge has been criticised by the materialist school of disability studies.[88] 'Disadvantage' is contrasted by Golledge with 'disability', in that disadvantage is what people face who are not physically impaired, but who are perceived to be different due to social, cultural, ethnic, economic, political, religious or legal constraints.

Besides Goffman, one of the most important theorists has been, of course, Michel Foucault. Foucault's importance for theorising the body cannot be denied. It was, after all, he who pointed out that the difference between for example 'man' and 'woman' is the effect of discourse, and not purely a natural and obvious fact of biology. Biological difference has a socially qualified objectivity; that is, it is precisely *not* objective outside of a specific historical context. All of this is very useful to body theorists. However, Foucault can at times play down the role of physical difference in favour of the discursive element.[89] Since disability is by definition linked to the actual, physical impairment of a body, playing down the physical can lead to what some critics[90] have called the 'vanishing bodies of postmodernism' – an imaginary *reductio ad absurdum* would allow us to discursively theorise away the body to the point where no body (or nobody) is disabled. Or to quote Brendan Gleeson: 'The epistemological repercussions of this [Foucault's vanishing bodies] are profound: to deny or underplay the materiality of physical difference is ultimately to reduce the general notion of somatic diversity to a mere ideological epiphenomenon.'[91] In effect, the body, disabled or otherwise, has been collapsed into language, bringing about a 'theoretical elimination of the materiality of the body',[92] which renders it highly problematic for disability theorists.

Another theoretical approach taken by disability studies has been a materialist analysis of disability. Vic Finkelstein[93] argued that disability results primarily from Western industrialisation. Finkelstein regarded the pre-capitalist or pre-industrial phase of production as one where impaired people were not automatically excluded from participation in economic activities; in such societies, according to Finkelstein, impaired people were dispersed in the community and not segregated in institutions. Some recent theoretical approaches, then, which look at disability both from a social point of view and from a view critical of the more discursive aspects of Foucault have, interestingly, come not from the discipline of history but from geography.[94] Here greater emphasis is placed on the socio-spatial conditions of impaired people, within an overall framework of analysis coming from the social constructionist school. Regrettably, the attempt by one such scholar, the aforementioned Brendan Gleeson, to provide a historical dimension to an other-wise materialist investigation of disability in rural medieval England, among other things, fails completely.

In a nutshell, Gleeson's arguments are as follows: his thesis, entitled *Second Nature? The Socio-spatial Production of Disability*, argues that disability is a socially imposed state of exclusion which physically impaired individuals may be forced to endure; this view is seen in contrast to the popular, or 'common sense' approach, that disablement is 'second nature' to impaired people.[95] Gleeson then proposes that a historical and materialist analysis will provide the explanatory foundations for a social theory of disability. He uses the elements of space and of social organisation as criteria to theorise disability. He concludes that while impairment was probably a feature of what he terms 'feudal'[96] England, disability was not. As he suggests, the non-disabling character of 'feudal' society may be attributed both to a confined realm of physical interaction (people live in a face-to-face society) and to the relatively weak presence of commodity production (advanced capitalism). So far so good. Unfortunately, his 'carefully designed empirical case-studies' relating to rural England in the Middle Ages are, in fact, data sets of Poor Law Records from Norwich (1570) and Salisbury (1635) – evidently neither rural nor medieval. He grossly underestimates the possibility for mobility of English peasants, stating that they were bound to the manor so that they never travelled more than a radius of five miles distance in their entire lives,[97] and asserts that rural production was geared up purely towards a subsistence economy,[98] which begs the question how he thinks medieval English towns could have existed at all, since according to his views there would not have been any surplus produced in the countryside. Gleeson's thesis, nevertheless, is important, since he went on to publish a much-discussed article[99] based on his research, and his theories later resurfaced in the foremost English-language journal dealing with disability issues.[100]

The central question he poses is: 'How have changes in the socio-spatial organisation of society affected the lived experience of physical impairment?'[101] His research intends to demonstrate that socio-spatial changes affect the lived experience by transforming the material structures of everyday life; therefore past transformations in the mode of production have social consequences for impaired people. In itself, this is an interesting, and, I think useful, approach. It is connected with the idea that prior to industrial capitalist modes of production, and the capitalist structuration of time in general and the working day in particular, the individual person had a far greater control over how they spent their day, and earned their living. Historians of the Middle Ages such as Jacques Le Goff[102] have substantiated this theory in principle: the flexibility of time in the Middle Ages allowed most people, including the peasantry (but with the notable exception of members of the church and the inhabitants of monasteries and nunneries[103]), to structure their working day as they saw fit. By implication then, as Gleeson argues, impaired people could still contribute to the labour-process, in their own time and at their own rate of working speed, and their disability became negligible in this context.[104] Mike Oliver, similarly, argues that 'feudal' society 'did not preclude the great majority of disabled people from participating in the production process, and even where they could not participate fully, they were still able to make a contribution'.[105] Again, in a non-Western, non-capitalist context, ethnographic data suggest that in traditional societies a 'single personal characteristic, such as the ability to hunt successfully or grow abundant crops, does not seem to define one's total identity.'[106] The wider range of economic activities and occupations available for all people, irrespective of physical capability, in such traditional societies, allows for greater options for the impaired as well, in contrast to industrialised societies, where specialisation is paramount. It is due to the prejudices and ingrained stereotypes surrounding disability now that some modern scholars imagine all impaired people to have been disabled, useless, and segregated at all times from the rest of society: '...social scientists too often assume that disability automatically causes an individual to become marginal to his or her social group. This bias perpetuates the belief found within our own society – that people with disabilities have always been peripheral to the social life of our species.'[107]

However, the position and status in society of a physically impaired person does not constitute itself in the working ability alone of that person: religio-cultural attitudes, among others, influence the way an impaired person is perceived. Economic integration into a society, as the modern scholars cited above do manage to argue quite convincingly, is equal neither to social acceptance nor to tolerance. For Western medieval Europe, notions of both impairment and disability would be impossible to explain without reference, for example, to the Church, charity, miracle healings, punishment or sin. Oliver has managed to hint at these other factors by emphasising the individuality of impaired persons. With regard to the Middle Ages, Oliver says: 'In this era disabled people were regarded as individually unfortunate and not segregated from the rest of society.'[108] It is one of the aims of this book to examine how 'the rest of society' treated disabled persons in a cultural context.

Materialist interpretations, as advocated by Gleeson and others, of disability in Western society are not sufficient as an explanation. Materialist theory has been criticised as 'an aid to understanding rather than an accurate historical state-ment'[109] which is therefore 'simplistic' in that it assumes simple relationships between the mode of production and the perceptions or experiences of disability; the impact of ideology or culture is just as great as (if not greater than) the mate-rialist situation. The adoption of a cultural angle aids an analysis far more. 'Culture' is here used in the sense Mary Douglas[110] described, as a 'communally held set of values and beliefs'.[111] It is cultural ideas that create the myth of bod-ily perfection, or the discourse of the able-bodied ideal, if one so prefers, whereas the materialist approach completely ignores such notions. Tom Shakespeare argued that what able-bodied people dislike or fear is not so much disability, but the fact that 'disabled people remind non-disabled people of their own mortal-ity';[112] therefore disabled people are a threat to order or to the self-perception of the able-bodied in modern Western society. One could criticise here that Tom Shakespeare is too stringently adopting a phenomenological approach which implies that all cultures essentially respond to impairment in negative terms.[113] Prejudice against impaired people could therefore be argued to be inevitable and universal. However, not all societies respond to impairment in the same way.

Anthropological evidence shows, for example, that even societies living in precarious economic circumstances still care for and support economically non-productive members (such as the sick, elderly or impaired).[114] Much work still needs to be done on cross-cultural studies of impairment, as many scholars of disability studies realise,[115] which entails examining not just different contemporary cultures (the ethnological approach) but also diachronic study of single cultures (the historical approach).

One more branch of modern theory on disability needs to be addressed. As full of problematic implications as the materialist theory is the 'politics of identity' approach to history (and disability studies): there the argument is made that each group in society creates their own history as a means of building their own identity. As criticised in this excerpt from American historian Laura Lee Downs:

> The politics of identity, feminist and otherwise, rests on a disturbing epistemological ground, in which the group's fragile unity, rooted in an emergent sense of identity as an oppressed other, is shielded from white male colonization by asserting the inaccessibility of one's experience. Only those who share the group identity and have lived its experience, whether seen as biologically given or socially constructed, can know what it means to be black, a woman, blue-collar, or ethnic in an America constructed as white, Anglo-Saxon and Protestant.[116]

The implication of identity politics for disability studies is that nobody can legitimately write about disability who is not themself disabled, since only bodily experience is the sole arbiter of 'truth'. Even more disturbing is the historical implication, resulting in the absurd proscription for medieval history, for example, that nobody could write about medieval peasants who was not a peasant in, say, thirteenth-century England.

Having taken issue with historians who fail to mention disability or at best regard disability as a human constant, it is also necessary to criticise some of the disability studies scholars for their failure to take into account historical matters. I have already pointed out the distinct lack of a sense of historic period evident in some disability studies work[117] and I am not alone in observing that scholars of disability studies, traditionally coming from a sociology or (modern) cultural studies background, need to familiarise themselves more with history. As Jessica Sheer and Nora Groce pointed out, 'the diverse range of social responses to physical disabilities is not well appreciated or understood by social scientists, policy makers, nor disabled people themselves'.[118] As a consequence 'social scientists and others have frequently assumed that disabled individuals born outside the industrialized world were either killed at birth or died when young'.[119] Bearing in mind that many impairing conditions, such as mental retardation, deafness or blindness, are not immediately noticeable at or near birth and require a certain amount of development in the infant before any difference becomes apparent, it does not seem logical to assume that such infants were killed straightaway. Such blanket statements therefore are more of a reflection on modern prejudices than they are potentially useful statements about disability in, say, medieval times. Social studies, and disability studies practised from within that discipline, have tended to ignore (pre-modern) history, to the point that 'disability studies are largely an ahistorical field of enquiry',[120] and conversely most mainstream historians have failed to take issue with social theory regarding disability.

Historical accounts of disability have tended until fairly recently to come from authors who were writing from the perspective of the development of institutions and treatments for the disabled.[121] The more recent disability studies authors have still included such clinical history, partly because they are interested in the oppression of impaired people, partly because the source material given in institutional histories is easily accessible – unlike the medieval material. Since (most) disability studies authors are not trained historians, the interpretation and analysis of material from other periods becomes more neglected and haphazard the farther it is removed from the author's own time. As Elizabeth Bredberg has pointed out, 'the quality of historical research and interpretation found within disability studies remains uneven',[122] sometimes even manifesting unfortunate factual errors. The interpretation of primary sources has posed yet more problems, so that even Foucault was out of his depth when he discussed the *Ship of Fools* in his seminal *Madness and Civilisation*,[123] and thereby regrettably led others whose work cited his study to perpetuate such interpretative misconceptions. The history of disability needs to take more account of earlier periods, and involve itself more with primary material from such periods, which entails 'a more thorough grasp of its historical setting and of the textual (or representative) convention in which it is presented'.[124] One may summarise that both histories of disability and disability theories have aligned themselves to a 'grand recit' or 'foundational narrative', whereby such histories or theories follow an established pattern: in the case of histories of disability, this most commonly takes the shape of a chapter on antiquity, then a paragraph on the entire medieval period, another chapter on the early modern period, with the rest of any book dedicated to the modern period and institutional history. If disability theorists only have such grand recits to rely on, then one cannot be too disappointed in the lack of historically applicable disability theory, either.

Some of the most useful theoretical approaches of analysing disability have in fact come from anthropology and ethnology. Within the wider field of medieval studies, too, anthropological and/or ethnological approaches are not entirely unheard of, important work having been done first and foremost by the Russian scholar Aaron Gurevich.[125] Ethnologists try to understand and analyse a culture different from their own, and to do so they have had to develop a theoretical framework that allows them to discard (as much as possible) their own cultural assumptions. Ethnology as a discipline, therefore, by dealing with different manifestations of 'culture' developed transcultural theories. In direct relation to the present work, this means that the theories of disability which ethnology, as an academic discipline, has constructed are far more appropriate than either the theories of disability studies or those of (medical) historians. As was demonstrated, disability studies tend to have an ahistoric approach to disability, while medical history has an almost exclusively progressionist perspective.

Anthropology has also shown that impairment can carry widely differing notions of disability with it. Potentially stigmatising conditions which are formally identical can have different meanings to people from different cultures around the world, and by implication to different cultures in time as well. In many cultures, 'disability' does not exist as a recognised category. From a compilation of anthropological data in the 1970s, the Human Relations Area Files, it is suggested that crippled and maimed people are treated as sort of lesser human beings by cultures in Tibet, Burma and Turkey, whereas people with the same physical conditions in Korea and Afghanistan are seen as possessing unusual, culturally valued abilities for which they are accorded special and superior status by their culture.[126] That acceptance or rejection of perceived disabilities is culturally specific, and also linked to its prevalence in a given society, can be seen from the following example. Ann Shearer cites an isolated tribe in West Africa some of whose members have a genetic 'abnormality' whereby large numbers of children were born with two large toes on each foot instead of five, a kind of 'claw' foot, and sometimes had webbing between their fingers as well. These children were not regarded as disabled, but were accepted by their society, seeing it as normal that children could come in all shapes, with either four toes or 10. According to legend, when the first child was born with 'claw' toes, it was killed, as also happened to the second child born with these features. But by the time a third such child was born, the tribe decided this was meant to be. 'So it extended its concept of the "normal" to accept it and the others who were born later.'[127]

An analysis by Dieter Neubert and Günther Cloerkes[128] of different ethnological studies concerning disability in 24 cultures has produced an immensely useful theoretical structure, which it is worth reiterating here in outline, since many of the authors' conclusions with regards to disability and the disabled in ethnology are equally valid when applied to medieval Europe. In ethnology, four competing basic theoretical assumptions have been made with regards to disability. It is disputed as to whether the social reaction to disability is universal, interculturally varied, culturally uniform, or intraculturally varied, or even whether all these theories have similar value.[129] Theories around universal and interculturally varied reactions compare different cultures, while theories of cultural uniformity and of intracultural variance look at one specific culture's reaction to disability. Based on analysis of empirical evidence from the cultures they studied, Neubert and Cloerkes conclude that a large part of the physical differences manifested by impaired persons, especially those which severely restrict or hinder bodily function (extreme deformations, total blindness etc.), are interculturally uniformly valued as negative, and are thereby deemed as disabilities. Differences with less obvious restriction on bodily function are interculturally more likely to be valued variably.[130] With regards to most forms of somatic differences the reaction to such persons varies interculturally; one can therefore speak of a tendency to variation in the social reaction to disabled persons.[131] Both intracultural uniformity and intracultural variance can be found in human societies, though there appears to be a tendency to intracultural uniformity (individuals with identical or similar impairments are reacted to similarly in one given culture).[132]

However, intracultural variance in reaction may be possible,[133] and the social reaction then depends to a great degree on the individual impaired person, what specific impairment they manifest, what their status is, and so on. With regards to the medieval period, one may first of all treat the 'Middle Ages' as a distinct and separate culture to modern, Western industrialised society, and so one may avoid the pitfalls of having to rely either on medical history or on modern disability studies. One may further use these theories to try and establish whether medieval reactions were culturally uniform or varied intraculturally. So, for example, this book investigates whether the reaction to impaired people in religious discourse was significantly different to the reaction in medieval medical discourse; religious and medical discourse could, following the ethnological model, then be treated as two facets of a single, medieval culture, in fact as two intracultural sub-cultures. One may thereby look at the question of whether there was intracultural variance in the reactions to impairment, and how such variance manifested itself.

Anthropological studies have emphasised the need for cultural relativism when analysing disability. Questions have been posed centring around what disadvantages might be accrued by a specific disability in a particular context. The relation between the biological and the social order can be transcultural, in the sense that everywhere and at all times, it is an individual who is sick, or impaired. Yet this individual is sick or impaired in the eyes of their *society*, in relation to it, and 'in keeping with the modalities fixed by it'.[134] How an impaired or sick person is treated, then, by their society, varies interculturally.

> ...at different times the sick person's identity is structured around different forms of pathology, in keeping not only with the state of medical knowledge and with the institutional system that takes charge of the sick, but also with society's dominant values and schemes of reference.[135]

Generally, anthropological studies have shown that most human societies have concepts of illness and impairment that oscillate between two poles, two extremes of thinking. Exogenous concepts embody illness/impairment in external factors, so that illness/impairment can be regarded as an external aggression affecting an individual person. In contrast, endogenous concepts position illness/impairment such that in various ways these afflictions are seen to reside within the individual person, and are connected with that person and their identity.[136]

With regards to 'identity', or basic assumptions on what it is to be a person, some anthropologists have asked what kind of identities can exist in a given society. The issue of personhood has been addressed by Ingstad and Whyte,[137] where personhood is about being human not just in the biological sense, but about being human in a way that is valued and meaningful. They have looked at difference and personhood (asking how biological impairments relate to person-hood and to culturally defined differences among persons) and pointed out the need for a distinction between humanity and personhood (at times a person's humanity may be in doubt, as in early infancy when personhood has not yet developed). Ingstad and Whyte have also drawn attention to some important theoretical questions, such as how impairment interacts with factors like age, gender and economic standing; what ability the family may have to care for an infirm member (bearing in mind that 'family' and 'care' are historically and culturally specific); how the occupational structure of a society incorporates people with impairments; and to what extent there are special programmes, institutions and organisations of and for disabled people.[138] Most interestingly for the theoretical basis of my research, they have emphasised the importance of the point in the life cycle at which impairment occurs, a point which 'may well be crucial',[139] as sustaining an impairment later in life has less of an impact on personhood and societal relations than sustaining an impairment earlier. In their ethnological studies of disability, Neubert and Cloerkes have also identified certain factors which can strongly influence the societal reaction to disability, namely the type of impairment, the economic circumstances of a given individual, the magical and/or religious beliefs of a society, the presence of xenophobia, and a variety of other values held in common by a given society (e.g. health, functional ability of a person, intelligence, physical integrity). The impaired are only perceived as disabled in *some* respects of social functioning overall, and equally they may be perceived as a threat to *some* of the values a society holds. 'The more central these values are, however, for the societal value system...and the greater the deviance [from them], the more powerfully the threat is felt.'[140] In other words, in a society which values manual work very highly, inability to perform such work would be regarded as more of a threat to the established value-system than in a society which, say, values social skills higher than productivity in manual work; a hypothetical extrovert but one-handed person would therefore be valued quite differently in these two societies.

Anthropology has also raised the issue of liminality. Robert Murphy, himself disabled, uses the concept of liminality to explain the relative position of impaired peoples in *all* societies. According to Murphy, disabled people are 'neither out of society nor wholly in it...they exist in partial isolation from society as undefined, ambiguous people'.[141] As such, disabled people 'lived in a state of social suspension'[142] where they are neither termed sick nor well, neither dead nor alive – this being in-between of disabled persons is of crucial importance for the discussions of notions of health, illness, medicine and the body. These issues will be addressed below with regards to such medieval notions in Chapter 4.1, and with special reference to liminality in medieval miracle narratives in Chapter 5.3. Perhaps the most interesting remark by Stiker, in his *History of Disability*, is made about the disabled as being liminal even to recognised excluded groups (heretics, Jews, Muslims, vagabonds): 'It is, perhaps, just their position – *on the border* [*sic*] of other groups that are fairly well recognized – that may furnish a vitally important but as yet unrecognized notion for understanding this society, one that has remained hidden to the eyes of historians.'[143] So the disabled may be liminal to medieval society as a whole as well as to marginalised groups within medieval society. The liminality of impaired persons is especially apparent in terms of gender, in that disabled people are deemed nowadays not to fit into the gendered male/female roles, so that severely impaired people are regarded as quasi-asexual.

Perhaps connected with the idea of impairment and disability as liminal are the notions of deviance and labelling. Deviance and liminality both pose challenges to established ways of thinking in a society. The liminal person, by being in-between categories, escapes categorisation, and does not occupy a fixed place. Similarly, the deviant person, by deviating from the 'norm', needs to be fixed into place through categorisation, in this case through labelling. The iconoclastic critic of modern medical practice Ivan Illich, though not strictly speaking an anthropologist, has expressed some important thoughts on deviance and how labelling renders the deviant harmless which are worth citing at length.

> Any society, to be stable, needs certified deviance. People who look strange or who behave oddly are subversive until their common traits have been formally named and their startling behaviour slotted into a recognized pigeon-hole. By being assigned a name and a role, eerie, upsetting freaks are tamed, becoming predictable exceptions who can be pampered, avoided, repressed, or expelled. In most societies there are some people who assign roles to the uncommon ones; according to the prevalent social prescription, they are usually those who hold special knowledge about the nature of deviance: they decide whether the deviant is possessed by a ghost, ridden by a god, infected by poison, being punished for his sin, or the victim of vengeance wrought by a witch...By naming the spirit that underlies deviance, authority places the deviant under the control of language and custom and turns him from a threat into a support of the social system. Aetiology is socially self-fulfilling: if the sacred disease is believed to be caused by divine possession, then the god speaks in the epileptic fit.[144]

If one applies these theories to medieval notions of impairment, one can demonstrate that two groups of people held 'special knowledge' about deviance: on the one hand theologians, and on the other hand medical authorities and writers on natural philosophy. Both these groups of writers produced texts which, in their various ways, and according to their specific criteria, fixed and labelled the position of impaired people, as shall be analysed in Chapters 3 and 4. In modern Western society, in contrast, it is purely the medical profession which lays claim to 'special knowledge' concerning the kind of physical deviance demonstrated by impairment. Furthermore, if one looks closer at how labelling 'tames' the deviant, another contrast between medieval and modern Western notions emerges: the absence of an umbrella term for 'disability' during the medieval period, as was discussed above, allows for the linguistic taming of *individual* crippled, blind, deaf or otherwise impaired people, whereas modern society, by referring to 'the disabled', places a *collective* emphasis on physical deviance.

Lastly, the ethnological model as outlined by Neubert and Cloerkes permits the continued distinction between the terms 'impairment' and 'disability', so that one need not disregard the theories of modern disability studies altogether. I am in fact proposing a synthesis here of disability studies and ethnological theories. The terms 'impairment' and 'disability' can be roughly equated with the ethnological concepts of 'evaluation' of and 'reaction' to physical difference. Many different cultures 'evaluate' physical difference, in that they recognise and describe such differences, and there are many intercultural similarities in the respective evaluations.[145] 'Impairment' then, in this ethnological model, is regarded as a 'fact' which exists independently of the social values attached to it, but which by virtue of being 'different' physically already becomes a 'disability'. The correspondence of this to the medical model of disability rests in the shared assumption of both models that an impairment is *eo ipso* a 'handicap'. The cultural or social evaluation of an impairment does not actually influence the physical condition of the impairment itself; it does, however, influence the concrete lived experience of an individual, in that the extent of social participation and the degree of consideration shown to an individual is constituted through the (e)valuation of impairment. Simply put, a fractured leg is a fractured leg in no matter what culture one looks at; practically every human culture would recognise the leg as 'fractured' and would deem that an undesirable state for a leg to be in. This would correspond with the 'impairment' notion, which, having its basis in medical and biological concepts, also lays claim to intercultural validity and cultural independence: 'impairment' is then essentially about the recognition of physical difference according to bio-medical criteria, without as yet attaching social judgements to that recognition. One could also argue that this represents an etic approach, in that it tries to state from an external (culturally independent) observer's position whether disability is present in an individual or not. Interculturally one can distinguish between impairments that are recognised as such in a given society, and thereby become 'disabilities', and impairments which are unrecognised. However, by making such distinctions, the definition of 'impaired' used by Western industrialised (i.e. modern European) society is transposed on to other cultures, and the Western cultural and/or medical categories are accorded absolute status.

In ethnology, the 'reaction' to people with undesired differences is, however, strongly dependent on many cultural variables.[146] This 'reaction' would then correspond to the notion of 'disability' as the culturally informed concept. In this model the social and/or cultural evaluation is crucial. A disability is only then present if a corresponding socio-cultural evaluation of an individual has taken place by their society. This evaluation takes place independently of the presence of any 'objective' (i.e. Western or modern medical or scientific) reasoning. The person with the fractured leg might then be reacted to in many different ways in different cultures, just as different cultures would not automatically regard this hypothetical person as 'disabled' if the culturally specific loss of function due to the fracture was insignificant (in our society somebody operating a computer keyboard does not need their leg to fulfil this function, hence in that situation the fracture would not position them as a 'disabled person'). According to this model, theoretically a disability is therefore possible without the prior existence of an objective impairment but in the process of evaluation by a society a disability is ascribed. A flow chart, devised by Neubert and Cloerkes, demonstrates the range of possible reactions to impairment (see Figure 1). The emphasis on

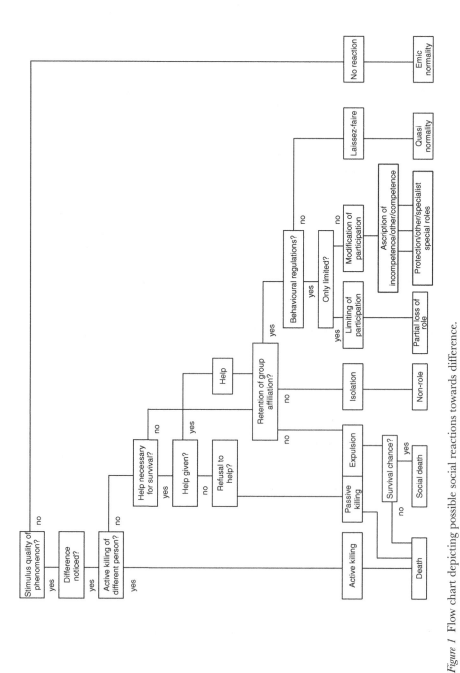

Figure 1 Flow chart depicting possible social reactions towards difference.

Source: Adapted from D. Neubert and G. Cloerkes, *Behinderung und Behinderte in verschiedenen Kulturen. Eine vergleichende Analyse ethnologscher Studien*, Heidelberg, 2nd edn, 1994, p. 55.

socio-cultural evaluation in this model lends it an emic approach, in that concepts are studied and analysed from within a society's belief and value system.

Making conceptual distinctions between 'evaluation' and 'reaction' (or 'impairment' and 'disability') is more or less making distinctions between the assessment of a factual circumstance and the assessment of a human as an individual person; attaching value judgements to a person does not concern just that person's physical, mental or psychological state, but also entails the person's social interactions and more.[147] Nevertheless, both ethnological models have only limited usefulness for intercultural comparisons. This is mainly due to problems of different socio-cultural concepts in describing, naming, categorising and labelling physical conditions. For example, in some non-European cultures somatic impairments like hermaphrodism and infertility are regarded as 'disabilities', whereas the modern Western medical model does not recognise these as such. In fact, as was demonstrated, the recognition of an impairment does not automatically lead to a view of that condition as disabling. For example, in modern Western society strong visual impairment is regarded as a 'defect', but it is not deemed a 'disability' (there are spectacles and contact lenses to correct impaired eyesight); instead it is down to the verdict by a professional (physician, social worker etc.) which manifests a disability: a disability has to be 'accredited' by a recognised authority.

How, then, to proceed from here in discussing disability in the Middle Ages? Having taken issue with modern disability theories, it is necessary to separate the wheat from the chaff. Since not all theories outlined above even address historical or transcultural issues, and of those that do, not all are applicable to the medieval period, selectivity is of the essence. Those theories or theoretical approaches that deal with culture as well as economics, with gender, liminality and personhood, will be found most useful. Jacques Le Goff's work had already transformed the body from a 'natural or banal given into a historically and discursively constructed entity'.[148] As argued above, the bodily discourse of otherness is based on definitions of identity which are grounded in the body, so that the production of identity and the experience of identity are both situated in the body. In this context Miri Rubin spoke of the body moving through a state of 'transcendence or liminality' as the body is transformed by a given cultural ritual, until the body is then remade into a recognisable part of the community. This may be applicable to bodies moving from young to old, or from sickness to health, or from layperson to consecrated priest. However, impaired bodies can be characterised by *remaining* liminal, as the anthropological theories discussed above have demonstrated. Medieval bodies possess a fluidity, according to Rubin, and resist fixity; they are unstable, changeable and not able to be fixed in categories. The medieval body as a body is made up of parts, it is a 'corps morcelé', so that the body is not a whole but a concentration of parts, made up of combinations.[149] Therefore an impaired body is also a female body, or an aged body, or a sacred body. Colin Barnes has suggested that attitudes to impairment are not simply explained by a single factor, but are 'culturally produced through the complex interaction' of economy, belief systems and central values of a given society.[150] This multifaceted analysis therefore is the theoretical approach that is most appropriate for a historical study of disability, which, in the case of the Middle Ages, allows for a positioning of disability within reference points of contemporary religion, scientific and medical knowledge. Though the distinction, made by the modern disability movement, between impairment and disability will be adhered to, it will not be forgotten that impairment, too, is not a purely medical, unchanging, ahistorical 'fact'. The next two chapters will therefore explore medieval notions of the body, of the states of health and illness, and of medicine and its role, within the context of the religion and natural philosophy of the period.

2.3   Summary

Disability has been a theme neglected by historians. In part this has been due to assumptions about the unchanging 'nature' of disability, in that disability was viewed as always having been part of the human condition. When disability was the subject of historical writing, the emphasis was placed on more recent historical periods, such as the nineteenth century. Much historical writing on disability, concerning various epochs, has been produced by medical historians, who tended to describe disability as an aspect of the development of medical facilities in general, taking a progressionist approach. In such histories, the medieval period is generally portrayed as medically backward, so that these secondary sources have, in fact, very little to offer with regard to disability in the Middle Ages. Other periods, such as classical antiquity, have had more interest devoted to them by historians.

The 'linguistic turn' in more recent history writing, that is writing influenced by postmodernist and post-structuralist theories, at first sight would appear to have opened up different avenues of historical enquiry, but conversely, has actually done very little to further the study of physical disability in past societies. Going back to the primary sources themselves, one finds that medieval historiographical writing was following conventions that prevented the inclusion of disability into historical writing, since the powerless, the *impotentes*, which encompassed the poor and various marginal groups, as well as the physically disabled, were not deemed to be suitable subjects for texts about the deeds done by the powerful in society.

It was hoped that the relatively new discipline of disability studies would provide a theoretical framework that would allow one to investigate disability in the Middle Ages. The key theoretical notion expressed by disability studies is the distinction made between impairment (the anatomical or biological 'fact') and disability (the cultural construction imposed on to impairment). Such a distinction allows a culturally independent analysis of impairment which does not automatically assume that impairment inevitably leads to disability in all societies at all times. However, some sociological theories had placed too much emphasis on the individual's stigmatised identity (as in the case of Goffman), while other theories emanating from a materialist viewpoint of disability failed to grasp any ideas about historical periods (notably the much-publicised work by Gleeson). The main problem of most work by scholars from the discipline of disability studies is its complete lack of any sense of historicity – disability studies is essentially an ahistorical field, due to the authors' lack of familiarity of working with primary sources dating to periods more than a hundred years removed from their own.

Anthropological and ethnological theories were found to provide by far the most useful theoretical apparatus for discussing disability and/or impairment in a historic period such as the Middle Ages. Anthropologists and ethnologists, as academics, are used to discarding their own cultural assumptions when examining cultures other than their own. The theoretical framework built up by these disciplines is therefore of far more use to a discussion of disability in the medieval period than either disability studies or medical history. Essentially, anthropology and ethnology allow scholars to recognise the great variance in how disability is perceived, and how the impaired are treated, by different cultures (both geographically and historically) as well as what variations might exist within a single culture. These differences were expressed in terms of intercultural and intracultural variance. Lastly, anthropological theories also raised the point with regard to the concept of 'liminality': the physically impaired are neither truly healthy nor truly ill, for example, and therefore cannot be easily categorised, but sit uneasily in-between conceptual roles.

Simplistic attempts to explain reactions to impairment are those which follow the principle of a genetic reductionism, whereby human repugnance of impairment is positioned as 'inborn' or 'instinctive'. Against such argumentation one can point to the incredible variety of human behaviour, as well as to the different evaluation of impairment in different cultures. Values, norms and the respective reactions to impairment can be universal, culturally specific or even specific to a sub-culture. It would be the aim of future research to establish the relation of these to one another (in history as well as in ethnology this may be done by intercultural comparative studies). Also, certain aspects of attitudes and behaviour to impaired people can be culturally specific, situationally specific, specific to the object or even specific to a personality. So the reaction to people who do not correspond to generally accepted values, like the impaired, can be culturally determined and intensely variable. Even if one thinks of impairment in terms of a 'stigma' (as Goffman did), then one can still regard stigma as being incredibly variable in historic and cultural terms; a stigma can change within one culture from one historic period to the next, and can also be different from culture to culture in a contemporaneous setting.[151]

3 Medieval theoretical concepts of the (impaired) body

3.1 Thisworldly: notions of health, impairment and sin

This chapter will locate the disabled body within the spiritual framework of the Middle Ages, that is within the prevalent discourses of theology and philosophy current between the end of Antiquity and the onset of the Reformation. Particular emphasis is placed on the distinctions made by medieval thinkers between the impaired body in this world, and the impaired body in the afterlife. As mentioned in the preceding chapter, bodies are never *just* physical objects, to be described in a neutral, 'scientific' way, but are objects whose understanding is determined by the intellectual culture of the day. What a body is or what meaning it may have is therefore subject to cultural change. Hence, the following section will examine concepts of the body as a vessel of spiritual and/or religious meaning,[1] plus concepts of what is 'natural' or 'normal' in a body. Since no discussion of medieval bodies could be complete without reference to sin, the question of whether a deformed body reflects a deformed soul will also be addressed.

The Bible as *the* basic text of Christian thought should be the starting point for an investigation of what religious notions circulated in the Middle Ages with regard to disability.[2] Few impairments are mentioned in the Bible overall. In the Old Testament, impairment is mentioned mainly in connection with prohibitions or punishment, and in the New Testament in connection with the healing miracles performed by Jesus and the apostles. In the Old Testament, the main instances are oft-quoted passages from Leviticus and Deuteronomy, which will be discussed more fully later. Other mentions are sporadic and seemingly random. Some examples follow:

- Genesis 19:11: Sodomites trying to attack Lot are smitten with blindness.
- Exodus 4:11: The deaf, dumb and blind are God's creation, as Moses is told: 'Who hath made man's mouth? or who maketh the dumb, or deaf, or the seeing, or the blind? have not I the Lord?'
- Deuteronomy 32:35: 'Their foot shall slide in due time; For the day of their calamity is at hand, And the things that shall come upon them make haste.'

This passage in the 'Song of Moses' has been interpreted to mean that the enemies of the Israelites are cursed, so that they will suffer the accidents or illnesses of old age prematurely.[3]

- 1 Samuel 4:15–18: Aged 98, Eli is practically blind; he dies by breaking his neck due to a fall. This event is reported in a neutral fashion, without appending any metaphysical importance to Eli's physical condition.
- 2 Samuel 4:4: When five-years-old Mephibosheth, the grandson of Saul, was picked up in haste by his nurse trying to flee so that he fell and subsequently became lame.
- 2 Samuel 5:6–8: 'And the king and his men went to Jerusalem unto the Jebusites, the inhabitants of the land: which spake unto David, saying, Except thou take away the blind and the lame, thou shalt not come in hither: thinking, David cannot come in hither. Nevertheless David took the strong hold of Zion: the same is the city of David. And David said on that day, Whosoever getteth up to the gutter, and smiteth the Jebusites, and the lame and the blind, that are hated of David's soul, he shall be chief and captain. Wherefore they said, The blind and lame shall not come into the house.'[4]
- 2 Samuel 21:20 (and 1 Chronicles 20:6): Goliath's son is also a giant, plus he has an extra digit on all his hands and feet, emphasising his 'freakishness'.
- 1 Kings 13:4: Jeroboam's hand withered ('dried up') in punishment.
- 2 Chronicles 16:12–13: King Asa is 'diseased in his feet' in the thirty-ninth year of his reign; he seeks help not from the Lord but from his physicians, and dies two years later.
- Psalm 38: The entire psalm deals with the theme of the sinner plagued by illness, losing 'the light of mine eyes' (38:10), and being deaf and dumb (38:13).[5]
- Zechariah 11:17: Impairment (shrivelling of right arm and blindness in right eye) is threatened to the shepherd as punishment for neglect of duty.

A medico-historical analysis of physical impairment mentioned in the Old Testament led Ohry and Dolev to conclude: 'Our observations show that disabilities are presented as divine punishment for human misdeeds, while compliance with the religious and moral laws will improve or heal physical handicaps.'[6] In addition, disability is more often than not used as a metaphor,[7] as in Psalm 38, for a physical manifestation of an undesirable spiritual state.

Deuteronomy and Leviticus, as mentioned earlier, contain the most relevant passages. Among general injunctions concerning proper sacrifice and worship,[8] Deuteronomy chapter 28 has verses connecting the character of a person, sin and physical imperfection, in that those who disobey the divine law are afflicted with various illnesses and impairments, such as blindness[9] and leg ailments.[10] Just to make sure and to keep all eventualities covered, the sinner or enemy of Israel is further threatened with 'every sickness, and every plague, which is not written in the book of this law'.[11] The book of Leviticus treats illness and impairment after a more precise fashion, listing very specific ailments. There are some protective injunctions, such as leaving part of the harvest for the poor to glean,[12] and not cursing the deaf or deliberately tripping up the blind.[13] The most (in)famous passage[14] relates to proscriptions regarding the priesthood, on who is allowed to become a priest and who not, and is worth quoting in full:

> Whosoever he be of thy seed in their generations that hath any blemish, let him not approach to offer the bread of his God. For whatsoever man he be that hath a blemish, he shall not approach: a blind man, or a lame, or he that hath a flat nose, or any thing superfluous, or a man that is brokenfooted, or brokenhanded, or crookbackt, or a dwarf, or that hath a blemish in his eye, or be scurvy, or be scabbed, or hath his stones broken.

A manuscript illumination from the Wenceslas Bible, dating from around 1400, neatly illustrates the scene where Moses prohibits the priesthood to some of the impaired persons mentioned in this passage.[15] This passage relates purely to prospective priests, and on its own does not imply any negative attitudes to disabled persons in general, though it has often been cited to emphasise the supposed disadvantaging of the impaired in ancient Jewish society by modern scholars. The 'blemishes' mentioned in Leviticus could be considered to be 'canonical irregularities' and, as modern commentators point out, 'The persons affected were not unclean and therefore were not excluded from a share of the sacred offerings,'[16] so that the injunctions against disabled people can be interpreted to mean only that the disabled should not approach the sanctuary, not that they are excluded from *all* sacred ritual, let alone cast out from society altogether (even if the prohibition against becoming priests means they cannot join the elite of society).

The passage from Leviticus relating to the prohibition on 'blemished' men becoming priests has always been over-emphasised, in that there has been an assumption by scholars that this prohibition against disabled people was always strictly adhered to throughout the Middle Ages. Theoretically, of course, such a ban existed, but in practice medieval priests could have been able to obtain a dispensation, though it may have been rarely applied for. Most of these dispensations date from the thirteenth century, and there is also some interesting canon law material which effectively cancels out the prohibition in Leviticus. Some earlier material also exists. The *Apostolic Constitutions*, dated to the fourth and fifth centuries, include a passage[17] stating that bishops must not be prevented from holding their office because of physical impairment or deformity.[18] The implication seems to be, perhaps, that people who had an impairment prior to applying for the priesthood were discouraged from doing so, but once someone became impaired after they had become a priest, they should not be prevented from carrying out their duties. In the Middle Ages proper, the *Liber extra*,[19] a collection of canonical documents promulgated in 1234 by pope Gregory IX, and which was designed to be authoritative throughout the Church, contained an entire *titulus* (XX) on the subject of physical intactness and perfection. Most decretals included there dealing with bodily defects and mutilations dated from the twelfth century, and six decretals confirmed that physical deformity mutilations and serious blemishes morally disqualified a person as a candidate for *higher orders*. One may surmise that lower orders, in contrast, did not warrant such disqualifications. In the case of disqualification, a dispensation was required, and commonly received; however, frequent dispensation did not diminish the overall significance of these prohibitions.[20] What does become apparent is that there is evidence that impaired people *can* have been in holy orders during the medieval period.[21]

In the context of whether impaired medieval people could become priests one may also look at the presence of impaired people in the institution that by the later Middle Ages became primarily involved in training future priests – the university. In theory, one needed to be, or intend to be, in minor clerical orders to attend a university (hence also the barring of women from university attendance), therefore one could assume that universities would enact similar prohibitions against the physically impaired as the Church did. If one looks at university or college admission policies in medieval England, no picture emerges of uniform legislation. There is occasional mention in college statutes of students who were refused admission on the grounds of physical impairment. For example, at New College, Oxford, the statutes of 1400 said that no scholars, including undergraduates, were to be admitted who had an incurable disease or a 'grave bodily deformity'.[22] However, short stature ('dwarfism') was not a reason to bar students. In the mid-fifteenth century two students at Oxford were allowed to determine as bachelors in their own halls (as opposed to in a public place), because the university authorities wanted to spare them the embarrassment caused by their diminutive height.[23] From continental Europe one may even find the example of a medieval 'supercrip' at university: Nicasius Voerda. Voerda had been blind from birth, but nevertheless was allowed to enter Louvain University in 1459, where he qualified in arts and theology; he then enrolled at the University of Cologne in 1489 and received a doctorate in canon law.[24]

Having discussed attitudes to impairment in the Old Testament, with particular reference to proscriptions that may have impacted on the physically impaired in the medieval period, I will explore impairment in the New Testament. There, the description of impairment shifts from punishment to healing. In most instances, disability is mentioned in the New Testament in the context of a healing miracle performed by Christ or one of the apostles, although the metaphorical meaning of disability as punishment does not disappear completely. The most well-known case of sin and impairment relates to the healing of the man born blind, where Jesus is asked by his disciples as to who sinned, the blind man or his parents, 'that he was born blind', and Jesus replies it was neither, 'but that the works of God should be made manifest in him', and proceeds to heal the man.[25] All of the ninth chapter of St John's Gospel is taken up by the story of the man born blind. This was a popular scene with medieval artists; so for example, among many representations, the Echternach Gospels of around 1030 contain an illumination depicting the healing of the man born blind,[26] and this scene also features in a mural, produced in the mid-twelfth century, for the Hermitage of San Baudelio de Berlanga (Soria), Spain.[27] It emerges that blindness is a metaphor for the stubborn refusal of the Pharisees and others to 'see' the truth, as Jesus tells them.[28] As one modern scholar of religion pointed out, Jesus broke with the traditional notion that illness was a result of sin, citing Jesus' statement to his disciples (John 9:3) that neither the man born blind nor his parents had sinned; in like fashion, Jesus did not regard the sick or disabled as (ritually) unclean and therefore untouchable.[29]

One other episode also refers to sin and impairment, in this case the healing of a man suffering from palsy, mentioned in three of the four Gospels.[30] Like the healing of the man born blind, this was a popular theme in medieval art, especially of the earlier period. As representative among many depictions I draw attention to two ivory carvings, one part of a diptychon dating from the early fifth century,[31] the other a book cover from the court school of Charlemagne dating from the early ninth century;[32] in manuscript illuminations we find an example in the *Hitda-Codex*, produced at Meschede around 1020,[33] and even by the late Middle Ages, such as in a miniature in the *Meditationes Vitae Christi*,[34] the iconographic convention of how this scene was portrayed seems to have hardly changed. The man is healed when Jesus sees his faith, and that of the 'multitude' who brought the man to him, and subsequently forgives the man his sins. There is a causal link between sin and ailment here, in that only *after* the sins are forgiven does the impairment disappear, in other words first the cause (sin) has to be removed, then the symptom (illness) will be cured.[35]

However, in the New Testament there is not always a direct causality between sin and illness, or impairment. Illness is not always *necessarily* the result of sin, as was the Old Testament view, but now it just *maybe* the result of a sin.[36] Many instances of the healing of impairment or illness occur in the New Testament where the status of a person as sinner or repentant is not mentioned at all – the question of sin in connection with the healing of an afflicted person is not always an issue. For example, Jesus heals possessed people,[37] a deaf and mute man,[38] a blind man,[39] and the blind beggar Bartimaeus[40] – none of whom are asked about their sins. At the pool of Bethesda Jesus healed a man who had been orthopaedically impaired, waiting there for a cure for 38 years.[41] This scene is illustrated as part of a series of panels, dated to around 1160, depicting events from the Bible, including the healing miracles of Christ, at the church of St Martin in Zillis.[42] The apostles carry on the healing activity, such as Peter who healed people with his shadow alone.[43] A fifteenth-century fresco by Masaccio shows this scene.[44] Philip healed the possessed, people with palsy and lame persons by preaching about Christ,[45] and Paul cured a man crippled from birth.[46] Peter, accompanied by John, heals a man lame from birth, through the power of the name of Jesus.[47] In medieval art, one can find representations of this last episode from three centuries: a mural from the early twelfth century at Idensen church in Lower Saxony, a fresco by Cimabue, produced after 1278 at Assisi,[48] and a fresco by Masolino from the first half of the fifteenth century in Florence.[49] In the biblical text, yet again there is no causal link made between the outward appearance of the body and the possibility of sin.

In summary, biblical references to disability are not of a uniform nature. Some Old Testament references link sin and physical 'blemishes', one very specific occupation (the priesthood) is barred to some impaired people, and some instances of impairment are mentioned without any qualifying moral overtones. In the New Testament, on the whole, the emphasis is on healing, and, with two exceptions, the spiritual condition of the healed person is not of importance. Faith of the supplicant is of far greater consequence for a successful healing than their sin.

Disability in the Bible appears to be of far less concern to the text itself than to modern interpretators. The problem relates mainly to misconceptions of modern disability studies writers, coupled with a belief that the treatment of the disabled in virtually all societies other than the present was linked to religious notions of sin. So, for example, Mackelprang and Salsgiver can state bluntly: 'Judeo-Christian tradition, prevalent among Europeans during and after the Middle Ages, taught that people with disabilities were expressions of God's displeasure.'[50] The authors reiterate the stereotype of a link between disability and sin, and combine that with a further stereotypical interpretation of the (in)famous passage in Leviticus; according to them, disabled people in general are forbidden to enter a temple, which, however, is not a statement to be found anywhere in the Old Testament, and they misinterpret the passage from John 9 to read that people who were born disabled were so because of the sins of their parents, a reading, again, not borne out by the text.[51] Shari Thurer also makes the connection between sin and impairment. 'In the Judeo-Christian ethic, physical defect is just compensation for sin. Moreover, disability may imply a handicap to productivity, and this in a society that values accomplishment.'[52] Thurer oversimplifies and generalises in two instances: on the one hand by assuming that sin and illness/impairment are always linked in all cases, and on the other hand by referring to 'Judeo-Christian' society as a single, static, change and timeless culture. The link between sin and disability also creeps into the following statement by P. K. Longmore: 'It seems likely that in western societies, until the early modern era, disability was viewed as an immutable condition caused by supernatural agency.'[53] With the arrival of eighteenth-century, enlightened ideas, that author believes, the modern, scientific outlook dispelled the 'dark age' notion of sin and disease (or disability or illness) as inextricably linked. Similarly, Weinberg and Sebian argue that the threat of blindness in case of transgressing God's commandments (Deuteronomy 27:27) signifies the sentiment that physical illness and disability are punishments. This is in fact the case with regards to that particular passage in the Old Testament, but the authors also posit this sentiment for the New Testament, arguing that, where Jesus speaks of forgiving sins as well as healing the disabled body (e.g. at John 5:14 and Matthew 9:2), 'These teachings imply that the sick and disabled deserve to suffer as a punishment for having sinned.'[54] As was shown earlier, another interpretation of these passages lies in regarding sin and illness as being in an equal, rather than a causal relationship, so that Jesus does not invariably forgive sins as a prerequisite to curing bodies.

Sin and illness are linked together in a long tradition in Near Eastern communities. One can think here of Babylonian ideas of illness, which among other factors ascribed the causes of disease and ill-health to the 'hand' of various deities, or the 'hand of a ghost'.[55] Sin in many such ancient Near Eastern cultures was equated with ritual impurity, and substances like oil or water acted to cleanse not just physically, but spiritually as well. Ritual purification therefore was believed to bring about physical health in late antique Near Eastern societies such as among Hellenistic Jews, as well as early Christians. In the Bible, a New Testament passage deals with the calling of the church elders to visit a sick person, with the anointing of the sick person with oil, and with the prayer of the faithful which will save the sick person 'and if he have committed sins, they shall be forgiven him'.[56] In other New Testament passages, especially in the Gospels, a different stance is sometimes taken, so that for example in the healing of the man born blind (John 9:1–7) a connection of sin and impairment is rejected. Also, the late antique Roman Church did not dwell on the relationship of sin and illness.[57] Essentially, though, the New Testament demonstrates an ambiguous, incoherent approach to sin and illness. Jesus sometimes criticised such attitudes of linking sin and illness, 'but his healing miracles often included forgiveness of sins along with restoration of health, and in one instance he is said to have told a man whom he had cured not to sin again, or something even worse might happen to him'.[58] This ambiguous nature of Jesus' attitudes to sin and illness forms the core of later Christian views as they developed over time. Sometimes, in later Christianity, the emphasis was placed on the forgiveness of sins, sometimes on physical cures, and sometimes on both combined; to further confuse the issue, at other times the older (i.e. Old Testament) attitudes reappeared which regarded sin as bringing about illness, so that sometimes the ritual purification in the form of anointing was seen as ancillary to physical healing[59] – all these varieties ran more or less concurrently through medieval Christian thought.

In the early medieval period examples for this dual strand of thoughts regarding sin and illness can be found. Caesarius, bishop of Arles (d. 543), several times spoke in his sermons concerning ritual anointing of the sick. His focus in these sermons had changed away from earlier Roman, that is late antique, attitudes on the matter. Caesarius used the passages from James 5:14 to emphasise the *clerical* element in the ritual of anointing, so that he could emphasise the double character of healing by anointing, as both a spiritual (cleansing of sins) and physical (curing the body) action.[60] In Visigothic Spain between *c.*550 and 750 there was some reversal in attitudes towards a more late antique Roman notion of healing, with emphasis placed on the importance of physical healing as well, albeit still retaining the spiritual healing element. One of the Spanish *Liber ordinum* texts of that period includes the following prayer to be said over a sick person:

[O Jesus our saviour, who art the true health and medicine...] Extinguish in him, Lord, the heat of lusts and fevers, destroy the torture of vices and the sting of pains, dissolve the torment of cupidity and sickness, suppress the swelling of pride and tumors, empty out the rottenness of vanity and ulcers, calm the inside of the entrails and the heart...remove the scars of conscience and wounds...put in order the works of the flesh and the material of the blood and grant him forgiveness of his sins.

(Ihesu saluator noster, qui es uera salus et medicina...extingue in eum, Domine, libidinum et febrium estus, dolorum stimulos ac uitiorum obtere cruciatus. Egritudinum et cupiditatum tormenta dissolue. Superbie inflationem tumoresque compesce. Vlcerum uanitatumque putredines euacua. Viscerum interna cordiumque tranquilla...Conscientiarum atque plagarum abducito cicatrices...Opera carnis ac sanguinis materiamque conpone, ac delictorum illi ueniam propitiatus adtribue.)[61]

Here it seems that both physical and spiritual healing are accorded equal place. As Paxton says: 'This highly rhetorical language may indicate that its author drew a causal connection between specific sins and infirmities or simply that the moral condition of the patient was as important as the physical.'[62] If one accepts Paxton's argument that this text does not necessarily or invariably reflect an attitude of causality regarding illness and sin, it again appears there is no clear-cut link between the spiritual and physical conditions. In Ireland, between the seventh and the early ninth century, one also finds rituals for the anointing of sick persons. There the emphasis is placed primarily on the forgiveness of sins, but no causal link is made as to physical health being dependent on spiritual health, so that again the texts appear rather ambiguous in that respect.[63] In summary, among these earlier medieval attitudes towards sin and illness, Paxton surmises that the Visigothic sources tend to favour ritual approaches to the sick from a physical perspective, whereas the Frankish (Caesarius of Arles) and Irish sources 'seem to have moved toward increasing spiritualization'.[64]

Some changes in the state of affairs occur in the ninth century, so that with the monastic reform of Benedict of Aniane, the Frankish rituals also tend toward a quasi-return of old Roman practice and approach closer to Visigothic practice.[65] In the Carolingian texts dealing with ritual anointing examined by Paxton, only one makes a direct, causal link between sin and illness, making bold curative claims for the power of ritual. This is a canon from a synod held at Pavia in 850, which states that 'sins are remitted and consequently the health of the body is restored'.[66] Such a causal relationship was, according to Paxton, 'never the orthodox understanding of ritual anointing',[67] and he points out that of the two North Italian manuscripts which contain the text in question, one manuscript omits the word (*consequenter*) linking forgiveness of sin and restitution of health. In the later ninth century followed some consolidation and synthesis of the ideas outlined above, which more or less came to form the basis for later medieval ideas on the subject; there was, however, never a complete end to the diversity of ritual revolving around sickness (and death) in the Latin West.[68] This excursion into earlier material has been necessary to 'delve into the sources of ideas and customs',[69] as Shulamith Shahar put it, enabling us to trace the development of later notions.

The Venerable Bede, too, one of the most famous writers of the earlier medieval period, preoccupied himself with the question of sin and sickness (or illness/impairment). He discussed one of the healing miracles of Christ at length, namely the healing in stages of a blind man.[70] Bede states that Christ chose to heal this man in a series of stages rather than in a sudden, single miraculous event as in other healings, so as to teach us about the spiritual blindness we suffer; only gradually and in stages can we be brought spiritually closer to the light of divine vision.[71] Here impairment and subsequent healing are used as metaphor, *without necessarily* reflecting on attitudes towards the disabled as sinful *per se*. Bede tells us in a lengthy analysis that for a variety of reasons illnesses are caused by God,[72] but then qualifies these statements somewhat: the morally just are afflicted by illness to prevent them from developing the sin of pride, or to enable them to practice patience like Job, while the morally sinful are smitten with illness as a means of inducing repentance in them; however, sometimes illness 'has nothing to do with the spiritual state of the sick',[73] and the famous example of the healing of the man born blind (John 9:3) is cited at this stage.

The complexity, and ambiguity, of medieval attitudes towards sin and physical illness and impairment is borne out by the changes made within a single narrative, a saint's *vita*, as it was transcribed in the course of the centuries. The *vita* of St Ambrose of Milan exists in two versions: the first version was composed by Paulinus in the fifth century and is extant in several manuscript copies, the second version was written in Milan by an anonymous author and now survives only in a single manuscript, at St Gallen.[74] Clare Pilsworth, who has studied hagiographical texts of the early medieval period in northern Italy, has examined and compared the two St Ambrose-*vitae*. She concluded that in the earlier version, by Paulinus, a link between sin and illness was made, whereas the second version does not seem particularly interested in such a link. Instead, in the later *vita* illness is used by the author for political ends, in that the miracle healings performed by St Ambrose occur to aristocratic people, while the older version was more egalitarian, narrating the cure of people from all walks of life. Sin, illness and cures are therefore tied to the political and social situation of the author of a text as much as they are to prevailing theological notions. There is also a different narrative emphasis in different types of hagiographical texts.[75] The *passioni* (lives of martyrs) model themselves textually on biblical accounts of miracle healing, as found in the Gospels, and therefore mention miracle cures of the blind, the lame and other people one could term 'impaired'. The *vitae* cover a much wider range of ailments, with the healing of all kinds of diseases as well as of impairments.[76] As far as earlier medieval hagiographies, at least, are concerned, one may surmise that different types of texts possess different agendas, and the topos of illness and/or disability becomes subsumed and appropriated by the particular agenda a specific text is promoting. Hence a reworking of St Ambrose's life results in the new author incorporating what is important to him, politically and socially, in the context of miracles and healing, and equally, the martyrologies focus on the cure of impairing conditions because of their imitation of biblical precedent.

Sin, impairment or illness, and notions of a link between them did not cease to be an issue in the later medieval periods. The Fourth Lateran Council of 1215 enacted a canon, number 22 of the council, with the incipit *Cum infirmitas* (sometimes also known as *Quum infirmitas*), which soon after became part of Gregory IX's codification of canon law, the *Decretales*,[77] and hence acquired official status in the Church. In that text is stated with regards to the apparent link between sin and illness: 'Since bodily infirmity is *sometimes* [my emphasis] caused by sin ...',[78] the physician ought to ensure a patient hears confession first before the physician then applies medical treatment, so that the soul is 'cured' prior to the body. The canon does not, however, present an invariable causal link between sin and illness, it is only *sometimes* the case. One could argue that asking the physician to refrain from treatment until after confession is a way of hedging one's bets (in case the patient died, it would at least be with absolution), not a statement of immutable certainty.

In summary, medieval attitudes to ill-health were manifold and ambiguous. A common theme in medieval thought has been the imagery of human bodies as the microcosmos,[79] that is, the human body represents in the small scale the ordering and hierarchy of the wider world outside – the macrocosmos – on the large scale. For example, William of Conches (*c*.1090–1160) stated in his *Sacramentarium* that the human body from head to foot is likened to all of creation.[80] By analogy, what can go wrong with the macrocosmos, that is, the corruption of the world through sin, can also go wrong with the microcosmos, that is, the corruption of the body through illness. This idea was expressed very well somewhat later than William of Conches' statement, by Peter of Celle (1115–83) in his text *De puritate anime*,[81] where he compared the health of the body with the purity of the soul, and illness was seen as corruption of the body, as privation was a corruption of the soul. Refinements and additions were made throughout the high Middle Ages to such basic notions. Theologically, illness could be explained due to humanity's Fall: prelapsarian Adam and Eve did not suffer from ill-health. Postlapsarian humanity, however, incorporates the state of *homo destitutus*, characteristic of which is a deficient nature (*natura deficiens*), so that *destitutio*, *deformatio* and *degeneratio* are practically normal phenomena associated with the human condition.[82] Illness in general is a *modus deficiens*, an absence or shortcoming.[83] In this sense, then, *all* illness is due to sin, namely specifically due to Original Sin. Ill-health may be perceived of as punishment for an individual transgression, but this perception is expressed 'rather cautiously and never in a generalising fashion'.[84]

Conversely, illness (and potentially resulting impairment) could even have a positive aspect, in the sense that if an affliction was sent by God, and not something a person brought upon themselves through their own foolishness, then nothing could cleanse the soul as well as such an affliction. In this respect, sickness/impairment could bring spiritual healing. Such views are found exemplified in a passage of the thirteenth-century Middle English text *Ancrene Wisse*, where temporary (that is, thisworldly) suffering allows one to be 'a martyr's equal'.[85] Sickness (or impairment) could therefore sometimes connote holiness, in the 'correct' circumstances. Ailred of Rievaulx was regarded as most saintly, even when, according to his biographer Walter Daniel, he suffered from various illnesses, some of which, like malnutrition due to his refusal to eat ('holy anorexia') were self-inflicted, while others were not, such as the arthritis forcing Ailred to sleep and eat in the monastic infirmary, and to be carried about on a linen sheet because of his arthritic pains.[86] The effects of illness on holiness can be seen for example in the case of Alpais of Cudot (1150–1211), who became paralysed so that she was bound to her bed, immobile, for about a year.[87] During her sleep and her enforced bed rest she had religious visions, and became known as a holy woman. Being declared a holy person for being incapacitated but having visions was due to the greater religious importance by the high Middle Ages of the *vita contemplativa* (or *vita interior*) over the *vita activa*. Some visionary women actively prayed for disease as a gift from God, Julian of Norwich for example. Many medieval mystic women described their illnesses as an opportunity for salvation, women such as Serafina of San Gimignano, Villana de' Botti, Margaret of Ypres, Dorothy of Montau, Gertrude of Helfta, and the aforementioned Alpais of Cudot. The leprous Alice of Schaerbeke said that her illness 'could be offered for the redemption of one's neighbour'.[88] All of these religious women welcomed sickness on a voluntary basis. While most medieval writers regarded illness (and by implication impairment) as something unpleasant to be avoided, these female mystics saw something positive therein, bringing them closer to God. Their sickness becomes a condition to be endured rather than cured.[89] In fact, the offer of a cure is a 'temptation' for Alpais of Cudot (who in a vision sees the devil as a physician), and for Elsbeth Achler and Catherine of Siena. In similar vein a poem by a nun of Töss nunnery has Christ saying: 'The sicker you are, the dearer you are to me'.[90] There is of course a strong gendered difference here, as Caroline Walker Bynum has pointed out: if an illness was manifest in a woman (of the high and later Middle Ages), she was less likely to be cured in a miracle healing, and her illness was more likely to be seen as something to be endured, whereas men were cured through miracles of their physical afflictions.[91] However, these are 'extraordinary' cases, of physical conditions seen as positive in certain women who were regarded as quite special from the rest of their communities, and one can on no account surmise that such attitudes extended to the 'everyday' illnesses, including impairments, of ordinary kinds of people, of whichever gender. The diseased (or profane, or even heretical) may sometimes be transformed into the holy, and the identity of the saintly constructed against or intermingled with the identity of the diseased.[92]

Having discussed ideas surrounding impairment and sin, I will now take a closer look at medieval notions of the teleological meanings ascribed to physical appearance, that is analysing medieval systems of aesthetics. The impaired body is seen, by modern theorists, in antithesis to the 'normal' body. In general though, in any system of aesthetics where the norm is also that which is beautiful (by that culture's standards), the impaired body is profoundly 'ugly'. Medieval notions of beauty and ugliness were partly informed by the cultural traditions of Antiquity, partly by theology. Since a body never just exists as a material object in this world, according to theologically informed discourse, but a body also embodies spiritual meanings, it is necessary to explore some of the medieval ideas about beauty, ugliness and the body.

Ugliness is the antithesis to beauty. It is a 'discordance that breaks the rules of that proportion on which both physical and moral Beauty is based, or a lack of something that a creature should by nature possess', as Umberto Eco phrased it.[93] However, art has the power to portray ugly things in a beautiful way, therefore the ugliness existing in nature can be represented beautifully in art. For example, representing the devil beautifully in medieval art caused a dilemma. With regard to this, St Bonaventure of Bagnoregio (1217–74) wrote that 'we may say that the image of the Devil is beautiful when it well represents the turpitude of the Devil and as a consequence of this aspect it [the image] is also repugnant'.[94] The relation of beauty, ugliness and sin is therefore a multi-faceted and complex one.

Just as in the New Testament there is no consistent link between physical impairment and sinful state, so in medieval theology such a link is not consistently made. The foremost patristic authority, Augustine of Hippo, firmly postulated the possibility of a beautiful soul encased within an ugly body. Amongst other things, Augustine was occupied by the question where, if a good God created everything, did badness come from (*Si Deus est, unde male?*).[95] His solution was to regard badness and ugliness as a privation (*privatio bono*) from divine goodness and beauty.[96] Beauty and ugliness are also relativised. In a tract entitled *de natura boni*, Augustine argued that the beauty of the ape, which in itself is beautiful and follows the *ordo* appropriate for the ape, is ugliness compared to the beauty of a human.[97] Beauty and ugliness exist only in opposition to one another; without the one the other would be meaningless as an Augustinian concept. Badness (or ugliness), therefore, is the foil of goodness (or beauty). Badness is there so that one may recognise goodness *ex negativo* (out of its opposite), which then makes goodness all the more good in comparison with badness, and the same holds for the pairing ugliness/beauty. This binary pair also has a didactic purpose within the divine scheme of things. Ugliness and badness exist so that one may recognise one's own faults and thereby may be led to praise God. In direct relevance to impairment, Augustine expands this, saying that divine providence shows that corporal beauty is the lesser beauty, since providence also has such beauty accompanied by pain and sickness, deformation of limbs and loss of colour, so that thereby (by the mutability of the body) we are reminded to seek the immutable.[98]

Augustine's concept of beauty and ugliness remained influential, as can be seen in the work of the high medieval scholastics. Philosophically, further concepts such as proportion, form and the relation of the part to the whole were added to the discussion of ugliness. William of Auvergne in the thirteenth century wrote: 'We would say that a man with three eyes or a man with only one eye is physically displeasing; the former for having that which is improper, the latter for not having what is fit and suitable...'.[99] Whether something is deemed ugly or beautiful therefore is connected with ideas about proportion. Lack of proportion means ugliness, as St Bonaventure said: '...there is no Beauty and pleasure without proportion, and proportion is to be found primarily in numbers: all things must have numerical proportion'.[100] But according to medieval philosophy, beauty can also come about through the contrast of opposites, that is, no beauty is possible without ugliness, therefore even monsters have a place in God's creation.[101] Because of a system of symbolism, whereby physical things can lead to knowledge of spiritual things, a moral significance of the physical world existed for an understanding of the spiritual world, and as such this also entailed a place for ugliness and particularly for the monstrous in the providential design of God.[102] Hence Augustine, in his *City of God*, could state that even monsters are divine creatures and belong to the providential order of nature; and Rhabanus Maurus could differentiate between different kinds of providence in portents: monsters are not against nature, but against the nature to which they are accustomed, so *portenta* (which come into being to signify something superior) are different to *portentuosa* (such as children born with six fingers) which are bearers of minor and accidental mutations, out of a material defect but not out of obedience to a divine plan.[103]

Individual ugly things can therefore nevertheless be part of a beautiful creation, or beautiful nature, and by partaking of nature, can even become beautiful through association with the greater entity that is nature/creation. This type of viewpoint was expressed in the ninth century by John Scotus Erigena:

> For anything that is considered deformed in itself as a part of a whole, not only becomes beautiful in the totality, because it is well ordered, but is also a cause of Beauty in general...As true reason does not hesitate to state, all the things that in one part of the universe are wicked, dishonest, shameful and wretched and are considered crimes by he who cannot see all things, are, when seen from a universal standpoint, neither crimes nor shameful or dishonest things; nor are they wicked.[104]

Such ideas were further explored by Alexander of Hales in the thirteenth century. Alexander believed there was a definite and positive place for ugliness or the monstrous within the divine order: 'Evil as such is misshapen [. . .]. Nevertheless, since from evil comes good, it is therefore well said that it contributes to good and hence it is said to be beautiful within the order [of things]. Thus it is not called beautiful in an absolute sense, but beautiful within the order; in fact, it would be preferable to say: "the order itself is beautiful!" '[105] Ugliness is therefore mitigated by the beauty of creation, so that although indivudual elements of created nature may be ugly, nature as a whole is beautiful, and by implication everything *within* nature becomes beautiful.

But beauty also needs integrity and form. This is stated in the theology of Thomas Aquinas, where all things must have all the parts that rightly belong to them, therefore a mutilated body is ugly. For Aquinas, what is required of beauty is 'integrity or perfection: since incomplete things, precisely because they are such, are deformed. Due proportion or harmony among the parts is also required'.[106] Aquinas was retrieving ideas on harmony, proportion and integrity that had already been widely circulated since antiquity. According to Aquinas, the 'human body is an organism whose structure [biological shape] corresponds to the requirements of its form [philosophical shape]'.[107] Form, as in the Platonic sense of the word, that is, the ideal nature of a thing, determines the appearance of the actual, physical body. With this in mind, we can turn to Aquinas' theory of beauty. With regard to the human body he states: 'If the members of the body, such as the hand and foot, are in a state which accords with nature, we have the disposition of beauty.'[108] The way in which the parts of the body fit together to make the whole body defines 'beauty'. Furthermore, the harmonious union of body and soul, which is what makes a human, is emphasised: 'For a soul joined to a body imitates its makeup in point of insanity or docility and the like ...'.[109] For Aquinas, body and soul are linked, so that disharmony in the one (e.g. insanity in the soul) is perceptible in the other (the body). These aesthetic theories are particularly important for philosophical concepts of impaired or deformed people. Aquinas, unlike many other medieval writers, actually addresses the issue of physical deformity: 'There are two kinds of deformity in the human body. In one, there is a defect in some limb, so that we call mutilated people ugly. What is missing in them is a due proportion [of parts] to the whole.'[110] According to Aquinas's notion, some impaired people are ugly because they are not complete in their body, therefore they are lacking harmony and equilibrium, and thus are 'deficient in certain symmetries and correspondences'.[111]

Augustinian concepts are also found in the writings of the Dominican friar Ulrich Engelberti of Strasbourg (*c.*1220–d. 1277). He wrote a tract on divine goodness, *De summo bono*,[112] which also covers a theory of beauty and ugliness: ugliness is *deforme* because it lacks proper form, in other words ugliness, as *de*-formed form is a subversion of the proper shape of created things. He then, however, follows Augustine in saying that a universe which exhibits lower degrees of beauty and goodness is nevertheless a better universe than one which contained only equally good beings. Basically, Ulrich of Strasbourg believed that ugliness, through its very contrast with beauty, contributes to the overall beauty of the whole.[113]

Connected with notions of the beautiful, that is, the proper proportions of the body, and with related notions of the disproportioned impaired body, are ideas revolving around the body as a symbol of social or political hierarchies, and farther-reaching concepts of the body as a microcosm reflecting a wider macrocosm. John of Salisbury (*c.*1115–80) used the analogy of a hierarchy among different parts of the body to express his views on political hierarchies. The head, which governs the body, is, for example, likened to the prince governing a republic, while the hands of the body are likened to officials and soldiers, and so on, down to the feet which support the entire body, which in the analogy coincide with the peasantry. In his *Policraticus*, John of Salisbury describes what happens to the state-body if the feet are removed: 'Remove from the fittest body the aid of the feet; it does not proceed under its own power, but either crawls shamefully, uselessly and offensively on its hands or else is moved with the assistance of brute animals.'[114] The impaired body, then, in this analogy is equated with the 'disabled' republic, literally a disabled 'state'. Expanding on this theme, imagery of the body could also be used as a symbol of towns and urban privileges by late medieval patricians. In religious terms, the best-known body imagery is of course the imagery of Christ's body in association with the cult of the Eucharist. In all these instances, this imagery is 'the natural symbol of the well functioning and harmonious body'.[115] Therefore the body *per se* is to be harmonious and functional, which by implication contrasts the disabled body as a disharmonious and non-functional entity.

The microcosm of the body demonstrates what happens when the entire proper hierarchical order of the macrocosm becomes upset and disordered. The idea of the body as made up of a hierarchy of corporal 'offices' (*officia*) had already been expressed by Cassiodorus in the early sixth century, and was reiterated by Hugh of St Victor in the twelfth century, in *De institutione novitiorum*, where each part of the body performs its own function (*officium*), and must not trespass on the task allocated to another bodily part.[116] The hand should not, therefore, usurp the function of the mouth – which is an interesting statement, since a speech-impaired person is liable to do just that, by using sign language. An impaired person would be, according to this way of thinking, a person whose intracorporal hierarchy had been unbalanced. The body politic whose feet had been removed, in John of Salisbury's text, becomes a disordered body, where hands and knees take over the function of movement properly allotted to the feet. Taking such ideas to a logical conclusion, any impaired body becomes a disordered body, challenging and upsetting the proper hierarchy of the 'offices' within the body, and disorganising the correct function of the body as a whole. One of the more intellectual of medical writers, Henri de Mondeville in his *Chirurgie* dating to the early fourteenth century, also made use of the imagery of specific *officia* pertaining to specific bodily parts,[117] so that anatomically as well as philosophically the impaired body became a disordered body. The notion of disorder in the impaired body can also be encountered in the following example of an intersection between anatomical and conceptual bodies. In the vernacular of late medieval South Western Germany the term '*ungestalt*' (as both noun and adjective) referred to something hideous or hideousness, but which literally translates as formlessness, and metaphorically therefore, unlike hideousness, *ungestalt* has actually no appearance at all. A person in late fifteenth-century Alsace becomes '*gantz ungestalt*', that is completely disfigured, utterly hideous, when their face is mutilated, and also the mutilated wounded and dead on battlefields of the period are described as '*ungestalt*'.[118] One may take this further, and infer that an impaired body that is also disfigured or mutilated – note that a sensory impaired person rarely has an obvious visible physical disfigurement – is in effect *no* body, the *ungestalt* person thereby becoming literally a nobody.

Nevertheless, disordered, defective or impaired bodies need not always be viewed as symptomatic of spiritual defects during the high Middle Ages. That it is not necessary to have a beautiful, or unimpaired, body to achieve spiritual salvation is expressed by Thomas of Froidmont in the twelfth century, who says that God does not require a decorous body but a beautiful soul.[119] St Bernard, in his commentary on the Song of Songs, also mentions the importance of the inner beauty; this is in relation to the black bride,[120] who has an interior beauty contrasting with the exterior ugliness of her dark skin.[121] More strikingly, the Messiah prophesied in the Old Testament is to be thought of as disfigured, so that we can recognise in him neither form nor beauty.[122] The contrast between spiritual inner beauty and exterior corporal ugliness was further embellished by medieval etymology, where word-play and sound of words lend a deeper meaning to the simple understanding of words. So one finds the pairing of *pulchrum/ sepulcrum*, and *corpus/corruptus*, where the didactic message of the material world's transience is emphasised.[123]

Besides authorities who are playing down the importance of physical appearance with regard to the state of an individual's soul there are, however, a few texts which present negative attitudes to ugliness and/or impairment. Matthew of Vendôme regards ugliness as a mistake of nature; nature, when fashioning something to appear ugly, is *insipiens* (foolish) and temporarily incapable of the rationality normally ascribed to nature.[124] Matthew here has a concept of nature, namely that 'nature' (what we would call the natural world) is identical with *natura* (created nature), which is similar to that found in Alan of Lille's *Anticlaudianus*, where nature is described as the *vicaria Dei* (i.e. nature as the substitute or deputy of God).[125] Besides ugliness due to a whim of nature, one finds notions of ugliness manifesting itself in people due to their ethnic origin from the East, where the fabulous and monstrous races are located;[126] due to the disobedience of Adam's children who ate a forbidden herb, resulting in their giving birth to deformed children;[127] due to descent from Cain; or due to descent from the offspring of fallen angels and human women.[128]

In vernacular literary texts of the high Middle Ages the topos of the physically ugly person appears quite frequently, as Jan Ziolkowski's[129] study of ugliness in medieval literature demonstrates, especially in the courtly literature, where ugliness is often used as a parody of the canon of literary beauty. There many examples of ugly people are given, the vast majority of them being female (again, parodying courtly notions of the feminine ideal of beauty), with corporal ugliness taking many shapes, from the ugliness associated with old age, to the ugliness found in the similarity of a person to animals. However, none of the examples cited by Ziolkowski refer to any person as impaired: there are no instances of crippled, extremely short or tall people, blind or deaf persons to connotate 'ugly' in this literary sample. Similarly, in a study of ugliness in the German romances of the high and later Middle Ages by R. A. Wisbey,[130] impaired characters are practically non-existent. The examples cited by him are primarily dealing with giants or exotic figures, whose physiognomy includes composite parts from animal bodies, such as boar's tusks, or ears like an elephants, or a hairy body. The literary figure nearest to an impaired person is a wild man-like character with a long crooked back in the *Yvain* of Chrétien de Troyes, who is otherwise falling into the category of the animal-composite figure.[131] In the *Mabinogion* a herdsman is described as ugly, having only one eye and one leg,[132] and as such forming an exception, in that his features could be regarded as those of an impaired person. In *Wigalois* by Wirnt von Gravenberc (c.1200) the wild woman Rûel has a crooked back and crooked legs,[133] which features conform to the stereotypical description and catalogue, given in head to toe fashion, of a wild man or wild woman as contrast and thereby parody of the courtly beauty ideal. The literary characters may be perceived as ugly, but the features that render them ugly are not truly features associated with impairment: there is a notable absence of blind or deaf figures, for example, and the ugliness is so stereotypical as to be parodic of beauty ideals,[134] rather than to be a deliberate denigration of physically impaired people.

The concept of a mutual influence or link between body and soul found its expression in physiognomy. As a 'science', physiognomy has antecedents in classical antiquity,[135] where the character of a person and their physical appearance was seen to be connected. Many of these antique ideas, transmitted through the copying of classical texts, continued into the Middle Ages, becoming especially popular towards the later period, that is the fourteenth and fifteenth centuries. Albertus Magnus opined that the physical appearance of a person can influence their character, qualifying this remark, however, by adding that this does not make a person behave in a certain way *absolutely*. This means a person retains an element of free will, so that instead individuals should strive to overcome the negative effects of physical blemishes.[136] According to Albertus Magnus, the soul moves the body in many ways; conversely, the parts of the body can pervert or corrupt in different ways the activities of the soul.[137] These sort of sentiments pave the way for the view that there is an interplay between soul and body, and possessing an impaired, defective, disfigured or simply an ugly body can mean that such a person also has a defective, that is, evil, soul. In a way, therefore, such sentiments counter the older, Augustinian views on soul and body, which were far more tolerant in this respect, that were discussed above. By the fourteenth century such ideas were taken further, and had, at least in the textual transmission, filtered down to the level of 'popular' literature: the French poet Eustache Deschamps, thinking that one could have no greater misfortune than to have deformed children, said 'a man with deformed limbs is misshapen in mind, full of sins and full of vices'.[138] The rising popularity of astrology, as a method of predicting a person's character, in the later Middle Ages may have also influenced the growth in popularity of physiognomics.[139] The association of physiognomics with astrology brought with it a view of the 'correspondence and analogy between humans, the natural world and the heavens'.[140] By the fifteenth century, the link between appearance and character was in the intellectual domain again as well as in the popular, as Guy Marchant, a Parisian theologian, printer and librarian, scholar and humanist, exemplifies. In a section entitled 'The Judgment's of Man's Body' in one of his publications,[141] he said: 'First we advertise that one ought to beware of all persons that hath default of members naturally, as of forehead, eye, or other member, though he be but a cripple.'[142] This achieves the pinnacle of late medieval prejudice against the physically impaired, warning 'normal' persons against the bodily other. In popular physiognomics of the late Middle Ages a person's moral disposition was believed to be apparent from their facial features,[143] though it is unclear how much importance the appearance of the rest of the body held for a physiognomic assessment of character. As a sideline in the discussion of character and physical appearance one may mention the effect demonic possession was believed to have in the later medieval period. Johannes Nider (d. 1438) mentions in his *Formicarium* that while angelic possession was a sympathetic and pleasant experience, demonic possession made people 'develop deformities in their eyes, face, and gestures [which are] horrible for other men to look at'.[144] The popularity of physiognomics, growing throughout the later Middle Ages, actually peaked in the sixteenth century. The famous character description of Richard III by Shakespeare, whereby the deformed, 'unfinished' Richard, 'cheated by nature' and with dogs barking at him, symbolises the very idea of an evil mind in an evil body, is as much pure sixteenth-century attitude as Martin Luther's vision of the devil in the form of a severely impaired child. However, it is these sorts of post-medieval sentiments that are usually cited by historians and disability theorists alike as examples of medieval notions about disability.

Generalising stereotypes of impaired people can be read as being part of the same intellectual strand as physiognomy. Bland statements, such as that blind persons are always fatter, possess a stronger body odour, and are more astute than the sighted, or that a person whose hand has been amputated always feels cold on that side of the body as the amputation, crept into texts on what we would now call natural history which were popular in the fourteenth and fifteenth centuries. These sentiments regarding blind people can be found in an encyclopaedic compilation by an anonymous author, the *Lumen animae*, on natural philosophy and morality, which misquotes Theophilus's famous *De diversibus artibus* in that respect, erroneously ascribing the origin of these prejudices to Theophilus.[145]

The depiction in art of physical impairment can of course also reflect cultural and social attitudes. The massive study by Ruth Mellinkoff[146] of physical difference, in the sense of disease or deformity (though not necessarily impairment), as depicted in late-medieval northern European art indirectly sheds some light on such attitudes of the period. In the context of a particular painting 'evil' characters are very often recognisable by their ugliness, deformity, or just plain physical difference from other characters, ranging from the kind and colour of clothes they wear, to their hair, posture, skin condition or even skin colour. In religious art, for example, the tormentors of Christ are often shown with just such 'blemishes'. Mellinkoff explained that 'ambivalence characterised attitudes toward those whose physical appearance had been affected by disease or deformity. Although the pious preached that charity and sympathy should be shown these wretched, a more common viewpoint saw their afflictions as the outward signs of an evil character and sinful deeds'.[147] This summarises the ambiguity of medieval attitudes toward the physically impaired, although this statement does over-emphasise the sin aspect. What is striking, though, is that in the survey of paintings Mellinkoff had conducted, she noted that some types of deformed people were *not* depicted in a negative context, namely those persons we tend to think of as the 'classic' disabled people, that is mobility, visually or aurally impaired people. This may well be due to the fact that by the later Middle Ages there existed a long tradition of depicting the 'classic' impaired person as a 'disabled' person who is the deserving recipient of saintly healing or charity, and therefore not depicting such physically impaired as 'evil' characters.

3.2   Otherworldly: impairment and corporal resurrection

The medieval theological idea of physical perfection in heaven for all those resurrected appears to be based on a series of biblical passages. From the Old Testament's 'Neither wilt thou suffer thine Holy One [Jesus, that is, according to prophesy] to see corruption',[148] medieval theologians deduced this would refer to the fact that God would not suffer his saints to look on decomposition. The idea was then further extrapolated via St Peter in the New Testament's 'neither his [Christ's] flesh did see corruption',[149] to the idea that the whole body (*corpus totum*) is also an uncorrupted body (*corpus incorruptum*), at least as far as the bodies of the saints were concerned.[150] St Anselm (b. 1033) extrapolated even further that the bodies of anyone entering heaven are also whole and uncorrupted. Anyone becoming one of the elect and entering heaven would have to be very similar to the saints, anyway. He stated that the bodies of the elect in heaven will be perfect, irrespective of what their condition was in life: 'There shall be none blind, lame or defective'; only those physical imperfections remain, such as the scars inflicted on martyred saints, which were sustained in pursuit of a righteous life ('but such defects shall remain as would redound to the glory of the elect'), though in general everyone in heaven will be healthy, and will suffer 'no pain, discomfort or unease'.[151] This notion found expression in imagery as well, for example in a tenth-century depiction of an angel who at the Last Judgement is commanding those bodily parts that had been separated or mutilated to re-unite themselves into a whole body.[152] Another depiction exists in a manuscript produced around 1255 at Bamberg or Eichstätt.[153] There the resurrected are shown emerging from their tombs with a perfect body, and those who had been mutilated in life (by war or by wild animals) have their missing limbs (or other bodily parts) restored to them at this moment: that is the significance of the bear in his cave on the far right of the image, who is returning a human limb to its rightful owner. This sort of scene found its way into the Middle High German encyclopedic text *Lucidarius*, which posed the question of what would happen to a person who was eaten by a wolf, which in turn was eaten by a bear, and that by a lion, how could from all of that a person be resurrected? The answer was that that which was human flesh was resurrected, and that which was animal stayed dead, since he who had created it can differentiate well between the two. Like a potter who creates a new vessel out of broken shards, so does God create again a beautiful human being who has no impairments.[154]

The perfection of the body at the resurrection is, however, a well-established idea, going back to that most influential patristic authority, Augustine of Hippo. Augustine said that 'all human beings will rise again with a body of the same size as they had, *or would have had* [my emphasis], in the prime of life'.[155] It would not be a problem, though, if 'the form of that body were that of an infant or an old man; for in the resurrection no weakness will remain, either of mind or of body'.[156] Therefore 'all defects will be removed from those bodies'[157] who enter heaven. Augustine was not entirely consistent in his writings as to which age the resurrected would have, nor was he consistent on the question of which shape, that is height and weight, they would be.[158] The martyrs, however, will be resurrected with their physical marks and scars, since for the blessed 'in those wounds there will be no deformity, but only dignity... the defects which have thus been caused in the body will no longer be there, in that new life; and yet, to be sure, those proofs of valour [the martyrs's scars] are not to be accounted defects, or to be called by that name'.[159] Augustine's near-contemporary, the Syriac writer

Ephraim, states that unborn children who die in the mother's womb will be resurrected as adults, and women dying in childbirth will know their unborn, now adult, children in the afterlife; as to adults, they will bear the marks of their lived experience on their bodies, and saints and martyrs especially will bear the physical scars and signs of their sufferings.[160]

The Church father Tertullian (*c*.160–225) had already written *On the Resurrection of the Flesh*, saying that bodies, even if they were badly mutilated, would 'recover their perfect integrity in the resurrection',[161] so that, if a body had 'wholeness', it could not have disease or deformity, and therefore existed in physical perfection. Thus Augustine and his contemporaries are not exactly formulating radical new ideas with regards to bodily resurrection. Gregory the Great (540–604) also wrote on the resurrection as a physical resurrection. In his *Moralia*, according to Gregory, the resurrected bodies will be the same bodies as their lived-in earthly counterparts 'in nature' but they will be 'different in their glory'.[162] In other words, the characteristics of a body, which constitute the character and therefore the person, are retained, but with the notable exception of physical 'imperfections'.

In the twelfth century, Otto of Freising,[163] almost verbatim and at great length, quotes from Augustine. He feels compelled to add to this that, although Augustine said persons will be resurrected in the bodily shape they had in life, 'we must not suppose that giants are brought back in such great stature, dwarfs in such extreme littleness, the lame or the weak in a state so feeble and afflicted, the Ethiopians in an affliction of colour so disagreeable, the fat or the thin in their superabundance or their lack of flesh, to a life which ought to be free from every blemish and every spot'.[164] He bases his aesthetic value judgements on other passages from Augustine,[165] dealing with notions of beauty and ugliness. With regard to 'monsters and abortions', and 'hermaphrodites, and two-headed creatures, whom a mistake of nature has badly joined or badly divided',[166] Otto of Freising condenses several of Augustine's passages on the question of the rationality of such beings, concurring with him that since they are rational, the same rules apply as for 'normal' human beings. Augustine had written on human monsters:

> Concerning monsters which are born and live, however quickly they die, neither is resurrection to be denied them, nor is it to be believed that they will rise again as they are, but rather with an amended and perfect body. God forbid that the double-membered man [a conjoined twin, perhaps?] recently born in the East – about whom most trustworthy brethren, who saw him, have reported, and Jerome the priest, of holy memory, left written mention – God forbid, I say, that we should think that at the resurrection there will be one such double man, and not rather two men, as would have been the case had twins been born. And so all other births which, as having some excess or some defect or because of some conspicuous deformity, are called monsters, will be brought again at the resurrection to the true form of human nature, so that one soul will have one body, and no bodies will cohere together, even those that were born in this condition, but each, apart, for himself, will have as his own those members whose sum makes the complete human body.[167]

Augustine had therefore made it clear that irrespective of the physical appearance here on earth, no matter how 'unnatural',[168] in heaven, after the resurrection, everyone had a perfect, 'normal' body, and Otto of Freising reiterates these ideas.

Also in the twelfth century, Peter Lombard used the imagery of a statue being melted down and then reforged out of the same material to explain his view that the resurrected body is basically the same body but remade perfectly; physical defects, therefore, are eliminated at the resurrection.[169] The leading thinkers of the monastic school at St Victor, Hugh (d. 1142) and Richard (d. 1173) of St Victor, believed the resurrected body would be identical with the earthly body, but it would be 'transfigured',[170] so that the body in heaven would be free from death, sorrow, disease and deformity. The Cistercian monk Herman of Reun, writing between 1170 and 1180, distinguished a spiritual resurrection of the soul alone, happening now, from a corporal resurrection expected to happen in the future, at which there will be no 'defect or deformity' and no 'corruption and poverty and want and all unsuitable things'.[171] In the mid-thirteenth century the Franciscan Bonaventure returns to Augustinian ideas, stating that the blessed will be resurrected without any deformities, unless they are martyrs, in which case they will carry their scars.[172]

The majority of theological thought on matters of eschatology tended towards the physical resurrection. There are dissenting voices, though. One writer to differ from the essentially Augustinian position on the corporal materiality of the resurrection was the ninth-century Irish philosopher John Scotus Erigena. Erigena believed death separated body and soul, with the body returning to its, ontologically higher, constituents of the four elements, thereby negating the question of the somatic form of the resurrected: reward in heaven or punishment in hell is for the spirit only.[173]

The implications for impaired people of the concept of corporal resurrection in a perfect body pose some interesting problems, which have partly been addressed in the work of Caroline Bynum,[174] though without reference to disability as such. Bynum was interested in examining medieval theories of the unity of body and soul, and in that context also discussed how the notion of the physical resurrection impacted on notions of body–soul unity. However, though mentioning the medieval writers who insisted on the physical perfection of the resurrected body, and additionally discussing medieval theories of self and personhood, Bynum neglected to utilise these findings for a discussion of how such theories could impact on the physically impaired, which of course is the main focus here.

Ideas of the unity of body and soul are not unique to the Middle Ages. In early Christian thought the notion of σῶμα (soma) was already apparent as a term used to refer to a body together with its whole personality and character, the self, therefore meaning body *and* soul, and not just the matter, the flesh, so to speak, of the body. Furthermore, when it came to notions of spirit or soul (the *anima* and *animus* of medieval philosophy), in Jewish thought of the Hellenistic period, in the

New Testament, and among early Christian orthodox thinkers there was no clear distinction made between the terms for spirit and/or soul, πνευμα (pneuma) and ψυχη (psyche).[175] The orthodox Christians followed the Jews in stating that 'the human personality is a single psychosomatic unity'.[176]

In the medieval period as such, one finds similar thoughts on body–soul unity.[177] In Hildegard of Bingen's *Causae et Curae*, for example, human beings are said to exist with two natures, namely those of body and soul, just as the flesh does not exist without blood, nor blood exists without flesh, 'though they are dissimilar in nature';[178] the soul is therefore said in no way to exist without the body, '... soul and body are one ...'.[179] An expression and further development of such notions can be encountered in eucharistic theology, after the fashion in which it emerged between around 1150 and 1350. This theology was primarily an espousal of Aristotelian philosophy regarding matter, whereby the body was seen to exist as both matter and form. The substance of a body was the crucial element consisting of both matter and form, which were nevertheless separate entities in their own right. A body was extended from matter and took a form which was governed by a particular appearance, quantity and shape.[180] This begs the interesting but sadly unanswered question of what 'form' impaired bodies would have taken, or of what 'form' contributed to the 'substance' of an impaired body, particularly one impaired from birth. And it throws open wider questions surrounding possible 'identities' of medieval impaired bodies, which will be addressed here.

At the turn of the twelfth to the thirteenth century the notion gains credence, influenced by the Aristotelianism then gaining popularity, that the soul has powers that can only be realised in conjunction with the body; the soul alone has no identity, but the personality of a person constitutes itself from both body and soul. William of Auvergne (d. 1249), for example, said that the soul does not form the actual person, instead, in contrast to the angels, it is the nature of the human soul also to possess a body and to be united intimately with it, so that the perfection of the soul is only accomplished through its corresponding body.[181] By the fourteenth century, the teachings of Thomas Aquinas on the self, form and identity and continuity had become accepted. Aquinas had theorised a 'whatness' (*haecceitas*) of the self embedded in the soul, where the soul takes on a similar position to what psychologists would now term the location of identity. The soul does not just accidentally possess a body with a specific gender, skin colour, impairment or age, but the soul carries the structure of the self, of the 'ego', and this is what deter- mines the body which will be resurrected, with all its physical characteristics. A soul cannot just wander from body to body, but needs its 'own' body. If one can at all speak of a late medieval theory of identity, then part of what we would now ascribe to the body, that is physical characteristics, would then have been ascribed to the soul. According to Aquinas, the soul carries the body in it when that body is absent, and the 'ego' is apparent when soul and body are united, as in life or after the resurrection. So the 'ego' is neither just the soul nor just the body, the 'ego' is a 'person' with an identity. Aquinas expressed that the soul is not the whole person, nor is my soul my 'self'.[182] A modern scholar of medieval religiosity, Arnold Angenendt, also discussed the problems encountered by medieval theological authorities with regard to the corporal perfection at the resurrection, of bodies some of whose parts had gone missing in life, through maiming for example, and indirectly thereby touched on the issues of disability at the resurrection and the unity of body and soul. Summarising the high medieval view, according to Angenendt, one can state that the lived life is eternalised together with the potential of its experience; it is not a faceless soul that enters the afterlife, but one that has been impressed with its own, earthly life.[183] As Bynum similarly concludes, such Thomist theories are not very far removed from late twentieth-century theories of identity and personhood.[184]

> The materialism of this eschatology expressed not body–soul dualism but rather a sense of self as psychosomatic unity. The idea of person, bequeathed by the Middle Ages to the modern world, was not a concept of soul escaping body or soul using body; it was a concept of self in which physicality was integrally bound to sensation, emotion, reasoning, identity – and therefore finally to whatever one means by salvation. ... Person was not person without body, and body was the carrier or the expression (although the two are not the same thing) of what we today call individuality.[185]

This would mean, in modern psychological thought, that a person with an impaired body would have a sense of identity of which the impaired body is a part. However, as can be seen from the examples above, the impaired body is not resurrected in an impaired state (unless impairment was the consequence of martyrdom) but instead every person will be resurrected with a perfect, unimpaired body. Where does that leave, in modern thought, the identity of the impaired person? In a sense, the impaired person will lose part of their identity at the resurrection by losing their physical impairments. The contradiction between perfect body at the resurrection and impaired body in life throws up quite a few problems about the identity or personhood of impaired people, as far as modern disability theories are concerned.

One could argue that none of these highly abstruse theological concepts were of any concern to ordinary people, so that the question of resurrection, identity and corporeality is really only academic. Nevertheless, through preaching about the resurrection and imagery of the Last Judgement, where the resurrection is depicted very physically, ordinary people must have grasped at least a smattering of such theology, including of course impaired people. As an example of how theological notions of the bodily resurrection may have filtered down to popular level one can cite surviving sermon texts, the *exempla* collections[186] on which sermons were often based, and miracle plays. Sermons in particular would have been important tools for the dissemination of such theology, since the medieval pulpit, in the words of one medievalist, 'may well claim to be the parent of popular adult education'.[187] Sermons included not just anecdotal stories, but also a smattering of natural history, stories about foreign lands, and history.[188]

One sermon from a late-medieval English manuscript has the following to state about the resurrection:

> ȝiff thou ende in good liff... than thou shalte to heven bothe bodie and sowle, even as thu arte here. But thi bodye shall than be glorified. What is that thi bodie that is nowe so hevy and so hoge, it shall be than as bright as the sonne...[189]

In an English miracle play, too, one can find allusions to the perfection of the body after the resurrection: in the Judgement scene from the fifteenth-century York cycle, the character of First Good Soul says: 'Lofed be thou, Lord, that is so sheen/ That on this manner made us to rise,/ Body and soul together, clean [= wholly],/ To come before the high justice.'[190] Some notion of bodily resurrection and physical perfection therefore will have been present at popular, non-theological level.

So the question still stands: did this affect the identity of impaired people? Another approach would be to argue that the comparison with twentieth-century psychological concepts is exaggerated, that one cannot, in fact, speak of identity. Here, however, the texts of Thomas Aquinas are actually very clear: by the later thirteenth century, at least, the concept of the unity of body and soul, and the localisation of 'ego' in the soul and the body, do allow a comparison with modern notions of personhood or identity. So if we assume that people did have some, albeit maybe watered-down, notion of a perfect bodily resurrection, and if we also assume that notions of the body as part of one's identity were existent, we still have the problem of impaired people's identity. If we do apply a rigorous twentieth-century view of identity, we are left with having to conclude that a (high and later) medieval impaired person had some kind of 'schizophrenic' perception of their body: an impaired body in life, a perfect body after the resurrection, so that in some ways they would not have the same body after life, even though they were taught that a person was only what they were because of their body *and* soul. Could it be, in the medieval intellectual discourse, at least, that though corporeal identity was recognised, impairment as a form of corporeality was just not considered important? Though sex, age or skin colour may have been important, physical impairment was not? This seems to be the most fruitful approach. The patristic and medieval authors cited above mention again and again that sex of a person is retained at the resurrection as a physical characteristic of a particular individual, but physical impairments or marks of illness are not retained. I therefore propose that though the Thomist notion of body and soul may be reminiscent of a twentieth-century psychology of identity, this is not the case entirely or unreservedly. It needs qualifying to allow for the idea that although certain physical characteristics (such as sex) may matter, others do not. Among the latter, physical impairments must be grouped. In fact, re-reading in this light the eschatological statements that only saints and martyrs carry their impairments with them at the resurrection shows just how special these cases are deemed to be: ordinary folk do not carry their impairments with them, whereas impairments sustained in martyrdom are special to the saints.

One may cautiously infer from this that impairment matters to twentieth-century people with regards to shaping an identity but that to medieval people identity, though including a corporeal element, was constructed somewhat differently. The physiognomists, of course, come closest to a modern notion of 'identity' by insisting on the influence of bodily characteristics, including impairment, on the character of a person – but these are ideas not found in the eschatological treatments. In fact, both Albertus Magnus and his pupil Aquinas point out that physical defects are repaired because they are of no consequence morally; as Bynum phrases it:

> The restoration comes, however, not in order to conceal their past experience but because their bodily defects might be adventitious, not truly reflecting moral character. Thisworldly defects such as blindness or fever have nothing to do with guilt or merit.[191]

This puts into question the whole concept, as was discussed in Chapter 2.2, of a Goffmanesque 'disabled/spoiled identity' for the theological or intellectual discourse of the Middle Ages. Being physically impaired in the Middle Ages may not automatically be part and parcel of one's identity; one may have an identity as a 'woman',[192] a 'Jew',[193] an 'old' person, but not as a 'disabled' person.

One final topic about medieval beliefs in bodily resurrection needs addressing. So far orthodox views of the corporeality of the resurrection have been dealt with. However, among the unorthodox, divergent opinions were to be found, most notably amongst the Cathar heresy. Catharism had a very negative attitude to the body *per se*, believing the body, and the material world in general, to be the creation not of the divine but of satanic forces, while only the soul and the spiritual world were the creation of God. Cathars therefore did not believe strictly in corporal resurrection, only in a life of the spirit.[194] Within such a scheme of things, what impact did such ideas have on physical impairment amongst Cathars? Would a deformed or impaired body be regarded even more a sign of the Devil's creation than a 'normal' body? Or would this physical difference be, literally, immaterial, since if only the soul is important the body is so irrelevant that the physical appearance of it in this world just did not matter? If the latter was the case, and we do not know for certain,[195] then the entire scheme of linking sin and physical shape, as sometimes happened in orthodox Christianity, would not be an issue amongst the Cathars. What impact this may have had on the day-to-day treatment of impaired people is a matter for even more speculation.

3.3   Summary

The physical body in medieval thought is a vessel conveying meanings beyond the purely anatomical, since it also embodies spiritual, theological and philosophical connotations. The Bible as the starting point for Christian beliefs was therefore chosen for a preliminary discussion of physical impairment. It was found that, apart from key passages in the books of Leviticus and Deuteronomy, the

Old Testament portrayed a relatively indiscriminate set of attitudes towards physical impairment. Prohibitions from Leviticus against physically deformed people becoming members of the priestly hierarchy may not have been as stringently adhered to in the Middle Ages as such, as there were a number of canonical dispensations for such cases. In the New Testament, a shift from punishment to healing occurred with regard to physical impairment. Numerous instances of miracle healings by Christ and the apostles testified to this. Especially the perceived link between sin and resulting illness or impairment became of far less importance in the New Testament, while some modern scholars have still stuck with the notion of all impairment as being due to punishment for spiritual transgression.

In the earlier medieval period, links between sin and illness or impairment were not made consistently, or always rigorously applied – a variety of attitudes to connections between sin and impairment ran more or less concurrently through medieval thought. The power of ritual as an instrument of spiritual healing was never completely absent, though, even if sometimes greater emphasis was placed on physical healing. In the high Middle Ages, these ambiguities were, in a sense, enshrined and coded in canon law through an article passed at the Fourth Lateran Council of 1215, whereby illness (or impairment) was regarded as only *sometimes* being caused by sin. Theologically, all human ills were caused by sin, due to the primeval Fall from grace, so that all illnesses, without any hierarchical qualifications, were in a very wide sense due to sin.

Medieval notions of aesthetics, that is, questions of what is deemed beautiful and what ugly, were also discussed. Here again beauty and ugliness were seen to exist in a theoretical framework where deeper meaning was applied beyond the anatomical alone. One important observation has been that deviations from beauty, or deviations from the 'norm', in the body as microcosm related to notions of disorder and chaotic reversal of the scheme of things in the wider world as macrocosm. A brief examination of literary texts showed that although parodic ugliness was employed as a topos of courtly literature, physical impairment as such played a much lesser role. Finally, in connection with ideas about aesthetics, late medieval concepts of physiognomy were discussed. Physiognomic theories did make a link between a person's outward appearance and the condition of their inner being.

An interesting issue has been what implication medieval notions of the afterlife had for the physically impaired. In general, medieval theologians and philosophers advocated a genuine corporal resurrection, at which the body as well as the soul would enter the afterlife. The physical shape the bodies of the resurrected would have in heaven was that of perfect bodies, with no 'defects', therefore manifesting no conditions we would now term impairments. An exception might be the bodies of saints and martyrs, whose physical scars and deformities would still be present at the resurrection, thereby setting them apart from the average impaired individual. These notions of corporal resurrection with perfect bodies carry important consequences with them for medieval notions of what we would call identity and personhood, something the disability theorists discussed in

Chapter 2.2 have emphasised. It was found that by being resurrected with a perfect body, while at the same time body and soul were seen as closely linked, medieval notions of identity and/or personhood differed markedly from such modern theories with regard to physical impairment. In modern theories, physical impairment is seen to shape and influence an individual's identity, while in medieval thought, it appears, physical impairment was not regarded as a very important criterion for a person's identity. Lastly, such notions of identity and physical resurrection were briefly discussed in relation to unorthodox beliefs in the Middle Ages, with specific reference to the Cathar heresy.

4 Impairment in medieval medicine and natural philosophy

4.1 Impairment and the medieval 'sciences'

In the discussion of modern theories of disability, it has been pointed out that there exists a tension between the 'medical' model of disability and the 'social' model. In this context, one can further differentiate between 'disease' on the one hand, and 'sickness' and 'illness' on the other hand. Medical sociology looks at disease as an abnormal biophysical condition, whereas illness and/or sickness are looked at as social roles. Disability thus becomes a chronic illness. This model has been criticised by disabled people as too one-dimensional and too negative. Medical sociology treats all impairments as illness, whereas the social model of disability tries not to regard disability as an illness, but as a form of social oppression.[1] Taking as the starting point those modern theories of disability, which regard disability as a social condition and impairment as a biomedical one, this chapter will explore medieval medical notions of 'impairment', not of 'disability'. In this context, medieval impairment will be examined in its relation to the medieval 'sciences'. The causality of impairment in medieval thought will be discussed, as will medieval medical attempts to prevent the formation of impairments, lastly turning to what modern scholarship terms 'social medicine' and 'alternative therapies'.

When talking about medieval 'medicine', what historians actually mean is just one facet of a wide range of ideas about health and illness, physical and spiritual well-being and healing activities, namely those that have been recorded in writing, and preserved for the perusal of medical historians and medievalists. This automatically excludes from the historical record the vast majority of what has been called 'folk medicine', or 'traditional remedies', or magical medicine, unless instances of such practices happened to arouse the attention of a particular medieval writer, who then generally had an unfavourable opinion on it. Miracle healings, which we would now perhaps categorise as 'magical medicine', were of course perfectly acceptable within their religious context, and are documented in a vast literature, as we shall see in Chapter 5, which will explore impairment through a discussion of miracle cures. In its narrowest definition, the study of medieval medicine therefore revolves around the analysis of medical textbooks, written by literate, often university or medical-school educated, health professionals.

These types of texts were intended as manuals for the instruction of other medical professionals, sometimes with more of a theoretical, sometimes more of a practical approach to the topic. Both surgery and medicine proper were thus written about. Other sources, however, from literary texts such as romances, or chronicles, or encyclopaedias dealing with what we would now call 'natural history', or religious texts such as biblical commentaries, also contain evidence for medieval notions of medicine. Because of the scarcity of references to impairment in the narrowly defined medical sources (the textbooks, manuals, *regimen* instructions and such like) I have also cited examples of medical beliefs and practice from these other, strictly speaking 'non-medical' sources.

One may encounter a problem if one is speaking about 'medieval notions' of medicine, and as a historian, both of medical and medieval history, one concentrates mainly on that (narrow) body of sources composed of medical textbooks. Namely, it begs the question in how far, if at all, such a small facet of medieval culture can be regarded as representative of attitudes to, concepts, and notions of medicine of society as a whole, not even taking into account the question of regional differences (such as divergences between Northern European and Mediterranean culture) and diachronic differences (between early, high and later Middle Ages). Essentially, since the textbook medicine which forms the bulk of medieval medical sources is the product of medical schools or is university-derived,[2] this is a question revolving around the 'medicalisation' of medieval culture. From the twelfth century onwards, the world of the liberal arts developed channels of social diffusion which became well-established and institutionalised as time went on. This diffusion was helped by the popularity of 'scientific encyclopaedias' in the thirteenth century, by writers such as Vincent of Beauvais, Thomas of Cantimpré, Bartolomaeus Anglicus and Albertus Magnus. 'Scholastic society was thus capable of building routes of communication along which there flowed currents of ideas and values between university circles and the rest of society, and was also capable of creating suitable (or at least acceptable) conditions for a labour market attractive enough for university graduates.'[3] It is reasonable to assume that what happened regarding the interplay between scholastic culture and wider medieval culture would also be applicable to the medical realm. Precisely this interchange, between learned medicine and 'popular' culture, is what Michael McVaugh studied for one region of medieval Europe – Aragon in the early fourteenth century. McVaugh found that the growth of 'bookish' medicine was not just due to its promotion by learned practitioners, but also due to public enthusiasm for learning and public expectations of the medical profession. Referring to a 'medicalisation' of later medieval society is therefore a valid concept.[4] It then becomes possible, for the later medieval period at least, to use medical textbooks as evidence for notions of the causes of and therapies for impairments.

One of the issues that need to be discussed before having a closer look at what medieval medical texts had to say about impairment concerns definitions of 'medicine'. What was medieval society's concept of 'medicine', and how did it differ from modern concepts? As anthropological as well as historical studies have demonstrated, different societies had different ideas of what medicine revolved around. To overcome misunderstandings due to varied definitions of the term, one modern historian has devised the following definition of medicine, which is perhaps more universally applicable cross-culturally than many definitions espoused by medical historians:

> By 'medicine' we mean (1) the substances, mechanisms, and procedures for restoring and preserving health and physical wellness; and (2) those who employed such substances, mechanisms, in order to assist people who availed themselves of their expertise. So medicine's role has been like that of religion but much more limited: to restore to health those who were beset by sickness or hampered by dysfunction or injury; in some instances to succor those whose health medicine could not restore; and to preserve health through prophylaxis or regimen.[5]

'Medicine' then, according to this definition, can encompass a wider range of notions and activities than the more narrowly defined modern view of medicine, as a purely biomechanical model, while medieval 'medicine' would fit this theoretical model.

One of the main differences between medieval and modern notions of what constitutes 'medicine' lies in the respective inclusion or exclusion of the supernatural or religious: the medieval world-view (and this applies to the entire period, from late antiquity to the early modern) did not insist on the division between 'medicine' (or 'science', for that matter) and religion (or metaphysics) that the post-Enlightenment mentality does. Medicine and religion were closely connected, already in the ancient world. The ancient Greek thaumaturgic demi-god, the *soter* Asclepius, has been compared by at least one historian with Christ the *medicus salvator*, or with the pagan healing gods of early medieval Scandinavians: Christ as healer can be positioned in this view as a new variation of the old, and culturally diffuse, theme of a *deus medicus*, a healing deity.[6] In some ways, therefore, this chapter is only a distinct segment, an artificial separation from the following one which deals with miracle healings, due to the constraints imposed by modern notions of what constitutes 'medicine' and what 'religion'. Religious influence over 'medicine', or at least attempts to exercise some modicum of control over medical practitioners, is another example of the close connections between the realms of the religious and the medical in the Middle Ages. Modern historians have often cited the Church's insistence, dating from a canon enacted by the Fourth Lateran Council in 1215, that physicians should get the sick to confess their sins to a priest before the physician treated the disease. This has often been interpreted to signify that the Church saw a link between sin and illness, so that therefore confession, and absolution, was regarded as a prerequisite to a successful cure. This is a vastly exaggerated view, in my opinion, especially seeing as, ironically, in the same canon, the text also stated that 'bodily infirmity is *sometimes* [my emphasis] caused by sin . . .'.[7] That text therefore does not present an invariable causal link between sin and illness, it is only *sometimes* the case. Perhaps one should bear in mind the risks for the patient that medical intervention carried in the medieval period (and sometimes still does, today, as news reports on botched medical procedures testify). In the light of such risk, it would only seem sensible for a patient to make a confession, so that should things go wrong, and the patient died, they would not depart this world unabsolved and in a sinful state. A similar point has been made by Michael McVaugh. He thinks that doctors were aware that getting their patients to confess could lead the patients to think they had a mortal illness. Such a negative psychological state might then impede the patient's physical recovery. Medieval doctors, concerned with the mental outlook of their patients as much as with their physical well-being, knew how important it was to get patients to think positively about their recovery prospects. Interpreted from this angle, the frequent injunctions by the Church in the four-teenth century to remind doctors of their duty – to have the patient confess first – showed that doctors were in fact more concerned about their patients' corporal than spiritual health.[8] Connected with the question of how far physicians 'collabo-rated' with the Church is the issue of whether members of the clergy were permit-ted to practise medicine. This is an issue in the high and later Middle Ages, since to attend a course in medicine at one of the universities, one had to be in holy orders. The issue is further confused by the fact that not all of the differing ranks of the clergy were explicitly forbidden the practice of medicine, but only those in higher orders, from fully-ordained priest upwards. Additionally, dispute rages among med-ical historians over whether it was just surgery that was forbidden to members of the clergy, or whether this applied to both surgery and medicine. The only consensus appears to be that there were no hard and fast rules.[9]

Disability is a problematic state, existing in an uneasy relationship with 'medicine', as was evident from the analysis of modern disability theories. Does impairment, then, have the same problematic connotations with regards to medicine? In some respects the answer has to be 'yes', since impairment as a state is not easy to accommodate into a (modern) medical model that is basically split between the binary opposites of health and illness: one is either healthy or one has a disease, whereas impairment, as was suggested earlier, occupies a liminal position somewhere between these two. Medieval understanding of ill-health sometimes allows for a third category, expanding on the binary scheme of health and illness. According to such medical theory, the medieval body can be either in a state of health, of illness, or in a neutral state between these two categories.[10] It is tempting to assume that impairment would have been classified as belonging to the 'neutral' category, but I have not been able to find any explicit textual reference in the sources for this view.

When dealing with notions of ill-health, we are on firmer ground as far as medieval theories are concerned. Very often ill-health, or deviations from health, were categorised according to a tripartite model. This model was derived from Galenic medical theory, and was further expounded by Avicenna (d. 1037).[11] In one form, this model consisted of:

- *mala compositio*
- *mala complexio*
- and *solutio continuitatis*.

Mala compositio referred to malformations of the body, what we call congenital impairments, *mala complexio* meant, literally, 'bad complexion' and referred to imbalances in an individual's humoral system, while *solutio continuitatis* meant a break in the body's 'continuity', what we would term 'trauma', indicating wounds, fractures or dislocations.[12] The first category, congenital impairments, covered conditions that were by and large incurable, so that medicine could do very little with regard to the *mala compositio*, while the third category, *solutio continuitatis*, was considered in the main to be the domain of surgeons and bonesetters. This left the second category, covering humoral imbalances, as the proper domain of physicians. However, impairments would, according to this tripartite scheme, have mainly been categorised as *mala compositio*, if they were congenital, or the result of *solutio continuitatis*, if due to accident or injury.

Medieval medical texts have, in fact, very little to say concerning impairments. In that, medieval medicine is not very different from modern medicine, which also does not deal with impairments much – in modern medicine, impairments, once manifest, and disability are shunted into the sub-discipline of 'social medicine' or 'rehabilitation'. The main reason for this silence, both of medieval and modern medicine, lies in the incurability of impairment. One may assume that medieval reasoning followed a similar logic. Isidore of Seville (b. *c.*560–d. 636), in his *Etymologies*, had defined medicine as 'that which either protects or restores bodily health: its subject matter deals with diseases and wounds.'[13] Once an impairment is manifest, it is too late for the 'protection' of the body through medicine, nor can medicine 'restore' an impaired body to health, so that Isidore's definition does not accommodate impairment as a proper subject for medicine. Occasionally a medieval medical text actually addresses this issue, and provides evidence for the theory that because of the incurability of impairments, medical professionals did not concern themselves with treatments for impairment. Ricardus Anglicus (Ricardus Salernus, fl. late twelfth/early thirteenth century), an author connected with the medical school of Salerno, wrote a tract entitled *Micrologus*. This work follows the normal medieval procedure of discussing dis-eases and their treatment according to a head to toe scheme (*a capite ad calcem*), but at one point provides a justification for why the physician is not concerned with impairments:

> Let the reader note that I do not deal with certain afflictions, such as epilepsy, chronic toothache, paralysis, apoplexy, etc., because I think *they are incurable* and I could find nothing certain or the fruit of experience in the authors I have read, though there are some quacks who vainly try to cure them [my emphasis].[14]

Ricardus therefore believed that a responsible physician should not 'mess around' with patients in attempts to try and cure the incurable. He later provides another reason for not treating what we might term impairments, which this time is less patient-centred, but focused more on the physician's status as a professional with a reputation to uphold. He refers to gout, which, strictly speaking, is more a chronic disease than an impairment as such, although the effects of gout can in themselves be impairing – more to the point, gout as incurable disease can be used as an analogy for incurable impairments. Ricardus states:

> The *Viaticum* is silent about this [gout] and has nothing useful to say, so I will not burden my pages with it, for I boldly assert that surgery and physic are useless, and so consider it *incurable and unworthy of attention* [my emphasis].[15]

Another reason for not dealing with impairments can be found in a later text. The following passage stems from a fourteenth-century tract on physiognomy: 'Master Ypocras instructed his disciples that they should be on their guard against those . . . who are maimed in any member; because they are spiteful in all things, and evil-speaking behind those who in fact think they are their friends.'[16] The 'disciples' of Ypocras (Hippocrates) are, of course, physicians. The inference seems to be that impaired people, who stand little or no success of benefiting from medical intervention, react negatively towards medical professionals, perhaps because of unrealistic expectations which cannot be met.

In surgery, too, the practitioner may be advised against attempting to cure certain conditions. Guy de Chauliac (*c.*1298–1368) mentioned three cases in which the practitioner should refrain from medical intervention: first, when the sickness is incurable (such as leprosy); second, when the sickness is curable of itself but is nevertheless incurable in an '*vnbuxom pacient*' without causing great suffering to the patient (such as cancer); third, when the cure of that sickness engenders a worse sickness (what we might now call iatrogenic disorders).[17]

In his discussion of medieval miracle narratives, Ronald Finucane has looked at the attitude of miracle texts to physicians and their therapeutic abilities. He points out the bias of such miracle texts, in that the registrars at curative shrines and miracle-scribes would, apparently, naturally declare *every* medical condition to be incurable by human means, as a way of advertising their particular saint's powers. Finucane qualifies this statement somewhat, introducing a different angle, whereby he believes the medical professionals themselves would have shied away from difficult or incurable cases. 'Sometimes doctors, perhaps as much to pro-tect themselves as for any other reason, are said to have refused cases which they judged incurable, even when fat fees were offered', and Finucane calls this a discernment of 'a certain degree of professional ethics among medieval practitioners'.[18] In other words, in this view, doctors did not try to overreach themselves, nor did they try to experiment on patients. Doctors therefore did not attempt to cure what was beyond their means.

For the reasons outlined above, my discussion on medieval medical views of impairment will therefore centre on two main topics: aetiology of impairments, and prevention of impairments. Medieval medical and natural philosophy texts tried to explain how impairments came about, or they tried to describe measures which prevented the incidence of impairment. A third topic, social and 'alternative' medicine, will present the more practical side to complement the previous, more theoretical, themes.

4.2   Aetiologies of impairment

It has been stressed that impairment is a problematic condition in (modern) medical theory. One reason for this is the problem of its aetiology. Impairments can be caused by a variety of factors, ranging from congenital impairment (with its own sub-factors of causation), via the effects of diseases, to the effects of trauma (that is, accident or injury). This means that 'the differentiation between disability and illness is blurred.'[19] One criterion of disability, or impairment, has been its permanence as a condition, but this is an insufficient one. First, chronic ailments can be regarded as both impairments and as illnesses; second, many illnesses do not permit a clear prediction to be made as to how long those conditions will last for and what therapeutic hopes there might be; third, a number of impairments are themselves the consequences of illnesses, for example blindness, lameness or mental impairment; fourth, long-standing and serious illnesses are hardly to be distinguished from impairments in cultures other than modern, western society, and are often regarded like impairments, causing similar reactions in a society.[20] Ergotism, or 'St Anthony's Fire' as it was sometimes called, for example, was not an impairment as such, but an illness brought about by poisoning through a fungus present in rye under certain environmental conditions. The effects of ergotism, however, included symptoms, like gangrenous, painful limbs, which could eventually take on a blackened appearance, dry out and break easily at the joints, which would lead to mobility impairments.[21] Therefore one can only position impairment within the modern medical model in an ambiguous and imprecise fashion. If one wishes to analyse the aetiology of impairment in medieval medical theory, then the issue becomes even more complex.

Medieval notions of the origins of diseases, that is their causality or aetiology, are at times very different from modern medical opinion. The main difference lies in the theories of contagion. Modern contagion theory revolves around the transmission of a disease by an agent, such as a bacillus, virus or other microbe. Medieval notions were in some ways more wide-reaching, in that 'contagion' need not be restricted to a physical, corporeal thing, but could be metaphysical as well. So, for example, an Anglo-Saxon text, composed in the mid-seventh to mid-eighth century but extant in an eleventh-century manuscript, states that the '*spiritum infirmitatis* refers to wind as spirit, since many infirmities come to the body from contaminated air.'[22] By the time scholastic, university-based medical theories had established themselves, 'infection', 'contagion' and 'corruption' were terms employed by medical professionals, but still in a sense very different to the modern one. Tommaso del Garbo, in the mid-fourteenth century, may have spoken of 'infection', but by that he did not mean the transmission of pathogens, as modern medicine would. 'Contamination' and 'corruption' metaphorically implied a spiritual sense, as well as the physical contagion of bodies or objects. 'Contagion' in medieval terms did not necessarily mean physical contact. In short, as a modern historian has expressed it, medieval medical notions revolved around 'contingent contagionism', that is the transmission of a localised corruption of the air from person to person, not (as in the twentieth century) via a pathogen, but through general factors, of which corruption of the air was the most important.[23]

As was discussed, impairments can be caused, according to the modern medical model, by congenital factors, diseases or traumatic events. Medieval medical theories, too, differentiated between causes (such as *mala composito*, or *solutio continuitatis*) of impairment but these cannot be simply equated with modern understandings of diseases or pathogens, let alone modern theories of congenital disorders. Bearing this caveat in mind, the analysis will now focus on medieval explanations for the causality of impairments.

One extremely interesting medieval view on the causes of diseases was cited by the surgeon Henri de Mondeville (*c*.1260–1320). Mondeville was actually discussing not what educated medical professionals like himself regarded as disease aetiologies, but what 'ordinary people' believed to be the causes of disease – a rare case permitting us a glimpse at notions of ill-health outside of the environment of learned medical texts. Mondeville narrates these 'ordinary' beliefs thus:

> The common people customarily divide diseases . . . into those which arise from a cause and diseases which have no cause, or are caused by spells. They say that a disease has a cause when the latter is extrinsic, exterior . . . like a stick, a stone, a knife or something else of that kind . . . They say that the disease has no cause, or is caused by spells, when it results from an intrinsic, interior cause . . .[24]

What is so interesting here, is that this 'common' model of disease enables us to make assumptions of how ordinary people may have thought about the origins and causes of impairment. Primarily, this 'populist' medieval model allows us to draw analogies between modern notions of the causal differences between congenital and acquired impairment, and medieval popular notions of causal differences between intrinsic and extrinsic disorders. One can then argue that congenital impairments, according to medieval popular mentality, would have appeared to result intrinsically, while acquired impairments would result extrinsically; acquired impairments could therefore have a cause ascribed to them in the medieval popular model, while congenital impairments would have no discernible cause in the popular mind. An acquired impairment would have an extrinsic cause, because it could, for example, be the very visible result of an accident or injury. The causes of (most) congenital impairments are intrinsic and invisible, in the sense that generally no direct link between a certain action and a resulting congenital impairment can be made. How far this fits in with other medieval notions of congenital impairment will be discussed in the next paragraph.

In the work of Galen (*c*.130–200) explanations for impairments are sometimes given. Galen was not only, alongside the quasi-legendary Hippocrates, one of the most influential writers on medicine, but his texts had been made fully available to the medieval West by the early fourteenth century,[25] so it is worth to briefly examine some of his theories on impairment. Galen discussed a little the question of how physical deformations (η διαστροφη) could arise. Already in the mother's uterus, lack of space for the developing foetus could cause malformations; or the amount or inappropriate consistency of the matter from which the embryo develops was to blame, since it prevented the natural movement of the sperm. After a foetus was carried to term, post-natal deformations could be caused by problems during the birth, or by wrong swaddling.[26] But deformations could also be caused by incorrect movement of the infant by the nurse, or by standing or walking for too great a length of time.[27] Galen further observed that if thumb and forefinger, or the large toe and the second toe, grow together this was caused by a lack of growth in the affected body parts, especially if this happened in children before the child as a whole had started growing in height.[28] With regards to club feet, or feet bent inwardly, Galen explained the cause as follows: it seems obvious that the soft and wax-like bones of infants and children could be deformed through bad posture, in that the nurses place the infants incorrectly in their cribs, either by wrapping them in too many blankets or by squashing them with something.[29] The growth of a hunchback in children, according to Galen, could lead to spinal deformations. If children developed a gibbus before they were fully grown, then they did not develop a proper spine, but instead only their arms and legs grew after a normal fashion. The reason for this Galen believed to lie in the deformation of blood vessels and in the lack of movement of the limbs, as well as due to lack of strength of the limbs. Through these disorders, the already matured body parts became thinner, and those body parts still developing impeded the lengthening of the spine. Arms and legs could grow normally without restrictions, since they were located farther away from the affected area. In this type of hunchback, located above the diaphragm, the ribs would not grow towards the outside as would be the normal case, but instead the thorax became pointed. Because of this, people affected by such a condition also suffered from *dyspnoia* (shortness of breath).[30]

Some other Greek and Byzantine medical writers also mentioned impairments.[31] Hydrocephalus was discussed in medical texts by Leonides (second/third century), Oribasius (325–403) and Paul of Aegina (seventh century). According to Leonides, hydrocephalus was caused by a collection of watery, sometimes thick or bloody, substances; these substances could collect in three different places in the head, for example between the skin of the head and the skin of the skull's bone. In those cases where water collected between the meninges and the brain, the outcome was deemed always to be lethal.[32] Oribasius also differentiated three types of hydrocephalus. However, he reckoned that a collection of water between the brain and the meninges could not be called hydrocephalus, since those people with that affliction died from it before the large, swollen head typical of proper hydrocephalus could emerge. As to the causes of hydrocephalus, Leonides believed that the disorder could often be caused during birth, when the midwife touched the head clumsily and 'squeezes parts'; in this causality he was followed by Oribasius and Paul of Aegina.[33] Paralysis was described by Aretaios (first/second century). In his medical work, he differentiated between paralysis on the one hand, and apoplexy/strokes and paraplegia on the other hand. Paraplegia, according to Aretaios, referred to the lack of sensation or movement in one body part alone, that is in an arm or a leg. In paralysis, normally only the ability to move (but not the lack of sensation) was impaired, that is in the sense of being lamed.[34] He also drew attention to the link between the left and right side of the body, and the left and right side of the brain, pointing out that if a paralysis was effected by a disease in the head, then the right side of the head affected the left side of the body, and vice versa. He said this was due to the structure of the nerves, which on emerging from the head crossed over in the form of an 'X'.[35] He distinguished and described different forms of paralysis, emphasising especially the loss of motor faculties. As causes for paralysis he cited wounds, blows, colds, lack of digestion, carnal desires, intoxication, strong emotional reactions and in children, fright.[36] It is interesting to read in this list of causes about mental or psychological aetiologies of paralysis: 'emotional reactions' and 'fright'. In a way, this causality by Aretaios was anticipating the explanations for 'hysterical' paralysis propounded by late nineteenth- and early twentieth-century psychology; 'hysterical' paralysis is also, by some modern historians, believed to have been the cause of so many of the impairments of those medieval pilgrims who were apparently cured at miracle-working shrines (as will be seen in Chapter 5.3). Aretaios wrote that children were easier to cure of paralysis than adults, but, interestingly, he then did not suggest any therapeutic measures.

Apoplexy (or stroke) was described by Caelius Aurelianus (fifth century) as a sudden, acute event, which could be caused by strong heat or cold, digestive problems, baths, sexual intercourse (especially in older people), injuries to the meninges and concussion of the meninges in children.[37] The consequences of apoplexy were loss of voice (*amputatio uocis*), a dazed mind (*oppressio mentis*), complete immobility of the entire body and cramping of the face (*immobilitas perfecta totius corporis atque conductio uultus*) and also a cold numbness of the limbs.[38] Caelius differentiated between lethargy, epilepsy, loss of strength (*dissolutio*) and lameness (*paralysis*), and all these were in turn distinguished from an actual stroke. Deafness was described by several Greek authors. Galen explained deafness in terms of damage to the auditory nerve, which extends from the brain top to the ear;[39] elsewhere, he suggested deafness was due to a bilious humour affecting the auditory passages.[40] These explanations were taken up by Paul of Aegina, who suggested venesection as treatment for deafness due to a bilious humour.[41] Alexander of Tralles (525–605) thought deafness was due either to trapped air, or due to a viscous humour in the aural passages, again citing venesection as a possible remedy.[42] From the unusual source of an Anglo-Saxon biblical commentary (which was partly influenced by Greek medical writing) comes the statement that, according to the physicians, deafness (and dumbness) 'arise from contracted and dormant veins'.[43] Meletius, a monk living in the Byzantine empire in the late eighth/early ninth century, wrote a tract *On the Nature of Man*[44] in which he suggested that the faculty of speech may be linked to a specific area of the brain (in this case, the third ventricle); furthermore, he proposed that a diagnosis of brain damage could be made on the basis of observing which type of speech disorder a person had sustained.[45]

In the thirteenth century, the encyclopaedist Bartolomaeus Anglicus had described the symptoms of arthritis of the hands, which he distinguished from arthritis of the feet, calling that form 'podagra' or gout. Bartolomaeus defined arthritis as 'an ache and disease in the fingers and toes with swelling and pain'.[46] He also provided an aetiology for arthritic symptoms: 'Arthritis comes from the age of the patient and from the region in which he lives and from the climate',[47] and described the crippling effects of the disease:

> One form of the disease is worse for it makes the fingers shrink and shrivels the toes and sinews of the feet and of the hands. This form ... makes the hands dry and crooked and closed and incapable of being opened. Also it makes the joints of the fingers unsightly with knotty bunches and this sickness must be treated soon, for when it is old it is only curable with difficulty. ...[48]

Another English author, John of Gaddesden (b. *c*.1280), author of the *Rosa Anglica* written around 1314, divided arthritic symptoms into three types: 'sciatica' or pain affecting the hip area, 'podagra' for pain in the joints of the feet, and 'cheiragra' for pain in the hands and fingers. Causes for such symptoms could include windy foods, constipation and overeating before going to bed and gastric overindulgence followed by sexual intercourse (in this he echoed opinions by Galen, who asserted that eunuchs never suffered from podagra).[49] Guy de Chauliac in the fourteenth century ascribed gout (*gutta*), which he regarded as synonymous with arthritis (*arthetica*) and podagra (*podagre*), to humoral dysfunctions, as a rheumatising ache of the joints, to be differentiated from the cramp.[50]

In a text associated with the Salernitan school, the *Practica* of Archimataeus, possibly dating from the twelfth century,[51] paralysis was in one cited case caused by sleeping after taking a bath. A lady became affected by paralysis of the face, which the author attributed to dissolution of humours which in turn affected the muscles. The author described a series of treatments, consisting of potions, a purgative, pills and unguents, which apparently cured the lady.[52] Paralysis was also mentioned in the *Rosa Anglica* by John of Gaddesden, of which he distinguished various forms. 'Sometimes the entire half of the body is afflicted, from the head to the foot ... and prevents speech, that is called general paralysis, sometimes it affects one foot only, or the finger only and that is called partial paralysis.'[53] Paralysis was also differentiated from cramp. As causes for paralysis he listed 'falling, percussion [compression] of the nerves, attrition and cutting across the nerves, also anger, fear and excess of cold ...'.[54] Accordingly, both what we would now call physiological reasons, and what we would term psychological ones could lead to paralysis in John's medical theory. Guy de Chauliac discussed cramp and palsy (paralysis), differentiating between the two by pointing out that in cramp (like in palsy) the 'working' is lost, but there can still be change.[55] Palsy, according to de Chauliac, arose through wounds and being hit, mostly in the head and the back; palsy caused privation of feeling in the sinews (nerves, that is) and prevented movement. As apoplexy was a 'softness' of all the body, palsy was a disorder affecting a 'half part', sometimes the right side, sometimes the left side of the body, or sometimes just one part, like a foot or a hand; therefore he could differentiate between 'universal or particular cramp in the palsy', the universal being palsy of all one side, the particular affecting one limb.[56] Breaking of the neck or back can cause palsy (paralysis), which affects the hands if it was due to a break in the upper region, and the feet if due to a break in the lower regions.[57]

In the mid-twelfth century, William of St Thierry had discussed speech disorders in his tract *On the Nature of the Body and the Soul*. He had assumed that the voice is a form of physical function, whereas speech was a psychic function. Voice was therefore not essential to speech, in his view, because it was possible for people to communicate by signs or by writing as well as by using their voice. However, if a mute person was unable to communicate by sign language or through writing, then such a person could not be said to posses a proper reasoning faculty.[58] A Salernitan surgical text, known as the 'Bamberg Surgery', also from the mid-twelfth century, stated that injury to the dura mater produced lingual discoloration (i.e. discoloration of the tongue), and injury to the pia mater destroyed the voice.[59] Speech disorders ('default' of speech), according to a Middle English translation of Guy de Chauliac (*c.*1298–1368), were caused by palsy (paralysis) or cramp of the tongue, by ulcers and through humoral imbalances, that is by too much moisture in the nerves; especially in the case of stammering (*wlaffynge*) they could be accompanied by 'flux of spittle without will', and these disorders present in children sometimes cured themselves fully by adolescence.[60] Similarly, a fifteenth-century Middle English translation of Gilbertus Anglicus (who was originally writing around 1240) stated that speech disorders were caused by corrupt humours which blocked the nerves and made the tongue lax, and caused it to become paralysed.[61]

Having mentioned what medieval writers called the 'humours', it is worth turning now to have a closer look at how humoral reasons were believed to constitute a causality of impairment. For Isidore of Seville, in the early seventh century, a humoral imbalance was the underlying cause of paralysis, namely due to too much cold: 'Paralysis, *paralesis*, is named from a destruction, *inpensatio*, of the body brought about by much cooling of the body, either as a whole or in part.'[62] An imperfection in the constellation of the humours is responsible for some diseases, according to Hildegard of Bingen writing in the twelfth century. For example 'gout', which can signify a variety of afflictions of the limbs, not just what modern medical terminology calls gout, is caused by foamy and lukewarm imbalances in the humours; contradictions within the humours force the nape of the neck of a person to be bent, the back is bent, and the person is rendered completely gout-ridden, although such a person can still reach a very old age.[63] A similar explanation is propounded by Hildegard for lameness. If such humours involve the moist and the lukewarm (which form the 'livor'[64] of the dry and foamy) getting out of balance, so that 'like a dangerous gust of wind' they are driven beyond their boundaries, and the humours are as if shaken by winds, then they produce dangerous sounding noises 'like thunder'; such a noise sounds through the blood vessels and marrow of a person, as well as through their temples, therefore with such an ailment the person is lamed and loses their strength in their entire body.[65] This state of affairs lasts until the 'livors' have withdrawn themselves and have returned to their proper place; however, with God's grace such a person suffering from lameness can live quite a long time.[66]

Humoral causality seems to have been favoured in explaining cases of acquired impairments. A passage in the prose Salernitan questions (written around 1200) asked why some impairments were not present 'from birth' (i.e. congenital), but instead arose over time. Here a mixture of humoral reasons and the effects of what modern medicine calls 'trauma' were given as causes: dropsy could be caused 'from a lot of humidity and little heat, paralysis from a humour and great coldness, and similarly the scialgia illness [sciatica], and arthritis and mania and melancholia and lethargy and many other illnesses. A tumor also happens at different times externally from shattering, or from a blow or a wound or from tight and strong bandaging'.[67] The passage concludes by pointing out that tumours can also be caused through humoral imbalance, which in turn was originally brought about by cuts or incisions.

Humoral casuistry and the connection between the reproductive organs and other body parts are linked together in a discussion of the reasons for speech disorders in one of the *consilia* of Taddeo Alderotti (d. 1295). Alderotti composed one of his longest and most detailed *consilia* for Count Bertholdus, who had an unspecified speech disorder due to a 'softness of the tongue'.[68] This was caused either by problems in the brain, due to excess moisture which affected the nerves linking brain, tongue and genitals, or by a genital disorder from where an excess of melancholy vapours rose to the brain, in turn affecting the tongue.[69]

Speech impairments had also been explained as due to purely humoral reasons by William of Conches, in his *Dragmaticon*, of about 1145. He located the causality of mental and speech disorders in the brain. A dull wit, soggy memory and imperfect speech were due to humoral influences on the brain. The rational faculty was located in the middle ventricle of the brain,[70] so presumably damage to that area would lead to impaired speech. Speech impairments are discussed in a similar fashion in the prose Salernitan questions of around 1200. A certain stammerer, whose tongue was 'tied', had his speech loosened through his hand, and similarly his tongue was loosened by placing hands on him. Two kinds of stammering were thought to be responsible: one arose from slipperiness of the nerves, the other from debility of the nerves. Humidity of the stomach could be transferred into humidity of the nerves, which could cause slipperiness of the tongue, and hence an impediment to speech. Debility of nerves could be caused by humidity flowing from the brain, and since all nerves originated from the brain, stretching of nerves could lead to pain in the mind, which could affect speech.[71]

Ugo of Siena, born in the second half of the fourteenth century, wrote a *Regimen sanitatis* for Niccolò d'Este of Ferrara, in which he included some accounts of specific medical case-studies. One of these concerned a man aged 21, who because of excess humidity in the brain was *traulus* (i.e., he had a kind of lisp) but who was also *altecha* (which roughly means 'tipsy') and had large spots on his chest – again, both of these latter conditions were ascribed to humidity in the brain. For therapy, Ugo prescribed dietary regulations and massage of the patient's tongue with drying agents. As Galen had referred to the slurred speech of drunks, and since Ugo was a Galenist, maybe the diagnosis of *altecha* was used as a vernacular Italian phrase for this Galenic notion (the *Regimen* was, after all, written for a lay reader).[72]

Speech impediments, such as muteness, were also believed to be linked for humoral reasons with hearing impediments, such as deafness. The Salernitan observation that all mute people were also deaf prompted a question on this issue:

> Why are all mutes deaf? Response. The nerves which come to the tongue in their origin are continued by nerves which come to the ears. If therefore it should happen that a certain humour obstructs the nerves of the tongue about the beginnings, they are obstructed like those which come to the ears, whence simultaneously he may be mute and deaf.[73]

Why a person who was mute from birth was also congenitally deaf was also examined by another Salernitan question, which proposed that, again, it was due to humoral causes, in this case humidity flowing over the ears and stopping them up; additionally, the same question asked why every blind person heard well, and explained that through an inversion of the 'animal spirit', which normally crossed over to the eyes, towards the ears[74] – more nerves leading to the ears, it seems, caused better hearing.

Another Salernitan question explored the link between loss of vision and loss of hearing. The case of a man was cited who had fallen and been concussed so that for two hours he lost his sight, and his hearing became partially impaired. When he lay down, he could hear, but when he stood, sat or walked about, he was unable to hear anything. The explanation given in this Salernitan text stated that the seat of imagination in the brain had been disturbed, and the optical nerve had been dulled, while concussion of the ear had rendered the man deaf and debilitated the aural nerves. As to why he was able to hear while lying down, but not in any other posture, that was due to humoral reasons, for a supine position enabled the 'vapour' from the stomach to ascend and open the nerve of hearing, which a standing or sitting position prevented.[75]

Overindulgence in sexual activity could have a detrimental effect, especially on the eyes, often believed to cause blindness. The assertion by Aristotle that too much sexual activity affected the eyes was constantly reiterated in the medieval period.[76] Hildegard of Bingen, writing in the twelfth century in *Causae et curae*, warned that people who 'discharge their seed' in lust risked becoming blind, while those who had intercourse in moderation would not be harmed.[77] Albertus Magnus, in the thirteenth century, told the story of a monk who died after having desired a woman too much, and at the ensuing autopsy it was discovered that his eyes had been destroyed.[78] In the fifteenth century, the *Problemata Varia Anatomica* stated 'coitus destroys the eyesight and dries up the body.'[79] An alternative viewpoint can be found in a *Regimen sanitatis* written by the physician Konrad von Eichstätt (fl.1326–d. 1342), originally in Latin, but later translated into German in many editions. He says with regards to coitus and eye disorders that if someone does *not* engage in intercourse at all, their eyes would be darkened, they would suffer from vertigo, and a heavy head, since moderate intercourse sustains health:

> Es spricht der meyster Avicenna, wer das mynnen übergeet, dem werden die augen tunckel und macht den schwindel und macht das haubt schwer. Ir wisset, das die getemperirt mynne pringet dise ding alle wider und macht sy aber wol gesunt.[80]

However, yet again moderation was the key issue, for a little later Konrad warns against immoderate coitus, which, amongst other things, 'impairs hearing and sight', as well as taking away the body's strength and causing premature age-ing.[81] It is interesting to compare such notions with that found in one of the miracle narratives (which will be discussed more fully in Chapter 5.3), where a man, Guibert, repeatedly became visually impaired due to over-indulgence in sexual activity.[82]

The humours were also responsible for apoplexy, which in turn was seen to be connected with paralysis, according to a late fifteenth-century Middle English translation of Gilbertus Anglicus' *Compendium medicinae*. Apoplexy was caused through a stoppage of principal parts of the brain due to corrupt humours; effects were loss of all movement apart from breathing; of three types of the disorder, greater apoplexy was incurable and killed a person on the first day, while medium apoplexy killed within three days or could be turned into paralysis, and lesser killed within seven days or became paralysis; greater apoplexy (the incurable type) affected a person's senses, such as loss of sight, hearing, taste, smell and movement, while lesser apoplexy, just related to the nerves originating from the rear of the brain, affected only motion.[83] Apoplexy (and epilepsy) in infants could be caused by suckling spoiled and sour milk, which affected the nervous system, according to the influential views of Soranus (early second century).[84]

A disorder similar to paralysis or apoplexy was described in the prose Salernitan questions. A certain person was mentioned, who from the crown of the head downwards had withered limbs, and diminished ones, and who was destitute of voluntary movement and of almost all sense. The reason for this was given as 'obstruction' of the blood, which could no longer nourish the affected parts of the body; also, the obstruction adversely affected the operative nerves of motion, but not the nerves of perception, so that the senses were still partially functioning.[85]

A central aspect of causality of impairment revolves around ideas on inheritance factors and congenital impairment. The human procreative process, that is the conception of children, was one of the most important areas for medieval aetiologies of impairment. In the early seventh century, Isidore of Seville had reiterated theories of inheritance from classical antiquity. In his *Etymologies* he wrote: 'They say that children resemble their fathers if the paternal seed be stronger; the mother if the maternal seed be the stronger. This is the reason faces are formed to resemble others; those with the likeness of both parents were conceived from an equal admixture of paternal and maternal semen.'[86] The Galenic two-seed theory, whereby both male and female produced a 'seed' for procreation was very wide-spread during the high and later medieval period. In contrast, the Aristotelian single-seed theory stated that only the male provided generative matter, that is the life-spirit or soul, while the female provided the matter or body of a foetus. As a rule, physicians favoured the Galenic theory, while some theologians and natural philosophers (e.g. Giles of Rome in the thirteenth century) favoured the Aristotelian theory.[87] One of the prose Salernitan questions, written by an English hand around 1200, tries to provide proof for the existence of maternal seed, by pointing out that children are 'born similar to their mothers and contract their infirmities'.[88] Besides such general ideas about how and why children resemble their parents, more specific ideas circulated as to the reasons for congenital impairments. Already in the Hippocratic corpus the notion of a link between the quality of sperm and the quality of the body which generates it was made; weak sperm came from weak parts of the body, and strong sperm from strong parts (this is the pangenetic notion of procreation, whereby sperm production is situated not just in the testes, but can arise in all parts of the male body).[89] This theory, amongst others, was then used during the medieval period to explain how infirmities and impairments could be inherited. One of the texts from the Hippocratic corpus, *On Generation*, looked at how birth defects could arise even in the progeny of physically healthy parents: damage sustained by the womb, a deficiency of the womb or constriction of the foetus by the womb were all seen as causes.[90] During the medieval period, such instances of healthy parents producing impaired offspring were explained in a variety of ways, echoing Hippocratic notions: small and weak children were due to the inability of the womb to nourish the foetus properly; repeated births of small and weak children were due to too small a womb (which restricted foetal growth); and deformed infants could be explained by a deficiency of the mother's womb, or through external factors such as falls, blows or other violence sustained by the womb.[91] The prose Salernitan questions, asking why a boy had congenital impairments of his eyes and ears, answered that his condition may have been due to a blemish in the quality of the sperm or in the womb or at the first stage of generation.[92] In the thirteenth century, Albertus Magnus tried to explain the causality for a case of dwarfism in an 8-year-old girl from Cologne, who at that age was still as small as a child of one year. Following ideas advanced by Avicenna (d. 1037), he relegated the origin of this 'monstrosity' to badly practised coitus, in which only a very small part of the paternal seed had been able to enter the mother's uterus.[93]

It is interesting to note that such ideas about the quality and condition of sperm and the resulting child were not restricted to medieval European (or Classical) thought, but seem to have wider Indo-European antecedents, hence one can argue they are cross-cultural. Already in the sixth century BC Vedic texts known as the *Garbha-Upanishad* there are similar notions: 'An excess of the father's semen produces a male, an excess of the mother's semen, a girl and if there is an equal amount of the two semens, a eunuch. A troubled spirit produces the blind, the lame, the hunchbacks and dwarfs. When the sperm is crushed by the wind and split in two, twins are born.'[94]

Ideas revolving around the importance of the constituency, or material quality, of human generative matter appear in an analogy with different types of cheeses in a twelfth-century text by Hildegard of Bingen, the *Scivias* dealing with the creation and form of the world. She stated that there were people carrying vessels with milk from which they wanted to produce cheese. These were analogous to men and women, who in their bodies carried human seed. A part of that was thick and made a fat cheese, due to the right consistency of the seed, while another part was thin and made a weak cheese, because the seed was useless, not ripe and badly mixed. From part of the bad milk a bitter cheese was made, since this seed, in a weak mixture, carelessly issued and uselessly mixed, produced deformed people.[95]

Medieval writers on natural philosophy and medicine were also concerned with questions of the inheritability of impairments. William of Conches, in the first half of the twelfth century, in his *Dragmaticon* (a revised version of his tract *On the Philosophy of the World*) put forward the notion that certain disorders, like chiraga or podagra, can be inherited.[96] However, a man with a missing limb does not engender a child with a missing limb, because nature 'flees imperfections' and makes up the missing matter by 'borrowing' from other bodily parts.[97] In this William of Conches reworked notions expressed in texts related to the Salernitan tradition. For example, in the collection of prose Salernitan questions written around 1200, two questions following each other address precisely this problem. The answer to the first question states that a father would pass on any incurable infirmity, such as *ciragra* or *podagra*, onto his son;[98] the second question tries to answer why people born with impairments (such as blindness, or lacking the normal function of their limbs, ears or nose) nevertheless are born with those physical parts, even though they cannot use them.[99] The answer is given that 'nature fleeing imperfections' tries to substitute matter that was absent in the parents (in the case of inherited congenital impairment) so that even though the parents may lack a sense or a limb, in the child the 'matter' is formed even if the function is still absent.[100] Guy de Chauliac echoed these views, with particular reference to gout. This time citing Avicenna (d. 1037), de Chauliac said that aches of the joints are some of the sicknesses that are had by heritage, since sperm follows the complexion of the man engendering a child.[101]

Ideas about procreation, inheritance and humoral factors were often combined into one theoretical edifice. A pseudo-Galenic text, possibly composed in late antiquity, whose Latin version became well-known in the Middle Ages from at least the thirteenth century onwards, was *De spermate*.[102] This text dealt with theories of conception, embryology, and also tried to explain instances of birth defects and congenital impairment. Humoral influences were regarded as very important, especially on the quality of the male and female seed at the time of conception, which had a strong impact on the physical constitution of the resulting child.[103] 'Since the humours were seen as both the means by which inheritance occurs and as the origin of disease, it also became possible to determine the inheritance of those diseases to which particular complexional types were thought to be liable.'[104] For example, a black humour, that is a melancholy one, caused a person who was conceived at the time when such a humour dominated to be particularly prone in later life to paralysis, dullness of mind or irresolution and severe ache in all their bones.[105] For a particular combination of factors, such as gender of the child, humoral influence and humoral history of the parents, *De spermate* explains the reasons for some impairments:

> If conception takes place in the hours of melancholy, the father and mother have also been conceived in the same hours, and the sperm is in the left part, the daughter will be melancholic, epileptic, and afflicted with paralysis. She will suffer from disorder of the spleen and quartan fever. She will also be stupid, slow of mind, and similar to her parents, and she will not be able to temper her nature in any manner.[106]

In other cases, the mitigating influence (the ability to 'temper nature') of what we would now call 'environmental' factors exercised a counter effect to adverse humoral combinations.

Unlike the Hippocratic notions mentioned above of why healthy parents produced impaired offspring, *De spermate* relied purely on humoral reasoning.

> Sometimes healthy parents generate children who are crippled or have a misshapen mouth or nose, and thus the child appears to have a different form from its parents because of the overabundance of the humours. Sometimes this is caused by a change in the nature of the sperm, because sperm has in the matrix the nature of that power which it has in its own place. It happens that the child inherits different diseases from the father and the mother or from the milk which it uses for nourishment.[107]

The constituency of milk[108] was believed to be influenced by the humours, just like all other bodily fluids or any physical part, so that we should not think in terms of 'environmental' influence in this case.

Humoral imbalances were therefore widely believed to be inheritable, or rather, transmissible from mother to foetus, as the following example demonstrates. William of Congenis, who taught and practised medicine at Montpellier in the first half of the thirteenth century, commented on a disorder called tinea: 'Often well-bred and rich people are found to suffer from this, because their mothers have lived in idleness and bred superfluous humours with which the child is born when it is conceived in the womb. . . . It is quite otherwise with the children of the peasants and the poor, who are always born beautiful, even though afterwards, through excessive labour and neglect of hygiene, they become ugly.'[109] Not only did William believe in the inheritability of humoral problems, he also advocated a kind of 'lifestyle' prescription, where moderate amounts of physical labour were regarded as beneficial. Towards the end of the period being discussed, the various notions about the inheritability of disorders, the quality of the parental seed(s) and the physical and emotional constituency of the parents became more and more popularised and amalgamated into such 'lifestyle' prescriptions, as William de Congenis had proposed. For example, writing in a humanist dialogue in the 1430s, Leon Battista Alberti gave the following advice on how to achieve the best offspring: husbands should not have intercourse with their wives when the men were troubled by disturbing emotions, as those passions weakened their vital strength. If such weakening happened,

> it may often be found that a father who is ardent and strong and wise has begotten a son who is fearful, weak, and foolish. ... Again, it is unwise to come together if body and limbs are not in a good condition and health. The doctors say, and they give ample reasons, that if a father and mother are low and troubled because of drink or bad blood or weaknesses and defects of energy and pulse, it is reasonable to expect the children to manifest these troubles. Sometimes, in fact, they will be leprous, epileptic, deformed, or incomplete in their limbs and defective.[110]

Alberti even considers the question 'What wise person would not rather remain childless than have diseased and insane children?'[111] Considerations such as these demonstrate that quite some thought went into questions about the physical and mental condition of one's prospective offspring.

Planetary influences could also be a factor in the causality of impairment. A treatise attributed to Constantinus Africanus (d. 1087), *De humana natura*, provides what appears to be the earliest account in the western Middle Ages of the influence the seven planets were believed to have over foetal development.[112] This notion does not seem to have developed from any ideas current in classical antiquity, but became widely held during the high and later Middle Ages.[113] Each of the planets held sway over one month of the period of pregnancy. Saturn was dominant in the first month, followed by Jupiter in the second, Mars in the third, the Sun in the fourth, Venus in the fifth, Mercury in the sixth, and the Moon in the seventh month. By that stage the foetus was believed to be viable, should the baby be born prematurely. In the eighth month Saturn held sway again, and 'by its cooling power, introduces heaviness into the embryo and the womb, and by its dryness weakens the moisture and gives nourishment to the embryo more sparingly'.[114] The negative influence of Saturn was used to explain why babies born after an eight-month pregnancy tended to die, unlike those born prematurely at seven months.[115]

The prose Salernitan questions, too, addressed the issue of why eight-month babies were prone to die, whereas seven-month infants survived. 'In the seventh month all the members are completed and are ordered following their natural disposition. If the foetus is born in this month it is healthy because it is emitted by its natural strength from which it is lively and healthy. But if it is in the eighth, it is bad and subject to die.'[116] The astrological reasons, similar to those in the text attributed to Constantinus Africanus, were then cited, listing the planet-month scheme. The text then asked why offspring born in the seventh month are healthy, but why those born in the eighth were subject to die. The response linked the mortality of such infants to an inherent weakness, debility, or, as we would say, impairment. If the child was born not by 'natural strength' but was born by its 'weakness' or 'debility', it was subject to die, and if it should live, it lived 'wasting away'.[117] In the eighth month, Saturn brought heaviness to the embryo by cooling, and by his dryness the humours diminished nourishment to the foetus.[118]

Saturn, as we have seen, was regarded as a cold and dry planet, therefore, according to the humoral scheme, people born under the influence of Saturn were often sickly, pale, skinny, cold, rough, lethargic, slow, sad, or thieving and grasping. The planet was furthermore linked to a specific group of impaired people, that is the lame and crippled. From a fifteenth-century woodcut in a block-book[119] we find an illustration of Saturn as an old man leaning on a crutch, below whom are depicted his children, that is the people born under Saturn's influence: besides farmers (engaged in animal husbandry) and criminals (in the stocks, on the gallows and on the wheel) we can also see the aforementioned cripples. A similar illustration, this time coloured in, also depicts an orthopaedically impaired person as one of Saturn's children.[120]

The planets could also exercise a direct influence on the presence or absence of congenital impairments. As *De spermate*, widely disseminated by the thirteenth century, explains it,

> [i]t happens sometimes that a daughter is not like her parents, and that is because of the nature of the planets. Sometimes a child is born mute, without feet, without head, without eyes, without hearing, and so on. The reason for this is, as Hippocrates testifies, that all substance of animate bodies endowed with a soul is bound to the planets and signs, which are connected to the four elements.[121]

Astrological notions, in the sense of planetary influence, and ideas on conception are therefore closely linked in this influential text.

A further astronomical factor believed to influence the physical appearance and constituency of a foetus was the particular phase of the moon during which conception took place. The phases of the moon exercised an influence over all living beings, as Ælfric in the late tenth century had already pointed out:

> It is, however, according to nature in the created order that each bodily created thing which the earth brings forth is fuller and stronger in the full moon than in the waning. As also trees, if they be hewed in a full moon, are harder and longer-lasting for building, and strongest if they are worked on when sapless. This is no sorcery, but is a natural thing through the created order.[122]

In Hildegard of Bingen's twelfth-century medical writings, such general notions about the workings of the natural world were reiterated and applied specifically to human procreation. In her *Cause et cure*, she said:

> People sow seed when heat and cold are temperate, and it grows into fruit. For who would be foolish enough to sow seed during the extreme heat of summer or during the extreme cold of winter? It would perish and would not grow. ... The same is true for humans who refuse to take into consideration the time of maturity in their lives and the time of the moon but want to procreate according to their impulses. For that reason their children will suffer with much pain from physical debility. But however much and whenever they are physically debilitated, God gathers his young buds. Therefore a man must be aware of the time of his physical maturity, and he must examine the time of the moon with as much care as someone who offers his pure prayers. That is to say, he should procreate children at a time that might not lead to his children's devastation from a physical debility.[123]

The reference to maturity relates to the appropriate age at which it is best to produce healthy children. Hildegard stated that if a woman conceived a child before she was fully mature, that is before the age of 20, 'she will produce a child that is infirm and in some way weak', while if a woman was too old, that is after the age of about 50 (when the menopause was thought to set in), if she still had a child 'this child will then have a defect'.[124] Men should therefore approach young women, not girls, with a view to having children, and men, until they had grown a beard, should not touch women, and of course both should eat and drink in moderation. The relevance of the moon is explained by Hildegard at a later stage in *Cause et cure*. The blood in men and women waxed and waned with the phases of the moon, which had an effect on the quality of human seed. 'When the blood in a human being has increased with the waxing of the moon, then the human being too, whether woman or man, is fertile for bearing fruit, that is, for procreating offspring.'[125] However, when the moon was weak (waning), blood in humans, and therefore also semen, were weak too. 'Consequently it is then highly ineffectual for procreating offspring. If a woman conceives a child at that time, whether male or female, it will be infirm, weak and not virtuous.'[126]

Similarly, the importance of astronomical factors was emphasised by Albertus Magnus in the thirteenth century. He argued that deformed births could be caused by a particular cause, or by a general cause; particular causes would be related to the paternal seed and the maternal reception thereof, while general causes could include the location and the relationship of the stars at the time of conception.[127] Albertus was not exactly certain which one of these causes was responsible, but he did note that some planetary conjunctions are recognised as particularly malicious, and pointed out that conception and birth should be avoided at such times. Specific problems might arise with regards to children born under a new moon, as they might be defective in sense and discretion.[128] Albertus himself claimed to have seen the results of astrologically badly timed conceptions on two occasions, where human beings were born with truncated arms and legs who 'will not have the appearance of a human body'.[129]

Connected with notions of the proper astronomical time for conceiving children were notions of the proper personal time. In particular, this meant avoiding copulation at the time of a woman's menstruation. The idea that menstruation is a 'damaging' biological function is a common one, occurring interculturally. In the Old Testament, for example, a woman 'shall be put apart seven days'[130] during her mensis, and sexual intercourse at that time was a transgression punishable by ostracism,[131] although these passages do not make any statements with regard to the conception of impaired children. Menstruation was also regarded as 'unclean' by some medieval authorities. The seventh-century archbishop of Canterbury, Theodore of Tarsus (668–690), stated in his *Penitential* that any women, lay or nuns, who entered a church or had communion during their menses would be subject to three weeks fasting in penance.[132]

More particularly, menstruation was believed to have a detrimental effect on any conception which took place as the result of intercourse at that time. Children generated during menstruation could be affected by impairments and diseases. St Jerome had already warned of the dangers of conceiving a child at this inappropriate period. 'If a man copulates with a woman at that time [menstruation], the fetuses conceived are said to carry the vice of the seed, so that lepers and gargantuans are born from this conception, and the corrupted menses makes the foul bodies of either sex too small or too big.'[133] In a series of texts, known as the *Pseudo-Clementines*, translated into Latin by Rufinus around 410, which were very popular in the Middle Ages as such and survive in numerous manuscripts,[134] a passage known as the *Recognitions* states: sexual incontinence is accompanied by demons whose 'noxious breath' produces an 'intemperate and vicious progeny ... And therefore parents are responsible for their children's defects of this sort, because they have not observed the law of intercourse.'[135] Here, in late antiquity, we already have the main line of argument that was to be pursued throughout the Middle Ages. Basically, the argument can be summed up as follows: intercourse at the wrong time and in the wrong way will result in the birth of defective children (I use 'defective' loosely here, implying both physically different and having character 'defects'). Gratian in the mid-twelfth century cited a letter by the seventh-century missionary Boniface, suggesting that corrupt sexual unions would produce corrupt children.[136] In the late twelfth century, Lothario dei Segni, better known as Pope Innocent III after his election in 1198, wrote an influential treatise, *On Contempt for the World*. In a passage concerning the dangers of contact with menstrual fluid he echoed Jerome, and said about the menses: 'Which is said to be so detestable and unclean, that grains that come in contact with it will not germinate, shrubs will wither, plants will die, trees will lose their fruit, and if dogs then were to eat it, they would run mad. Fetuses conceived [during menstruation] contract the defect of the seed, so that lepers and elephantiasis are born from this corruption.'[137] The menses retained their danger even if a child had been conceived outside the time of menstruation itself, so that according to William of Conches the maternal blood had to be 'purified' by the liver before reaching the foetus via the umbilical cord.[138]

Theologians and canonists of the high Middle Ages regarded intercourse during menstruation as a mortal sin, precisely for the reason that it was likely 'defective' children were begotten at that time. Examples of these opinions can be found in the writings of Raymond of Penyafort (d. 1275), John Duns Scotus (d. 1308) and Thomas Aquinas (d. 1274).[139] More popular, that is, less learned, treatises also repeated such views. In Dan Michel's *Ayenbite of Inwyt*, translated from the French in 1340, reference is made to the times when 'sin is in spousehood', particularly when a man goes to his wife during a time when he should not go. This means during menstruation, the 'sickness which women commonly have', which would be a great sin since God forbade that a man should then have communion with his wife. Children would be imperilled, since during such a time children are often begotten who are crooked (i.e. lame), blind, leprous, deaf, dumb and scabby; in adulthood such people were prone to gout and boils and other 'wretched evils'.

> þet is huanne hi is ine þe ziknesse þet wyfmen habbeþ communliche. zuo þet
> he is na3t ne spareþ huanne he wot þet hi is in zuich stat. Zene3eþ gratliche
> and uor þan þet god uorbyet þet man ne habbe uela3rede mid his wyue. ine
> zuich stat and uor þe peril of his children. Vor ase zayþ saint gregorie. ine zuych
> stat byeþ ofte beyete þe crokede þe blynde and þe mezels. þe dyauue þe
> doumbe þe ssornede þe scallede. and men and wyfmen þet habbeþ oþere
> zyknesses in hare bodie þanne hi comeþ to manhod ase goutes and beles. and
> oþre ssrewede eueles.[140]

One final aspect of the perceived dangers of menstruation needs analysing. Menstruation was regarded as dangerous to conception by scholastic writers of the high Middle Ages, using arguments in part derived from Aristotle. Broadly put, according to ideas of natural science, the menses (or *menstruum*) accumulated gradually over each cycle as a kind of formless matter. Only the male seed had form itself (*homunculi*) and was pure maleness. The female simply received the seed and nurtured it, but did not generate. By extension of this reasoning, the female was of necessity already partially defective; an idea that was theologically backed up by the creation story, where Eve's creation out of Adam's bent rib made Eve herself deviant from the male norm. The idea therefore existed that the female *per se* was defective. The clearest expression of this kind of argument can be found in Albertus Magnus' *De animalibus*,[141] where, moving on from the premise of menses as formless matter, the practical advice given by theologians and physicians alike was reiterated, that semen had the best chances of 'forming' the menses in the earlier part of the cycle. If conception took place during a later stage of the cycle, however, there was a sliding scale of degradation and degeneration: having missed the ideal time for generating male offspring, the next best would be female children, that is only slightly 'deformed', followed by the severely defective (i.e. impaired) progeny, and lastly and worst of all no offspring at all[142] – the *horror vacui* of medieval philosophy.[143] It is worth just repeating this hierarchical list of value judgements: male, female, deformed, nothing.

Most discussions in medieval treatises centre on the method used in intercourse. Any deviation from the one prescribed method (the so-called missionary position) was seen to either avoid the main purpose of the act, that is procreation, or if a child was conceived by any other method, then it would 'suffer deformities because of its parents' aberrant practices'.[144] Such notions were not at all unusual. A popular work ascribed in the Middle Ages to Albertus Magnus, *De secretis mulierum*, mentions three main reasons why defective children are born. First, if the woman did not lie absolutely still but actually moved during intercourse, the male seed 'might be divided and a defective child conceived'.[145] Second, the woman should not let her thoughts wander during intercourse, but she should concentrate on what is going on, otherwise if at the critical moment she thought of something else, for example some animal like a cow, the child might turn out to resemble one.[146] And third, any non-standard coital position might result in birth defects in those children who were the results of their parents' 'experiments' in the conjugal bed,[147] such as a child lame in one foot and with a curved spine.[148]

Popularly disseminated notions along the lines of improper sexual conduct could also be found in religious literature aimed at what might be termed a vernacular audience: penitentials, preaching and sermon tracts. Here the argument based on sex and sin was expanded upon, and besides the actual practice of intercourse and the date of the act, other damaging factors such as pregnancy, lactation or menstruation were considered. Robert of Flamborough, author of a penitential (written between 1208 and 1213), warned that children conceived during pregnancy (now considered highly improbable), menstruation, or before a previous child was weaned, would be lame, leprous, given to seizures, deformed or short-lived.[149] Note that all three bad times for conception Robert refers to are times that we now know to be infertile or 'safe periods', in other words naturally contraceptive periods – one could speculate that precisely because of the lack of conceptions during such times, which medieval people, especially women, may well have been aware of,[150] they were forbidden by moralists, as intercourse then would have been for pleasure only and not for procreative purposes. Berthold von Regensburg, a thirteenth-century preacher, added to this list of physical deformities the dangers of deafness, meanspiritedness and demonic possession;[151] again, such potential impairment and moral defectiveness in many children was ascribed to their conception at forbidden times, to which Berthold added the six weeks immediately after childbirth (i.e. yet another 'safe period'), and furthermore, he noted that nobles and burghers were less prone to such sins than the peasantry.[152] A French Church synod of the thirteenth century proclaimed that children conceived from illicit sex would be born humpbacked, crippled or deformed in some way.[153] Furthermore, from a fourteenth-century manuscript we have the usual prohibition of illicit sexual activity, that is during menstruation, lactation and pregnancy, and the prediction that children born from such unions would be leprous, lunatic or possessed.[154]

Impaired children could also be born as the result of intercourse at religiously 'wrong' times, besides improper personal and astronomical times. For example, this related to avoidance on Sundays,[155] the feast days of saints and during Lent. Gregory of Tours (d. 594) told the story of how St Martin had cured a severely deformed boy, who had been born in that condition as a result of conception on a Sunday, that is, one of the forbidden days.[156] Gregory of Tours ended his miracle story with a moral: 'Be content to indulge your lust on the other days, but observe this day without pollution in praise of God. For if [intercourse] takes place, then children are born who are crippled or suffer from epilepsy or leprosy.'[157]

Patricia Skinner, who has studied evidence from southern Italy from the early medieval period up to the twelfth century, has reached the conclusion that there, too, congenital impairment in the child was often linked with sexual transgression of the parents. 'Anecdotal evidence suggests that there was a very strong feeling that malformed babies indicated sin on the part of their parents, particularly some kind of sexual deviation.'[158] Skinner, referring to the 'intergenerational responsibility' proposed by Christiane Klapisch,[159] continues by surmising that because of the association of congenital impairment with parental sin, 'the newborn might be abandoned or exposed rather than raised, particularly if it had a serious birth defect.'[160] However, in general this is not borne out by the evidence.

In the case cited in the previous paragraph, of St Martin's miracle healing of a congenitally impaired child conceived on a Sunday, which Skinner herself referred to,[161] Gregory of Tours says the exact opposite: '[The mother] did not dare to kill him; instead, *as is customary for mothers* [my emphasis], she raised him as if he were a healthy child.'[162] Many of the miracle healings discussed in Chapter 5, also dealt with congenitally impaired children, who were obviously not abandoned, exposed or otherwise killed, but raised by their parents, so that eventually they could be taken to a shrine in the hope of a cure.[163]

Although notions of links between sin and disease in general, and impairment in particular, have already been discussed to an extent, in the chapter dealing with medieval theological and philosophical concepts of impairment, it is worth taking a closer look at this stage at the presumed connection between congenital impairment and sin. In the Old Testament, the concept of children carrying the sin of their parents with them appears mainly in relation to illegitimacy, not in connection with transgressive sexual practices between properly married parents[164] – the passages from Leviticus concerning the uncleanness of menstruating women do not say anything about the conception of children at that time. The belief of some medieval writers, as was demonstrated, that menstruation posed the danger of engendering impaired children appears to have been derived from a purely Christian notion, as it does not appear in any of the Judaic writings, or the texts of the ancient anatomists and biologists.[165] The sin of the parents in Judaic thought for which children have to pay is being conceived extramaritally, and part of the punishment is that such children should not themselves 'take root' and procreate;[166] other than that, such children are simply the 'testimony' to their parents' crime. In some Patristic literature, even this is played down, and children are 'absolved' from the adulterous sins of their parents.[167] Nevertheless, according to Augustine, though God had given humans the capability for sexual intercourse, and in essence therefore the act was good, in practice every concrete act of intercourse was evil and therefore every child could literally be said to have been conceived in the sin of its parents.[168] Such ideas went a long way. By the high Middle Ages a bestiary compiler could say that all new-borns, of all species, are 'dirty': 'In fact, all recently born creatures are called "pulli", because they are born dirty or polluted',[169] and only the act of baptism 'cleans' the infant. More of the same can be found, for example, in a Middle English version of *Dives et Pauper* which looked at children afflicted by illness: 'Also God smytyght hem wyt sekenesse and myschef sumtyme for the fadrys synne and the modrys, for they lovyn hem to mechil and welyn goon to hell to makyn hem riche and grete in this world.'[170] Here it is not just the parents' sin (whatever it might be – original sin or specific transgression), but the excessive love of their offspring that is punished by illness.

It seems, then, that ideas about congenital impairment being due to transgressive sexual behaviour of the parents are so only in a very general fashion, in that *all* sexual activity, even legitimate, is sinful due to Original Sin.[171] Notions about specific sexual transgressions surface in the medieval period (perhaps influenced by rediscovered classical texts on natural philosophy), especially in relation to children conceived during menstruation, or resulting from non-standard sexual positions. By the early modern period, when the famous Shakespearean quote, 'the sins of the father are to be laid upon the children',[172] comes about, the concept of parental transgression, inheritance and sin had become popularised, and, one might say, through Shakespeare entered modern notions of parental responsibility and culpability. Cross-culturally, it seems, similar notions exist.[173] All one can state with certainty is that medieval views on sin, sex and congenital impairment were not uniform, but that instead ambiguous and at times even contradictory notions existed side by side. To illustrate such ambivalence one may look at how two opposing ideas about 'inter-generational responsibility' feature in the same source. In the late twelfth-century *Lais* of Marie de France, two narratives revolve around the consequences of adulterous unions: in *Bisclavret*, the apparent offspring of the sinful wife and her knightly lover are born with deformed noses, but the child from the equally adulterous affair in *Yonec* between a young wife and a knight becomes the eponymous hero.[174] One may conclude from this example that it did not necessarily follow that parental sin automatically impinged upon the children – congenital impairment need not invariably have been regarded as a consequence of parental transgression. Perhaps one can generalise by surmising that medieval sources stemming from a theological or philosophical tradition tended to view congenital impairment as the result of a *moral sin* (i.e. through transgressive acts by the parents), whereas sources coming from the medical tradition, or from natural philosophy or 'science', regarded congenital impairment as the result of *sin through stupidity or ignorance* (i.e. parents should know better than to have inappropriate intercourse).

Besides the influence of the humours, planets or the timing of conception, the 'maternal imagination' also had an impact on whether the child was congenitally impaired or not. The notion that what the pregnant woman sees, hears, feels and generally experiences or imagines, had a strong influence on the development of the foetus appears to be a cross-cultural and ancient idea. Soranus, in the early second century, had already written about the influence of 'maternal imagination' on the development of the foetus.

> What is one to say concerning the fact that various states of the soul also produce certain changes in the mould of the fetus? For instance, some women, seeing monkeys during intercourse, have borne children resembling monkeys. The tyrant of the Cyprians who was misshapen, compelled his wife to look at beautiful statues during intercourse and became the father of well-shaped children.[175]

Soranus continued by advising that during intercourse the women must be sober, as a drunken state amplified phantastic imaginings of the soul, which could cause 'misshapen' children.[176]

The collection of prose Salernitan questions compiled around 1200 also dealt with issues of the maternal imagination.[177] A pregnant woman, around the critical fourth month of pregnancy, may have desired something and touched her face or other body part, whereby later her child is born with a similar shape to that which she desired; the reason is given that the imaginative cell in the head shapes the spirit, and by touching her head, the pregnant woman transferred some of the humoral quality of the spirit into her body, from where the foetus picks up these qualities in its nourishment.[178]

Giles of Rome, in his tract *De formatione corporis humani in utero*, written around 1276, also made reference to the maternal imagination. He mentioned the case of a (presumably white) woman who gazed on an Ethiopian before having intercourse with her (white) husband, and subsequently gave birth to a black-skinned child.[179] This story had already been told by Vincent of Beauvais, in his *Speculum naturale* (written between 1247 and 1259), who says the orator Quintilian defended a Roman matron, who had given birth to a black child after seeing an Ethiopian, against charges of adultery. Vincent of Beauvais added a warning to pregnant women not to gaze at certain animals, like apes, to avoid similar mishaps.[180] A Middle High German poem, *Reinfried von Braunschweig*, written around 1300, cautions that when a woman has unnatural phantasmic images in her mind at the moment of conception, this can later on lead to the creation of deformed births.[181]

Perhaps ultimately these medieval notions of the impact of the maternal imagination on the foetus can be traced back to a passage in the Old Testament. The story in question actually revolves around striped or multicoloured sheep, but the principle whereby the sheep gain their patterned fleeces is the same as the effects of the maternal imagination in humans. Jacob and Laban, in the biblical narrative, reached an agreement whereby Jacob could keep any 'speckled and spotted cattle, and all the brown cattle among the sheep, and the spotted and speckled among the goats'[182] as payment for herding Laban's animals. Jacob took

rods of wood on which he had made striped markings, and placed these by
a watering trough, where the animals could see them. 'And the flocks conceived
before the rods, and brought forth cattle ringstraked, speckled and spotted.'[183]
A carved roof boss from the nave vaulting at Norwich cathedral, executed
between 1463 and 1472, illustrates this story, showing Jacob, surrounded by the
sheep, preparing his striped rods. Jacob even went in for some selective breeding,
because he started placing his striped rods only in front of the stronger animals,
but not in front of the weaker ones,[184] so that he ended up with the healthier
specimens and Laban with the weaker ones. Giles of Rome in the thirteenth
century mentioned this story in one of his works, in the context of his discussion
of the maternal imagination.[185]

Connected with notions surrounding the maternal imagination were beliefs in
the impact of food, and environmental influences, on congenital impairment.
In some sources it was presumed that the food consumed by a pregnant woman
could have an influence on the shape of the child. In a collection of Anglo-Saxon
medical, astrological and magical texts, originating from the tenth century, we
find the following notions:

> Again there is another thing: if a woman is four or five months pregnant and
> she then frequently eats nuts or acorns or any fresh fruit then it sometimes
> happens because of that that the child is stupid. Again there is another thing
> about this: if she eats bull's flesh or ram's or buck's or boar's or gander's or
> that of any animal which can beget, then it sometimes happens because of
> that that the child is humpbacked and deformed[?].[186]

It is worth pointing out that all the meat the pregnant woman should avoid
consuming is from male animals, that is animals which can beget, and only the
male of the species has the capability to beget, according to the single-seed theory
of conception outlined earlier. One might also speculate that the proscription
during pregnancy against human female consumption of meat from male animals
is based on notions of binary opposites, between male and female, begetting and
carrying. A transgression of such taboos could then explain the birth of an
impaired child. Regulation of a woman's food intake during pregnancy was also
advocated by Vincent of Beauvais in the thirteenth century. Following Arabic
writers such as Haly Abbas, Rhazes and Avicenna, Vincent pointed out that
improper food consumed during pregnancy could harm the foetus.[187]

In the *Parzival* of Wolfram von Eschenbach, a romance written in the early
thirteenth century, the notion of physical impairment as caused by the dangers of
ingesting the wrong kind of food can also be found. The hero of the story at one
point encounters a knave with the telling name Malcreatüre, a 'monster' (*ungehiure*)
who is the epitome of ugliness. The country, Tribalibot, where Malcreatüre
originates from has many such deformed inhabitants. The reason for their
appearance lies in an ancient transgression. Adam warned his daughters against
eating certain plants, which possessed the power to deform their offspring and to
change the form which God gave to humanity at Creation; some of the

daughters could not resist, ate the plants, and that is how defective people were born.[188]

Notions similar to the medieval maternal imagination, as well as notions about transgressive behaviour, can also be found in other cultures, as many ethnological studies have demonstrated. Ethnologists have termed such beliefs 'mystical retribution', which might be an appropriate term to apply to medieval notions, too. For example, among the Ojibwa of North America some hydrocephalic children were believed to be born with that condition due to homosexual relations their mothers had; also in America among the Navajo the belief existed that making a batten stick for the loom while pregnant caused the baby to be born with flat feet and only two toes on each foot; and among the Lepcha of Sikkim in India a girl who squinted was believed to do so because her father had squinted with one eye (perhaps to see if a roof line was level) during her mother's pregnancy.[189] Many cultures regarded accidents, physical aggression, inheritance and special psychological stresses as 'natural' causes for impairment. An interplay between psychological stress and somatic stress could readily be acknowledged as a factor in the aetiology of impairment.[190] In western Europe, beliefs in the concept of 'maternal imagination' were still alive and well in the later nineteenth century. One German medical professional even managed to draw particular attention to the dangers of exposing pregnant women to the sight of impaired people. As late as 1876, Karl Friedrich Heinrich Marx (1796–1877), physician in Göttingen, said that pity for cripples and other people suffering from nauseous ills should be restricted to ensuring that they stay in appropriate hospitals with gardens, which, however, they should never leave, since the repulsive sight of such unfortunates had to be removed from public view, as their impression on sensitive people, not to say pregnant women, was very disquieting.[191]

Besides causalities for congenital impairments, peri-natal aetiologies were sometimes alluded to in the texts. Bad posture of the infant during swaddling[192] was believed to be a factor in the cause of impairments, especially of the limbs. However, such admonishments were not necessarily intended purely as good paediatric advice, but also entailed a moral message. To an extent the entire business of engendering children, as was discussed earlier, and especially the new-born child, were focused upon as appropriate themes for the analogy of the corporal and the spiritual. We encounter the themes of religious analogy and potential impairment in *De proprietatibus rerum* by the encyclopaedist Bartolomaeus Anglicus (writing *c.*1230), who says: 'And for tenderness the limbs of the child may easily and soon bow and bend and take diverse shapes. And therefore children's members and limbs are bound with lystes, and other covenable bonds, that they be not crooked nor evil shapen . . .'.[193] At first reading this is an advice to child carriers to prevent deformity of a child's limbs, but in the light of the theological readings discussed in the chapter on medieval theories of impairment, there is also the second reading of the misshapen limbs being analogous to the misshapen soul. More explicitly, a tract by John Gori of San Gemignano (*c.*1260–1323), a Dominican hagiographer and moral theologian, compared the care that must be given to the new-born infant to the care that must be had for the soul of the *conversus*, the newly converted Christian; infants must be swaddled in order to straighten their limbs 'since they are easily malformed'.[194] From a social point of view, such exhortations could have severe implications for midwives and nurses. Not only did midwives have the duty to inspect the new-born for birth defects and marks (some of which may actually have been caused by the midwives' own intervention in parturition),[195] but they were also responsible for the correct swaddling of the infant, which if it was not done properly was believed to lead to crookedness of limbs in adulthood. In the Middle English translation, by John of Trevisa, of Bartholomaeus Anglicus' *De proprietatibus rerum* the midwife is advised to straighten and stretch out the infant's limbs before binding them with cradle bands to prevent deformed and crooked limbs from arising.[196] Similarly, '...if it [the infant] be crookedly handled it will grow likewise, and to the ill negligence of many nurses may be imputed the crookedness and deformity of many a man and woman which otherwise might seem well favored as any other', as Eucharius Roesslin put it in the *Byrth of Mankynde* in the fifteenth century.[197]

Within the topic of aetiologies of impairment, one final area to be considered is iatrogenic impairment, that is impairment caused by the actions of medical practitioners or through the therapies they advised. Iatrogenic diseases are today a recognised, if unwelcome and understated, fact of medicine.[198] It is interesting to observe that similar notions were present among medieval people. As was pointed out earlier, many medieval medical texts disregarded impairments, and practitioners shied away from attempting to treat what was regarded as incurable, so one may assume that incidences of iatrogenic actions making already existing impairments worse were relatively rare. However, where a condition presented that a particular doctor or surgeon believed to be curable, there was a chance of making matters worse, thereby leaving the patient impaired. In the corpus of ecclesiastical literature which was designed to help the confessor hear confessions, impose penalties and such like, mention is sometimes made of the obligations and failings of doctors. (One could argue that religious texts would naturally be biased against anything medical, but that is not necessarily the case – it is more an exaggeration of the modern historian to see a gaping chasm between medieval religion and medieval medicine than it is a reflection of medieval attitudes.) The physician, in one of these manuals, the *Baptistina* of *c*.1480, is deemed to have sinned mortally if due to his *imperitia* (inexperience, incompetence) the patient dies or is impaired. The *Baptistina* manual was the work of Baptista Trovamala de Salis, who pointed out that to avoid such a sin, the physician, if pushed to the limits of his competence, ought to consult with colleagues, other physicians, that is. An example is given, the case-study of a patient with a broken shinbone or arm 'who is disabled because of the physician's *imperitia*'.[199] The doctor was deemed responsible for damages, and if the patient, who had thus been impaired, had a family, the doctor must also compensate them for the patient's loss of earnings. It is interesting to note that here, in a late medieval *summae confessorum*, the notion of impairment as potential disability is found, unlike in the medical texts, which say nothing about the economic or social implications of impairment. The recognition of the possibility of iatrogenic impairment was not only expressed in religious texts, but, not surprisingly, also found its way into legal matters.

An English legal text of around 1290, the Anglo-Norman *Mirror of Justices*, had a little to say regarding medical practitioners who caused iatrogenic impairments. Physicians and surgeons who do not know how to perform the correct treatment, or who 'behave stupidly and negligently', or who are not careful 'especially in their cauterisings and amputations, ... then, if their patients die or lose a limb, they are homicides or mayhemers'.[200] If the notion of disability as a *consequence* of iatrogenic impairment exists, then it seems logical to take legal action against the person who caused the impairment in the first place, and sue the physician or surgeon. This is precisely what occurred in August 1320, when one Alice of Stocking filed a complaint against the surgeon John of Cornhill, who had persuaded her that he could cure a disease of the feet (*infirmitate in pedibus*) within 10 days; after 6 days, however, Alice could no longer put her feet on the ground and had become incurable.[201] A similar case occurred in the 1420s[202] in England, when William Forest of London sued the surgeon John Harwe, an 'enfranchised surgeon', for malpractice, after the treatment of William's wounded hand resulted in the permanent loss of use of the right thumb. The charge was made of '... an alleged mistake in the surgical treatment of an injury to the muscles of the thumb of the right hand ...'.[203] The evidence was heard by a panel of experts, consisting of four physicians and four surgeons, one of whom was William Bradwardyn, who had accompanied Henry V to Agincourt in 1415. Harwe and his assistants, the barbers John Dalton and Simon Rolf, were acquitted of the malpractice charge, the reasoning of the eight medical people being that William Forest had voluntarily succumbed to the treatment.

> William was thought to be in danger of death owing to the excessive loss [of blood] and quickly deciding that he would rather suffer mutilation of his hand rather than death the said John Harwe with the express consent of the said William, who was thus bleeding, when other remedies had failed stopped the bleeding with the cautery, as beseemeth, and saved his life and freed him from the bonds of death.[204]

The panel then blamed William's impairment and his 'ugly scar' on extraneous factors, such as malicious astrological influence: 'They declared that any defect, mutilation, or disfigurement of the hand was due either to the Constellations aforesaid [Aquarius and Gemini] or some defect of the patient or of the original nature of the wound.'[205] William Forest was obviously at a legal disadvantage vis-à-vis representatives of a professional body, including a surgeon with royal connections.[206]

Possibly to prevent legal action in cases of iatrogenic impairment, other regions of medieval Europe had devised a practice referred to as *desuspitatio*. The start of references to this term first emerged in Catalonia in the early fourteenth century. *Desuspitatio* consisted of 'a formal determination, accurate and objective, of the expected consequences of a wound. To be *desuspitatus* means, literally to be pronounced out of danger, whether of death or of the loss, mutilation or impairment of a limb.'[207] This term was peculiar to Catalonia, but a similar procedure for forensic medical testimony was already in evidence in Bologna in the 1250s. A detailed Catalonian account from 1338 of a surgeon's arguments for *desuspitatio* has survived from Gerona in the kingdom of Aragon. Guillem Guerau, who was a recognised surgical practitioner, was brought before a judge to determine whether the wounds or blows which had been inflicted on his patient were 'mortal or involved the risk of death or loss of members'.[208] The surgeon asserted that the wounds, 'which appeared to have been made with a club',[209] were moderate, and the man should not die

> inasmuch as neither in the head nor the arm did he have a broken bone and he had only good signs: he didn't have a swelling of the head, he wasn't vomiting or suffering from collapse [?*stratimentum*], which are all ominous indications. Therefore he stated that the patient was in no danger of death or disability and declared him *desuspitatus*.[210]

Skull fractures were regarded as particularly dangerous, so the absence of such an injury probably indicated that in this case the surgeon was making a valid prediction for the patient's health. In another case where a surgeon had made the wrong prediction, declaring the patient safe but the patient died the following day, he was accused of negligence and incompetence of the arts of surgery (*negligenciam et impericiam artis cirurgie*)[211] – evidence that notions of iatrogenic disorders and medical incompetence were not restricted to the realm of confessor's manuals. One way around the issue of whether to resort to legal action in cases of iatrogenic impairment was to enter into a contract with the medical professional prior to the start of treatment, setting out the details beforehand. This is what happened in 1318, when one Creschas de Torre of Gerona (in Aragon) dislocated his hip (*ancha*) and was unable to walk any more. He made a contract with a surgeon, Guillem Guerau of Besalú, specifying that the surgeon should receive the sum of 1,000 *sous* as soon as Creschas could walk again to the window (presumably referring to walking from his bed to the window of his bedroom) with the aid of a cane.[212] In England in the 1480s, similar 'pre-operative' contracts were also in evidence. The London surgeon John Brown entered into a contractual agreement to cure a priest of the palsy; part of the stipulations appear to have been that the priest should be able to walk again, albeit with a stick, and be able to say mass, which did not, however, materialise, since the priest withheld payments on the grounds that the cure had not been effected.[213]

Medical practice for other reasons than trying to cure or prevent impairments could also bring about iatrogenic impairment. Sleeping after a phlebotomy was considered very dangerous for a patient, as it could induce deafness or blindness. The prose Salernitan questions, written around 1200, try to explain why sleep was forbidden after phlebotomy. Patients should not sleep after this therapy because humoral problems related to heat and humidity block the nerves; the humours which are in motion may have obstructed the nerves and may have caused deafness and blindness.[214]

One final aspect of iatrogenic impairment needs to be considered. This involved the medical practice of 'cutting the tongue string'. Ostensibly a therapeutic measure for speech impediments, cutting the tongue string actually seems to have caused more harm than good. The practice appears to be derived from a passage in Celsus (first century), who advised on the need to cut the tongue string in a speech-impaired person:

> Again the tongue of some persons is tied down from birth to the part underlying it, and on this account they cannot even speak. In such cases the extremity of the tongue is to be seized with forceps, and the membrane under it incised, great care being taken lest the blood vessels close by are injured or bleeding. . . . Many, when the wound has healed, have spoken. I have, however, known a case where, though the tongue has been undercut so that it could be protruded well beyond the teeth, nevertheless the power of speech has not followed.[215]

However, fear that the neonate may have an impeded tongue, and hence impeded speech, for centuries often led to the practice of cutting the tongue string automatically after birth, whether or not the infant was mute. In one of the Salernitan texts, the *Second Salernitan Demonstration* from the first half of the twelfth century, cutting the tongue string was advised as a remedy. Speech disorders were seen to differ among individuals, so that in some cases surgery, that is severance of the ligaments, was mandatory where the ligaments were too close to the tip of the tongue; this then enabled the tongue to move freely in the mouth and over the palate.[216] Right up to the sixteenth century, medical treatises advised this as a precautionary method to prevent speech impediments, even if some physicians were critical of the procedure.[217] Midwives, parents or nurses in Italy in the seventeenth century were still cutting the tongue string to make it easier for the infant to suckle.[218] In fifteenth-century Germany, with the beginnings of regulatory measures for midwives, the *Heilbronner Hebammenordnung* stipulated that midwives are not allowed to 'loosen the tongue' of the neonate without consent of a physician, since through this practice and through ignorance great damage is done.[219] From a modern point of view, the problem with this remedy is that it can actually *cause* speech impediments, if not total muteness, in the first place; the 'ligaments' or 'membranes' the physician/surgeon was advised to cut are precisely those muscles a person needs to have control over the movement of their tongue, without which intelligible speech is impossible. Such a case, where cutting the tongue string only made matters worse, is encountered in the register of a foundling hospital at Florence, the Ospedale degli Innocenti:

> On the 18th September 1452 at the thirteenth hour a female child was brought and placed on the front. She was about eighteen months old, and the person who brought her fled and did not wish to say whose she was or what

her name was. She brought with her a note that said she had her tongue-string cut because she stammered, and that *afterwards she spoke badly* [my emphasis]. The abovesaid child is mute and crazy and therefore the wet nurse will be given thirty-five solidi per month.[220]

This neutrally voiced account screens the rather sad story of an individual, who was effectively abandoned, if not to say dumped, apparently because of their 'defect', which ironically was caused by probably well-meant therapeutic measures.

From exploring ideas about the generation of offspring and procreation as a whole, it was seen that the practice of intercourse itself could determine the outcome. Deviation from the prescribed practice might result in deformed children. Astrology, in the correct timing of conception, was also seen to play a part. Sometimes even factors such as the food consumed by pregnant women were regarded as influencing the well-being or impairment of a child. Furthermore, sexual activity during a woman's pregnancy, lactation or menstrual period was believed to be particularly dangerous: children conceived at such times were most likely to be born with a birth defect. Menstruation especially had a negative effect on the outcome of a conception.

Henri de Mondeville, in the early fourteenth century, had stated that the 'common' people differentiated between diseases which have causes, and diseases which do not, as was discussed earlier.[221] I had proposed that Mondeville's 'extrinsic' causes could be equated with what modern medicine terms acquired impairments, meaning impairments sustained in later life, through accident or injury, while his 'intrinsic' causes could be equated with modern notions of congenital impairment. Mondeville had furthermore asserted that the 'common' people believed an ailment had no cause known to them, if it stemmed from what he called an 'intrinsic' cause. However, as the many medieval aetiologies for congenital impairment, analysed in this chapter, demonstrate, medieval people at all levels of society must have had some awareness of what factors could cause the birth of an impaired child. Astrological beliefs were fairly widespread, and ideas about when and how to have sexual intercourse were promulgated by the Church, through instructions to confessors and through preaching.[222] Therefore one may readily assume that most medieval people did possess fairly clear ideas concerning at least some of the causes of congenital impairment.

4.3   Preventative medicine

Under the rubric 'preventative measures' I will discuss and analyse prescriptions, treatment methods and recipes in medieval medical texts which attempt to prevent particular physical conditions and dysfunctions from becoming impairments. A classic example would be the description of how to set a fractured leg in a surgical manual, which, if performed correctly by the surgeon, would allow the fracture to heal and, by not leading to complications, would prevent long-term, chronic or permanent damage. Henri de Mondeville, in the very early fourteenth century, had already alluded to the 'preventative' aspects of surgery: 'by a local remedy, or sometimes by a mere word, surgeons can save a finger, a hand, sometimes an arm, and thus the life of some poor sick artisan; if he died, his wife and children, whom he feeds through his labours, would die also.'[223] The surgical procedure would therefore prevent what one would now term 'impairment'. Similarly, recipes or prescriptions from textbooks intended for physicians which aim to prevent a specific condition from becoming an impairment will also be discussed. Rarely did medieval medical texts cover remedies for already existing conditions that we would now term 'impairments', although sometimes impairing conditions were mentioned in such texts. Gentile da Foligno (d. 1348, also known as 'Speculator'), author of medical commentaries and textbooks, as well as several *consilia* (books of medical advice), listed in these not just diseases following the customary head to toe sequence, but also some impairments. For example, he mentioned debility of the brain and nerves, epilepsy, apoplexy, cases of paralysis, eye and ear troubles, arthritis and hunchbacks.[224] In similar fashion, his near-contemporary John of Rupescissa (active in the 1340s and 1350s) wrote an alchemical and medical text, *De consideratione quintae essentiae* (Consideration of the fifth essence); in the second book of this text he dealt with remedies for various diseases, including some impairments, such as the impediments of old age, how to restore one who is nearly dead back to their senses, paralysis and spasm.[225] However, the vast majority of medieval medical texts gloss over conditions we would refer to as 'impairments'.

I found it more useful for the purposes of my argument to organise my source material according to the topic contained therein, rather than to discuss the texts according to type of source. So I will not discuss surgical, medical or natural philosophical texts as separate categories, but I will amalgamate the topics found in such texts, and pursue a thematic analysis of the evidence. Again, in my thematic structure I found it most useful to follow the precedent set by a large number of medieval medical texts themselves, and will therefore organise my material according to the head to toe description of afflictions and their remedies that such textbooks promulgated.

Head injuries can, of course, have very serious repercussions for the person concerned, which is why many medieval medical texts mention such injuries, and advise caution in the application of therapeutic measures. There is some evidence for the occurrence of head injuries and their treatment in Anglo-Saxon medical texts.[226] A group of remedies from *Leechbook III*[227] specifies what to do in case there is a wound on top of one's head and a bone is broken, and in case of a broken bone in the head which will not come out.[228] Obviously such wounds, probably, mainly the result of fights and accidents, must have occurred often enough to merit specific mention as a separate category of ailment that then requires specific treatment in the texts. If the bone pieces cannot be removed, the outcome of the injury is likely to be brain damage, leading to debilitating conditions, or death. In the *Leechbook* the treatment for a head injury leading to a 'folded-up skull', presumably a wound sustained from being hit on the head which breaks the bone, is described as follows: 'If a man's skull is folded up, lay the man supine, drive two stakes at the shoulders, then lay a board across his feet, then strike on it with a sledgehammer; it will come right at once!'[229] A similar remedy is mentioned in the *Petrocellus*,[230] where the physician is to put shingle at the sick man's feet and to hit it with a mallet until the man speaks. Both these treatments could, in fact, make the condition far worse;[231] the kind of motion incurred by hitting and beating, even if just at the foot end of the patient, could well cause further injury and possibly result in permanent brain damage, leading to impairing conditions if the patient survived at all.

Greater sophistication and an awareness of the importance of taking care when dealing with head injuries is shown in later medieval texts. Theories of the brain, its morphology and its functioning had developed, partly from empirical study, partly from the subsumption of medical, and especially humoral, theory. William of Conches' description of the brain, from the twelfth century, is an example of such theories. According to him, the brain is divided into three cerebral chambers he calls 'cells'; each cell has an appropriate quality, is located in a particular area of the head, and is linked with particular nutritional aspects. Here humoral theories and the importance of nutrition and lifestyle, as could be found in the *Regimen sanitatis*, are applied to a theory of how the brain works.

By the later medieval period the practical knowledge gained from performing surgery and from subsequent availability of practical surgical manuals allowed a greater understanding of how to go about curing head injuries, and preventing greater damage to the brain in the process. The *Chirurgia* (*c*.1180) of Roger of Salerno (Ruggiero Frugardi), and the Occitan verse adaptation of this text by Raimon of Avignon (before 1209), both mention trauma to the skull, in the form of fractures or wounds.[232] From a fifteenth-century manuscript[233] stems a recipe for removing broken bones from a head wound, instructing in how to prepare herbal remedies for curing the wound by making poultices to put on the head; the text also discusses prognosis, that is if such-and-such a phenomenon is apparent, then the patient will die, or live, as the case may be. There is great concern shown over preventing rupture of the dura mater, here called *tay*. This is evidence of a recognition by the author of the text that exposure of the layers of the brain that lie below the dura mater, the arachnoid layer (here called *spynnyng webb*), will lead to the inevitable death of the patient.[234]

Hydrocephalus was believed to be treatable by some late antique Greek medical writers. Leonides (second/third century), Oribasius (325–403) and Paul of Aegina (seventh century) all advised that if water had collected on the outside of the skull (but under the skin), then a surgical procedure could be made, in which the size of the incision was dependent on the size of the afflicted head. Surgical aftercare included placing a piece of wool soaked in egg on the head (recommended by Leonides). Special care was needed in treating infants when bandaging the head: because of the risk of pressure to the still soft skull, Leonides advised using a kind of cap instead of bandages.[235] In the fourteenth century, Guy de Chauliac briefly mentioned some cures for 'water in the heads of children', citing the earlier authorities William of Saliceto (1210–76/80), Lanfranc of

Milan (*c*.1245–1306) and Avicenna (d. 1037).[236] A miniature in a twelfth-century manuscript of Gerard of Cremona's *Chirurgia* depicts a surgeon trying to treat a child for hydrocephalus, by using incision.[237]

A case of head injury occurring in a real person is documented by several chroniclers. William of Malmesbury relates how Baldwin, count of Flanders sustained an injury to his head during the attack on Arques in 1118. Baldwin's helmet was battered repeatedly, so that he was injured in the brain.[238] A physician was sent to treat him, but could not cure him completely. He did not die immediately, though, but according to another source, Orderic Vitalis, he lived with his injury from September that year (1118) until his death in the summer of 1119.[239] It is highly likely that he sustained some form of brain damage, although the sources are silent regarding further details of his injuries.

Trepanation was one method, with a long ancestry,[240] that was used as a form of medical intervention in cases of disease or trauma affecting the head. A case of trepanation carried out as a form of medical treatment dating from the later medieval period may be found in the anecdote surrounding Geert Grote (1340–84), founder of the religious Modern Devotion movement. His skull was exhumed around 1450 and was discovered to show an artificial opening in it – possibly the result of a trepanation. The cryptic statement that Geert used to make during his lifetime, '*habeo caminum in capite*' ('I have a chimney in my head') may well have been a reference to this trepanation.[241] That Geert Grote's trepanation was not an unusual or isolated case of this practice during the medieval period can be substantiated by archaeological evidence. At the hospital of the Cistercian abbey of Øm in Denmark, the cemetery attached to the site yielded the skeletons of several hundred individuals, comprising men, women and children (so that it seems the abbey's hospital was catering for non-monastic patients as well as the monastic community). Some of the skulls found during the excavation showed signs with clear evidence of trepanation, and furthermore had new bone growth around the trepanning hole anterior to the death of the individual, proof that the patient survived the operation.[242]

Visual impairments, ranging from various degrees of sight disorders to complete blindness, were another commonly found topic in medical texts. Remedies for eye diseases occur frequently in Anglo-Norman herbals and leechbooks. Does this imply either a great frequency of such diseases among the Anglo-Norman population, or the greater concern of physicians to treat such diseases rather than other pathologies, possibly leading to quite some knowledge on the matter? Illuminations in twelfth-century manuscripts suggest that operations for cataract may have been performed, but the illustrations are not referred to or described in the accompanying text. An example of such a cataract operation can be seen illustrated in a late twelfth-century manuscript.[243] Since a number of prominent men were nicknamed *monoculus* it appears that not all eye diseases were curable.[244] Eye disorders and blindness could also result from wounds sustained in combat. Raimon of Avignon's verse version (before 1209) of Roger of Salerno's *Chirurgia* mentioned that 'It sometimes happens by chance, however rarely, that a knight is wounded in the head or nose by a dart, so that the eye is affected, or in the ears and other parts.'[245] Once a visual impairment had become complete blindness, however, there was nothing the medical texts could suggest as possible treatment.

Disorders of the ear are also dealt with by medical textbooks, although deafness is generally regarded as incurable. In medical texts, sometimes an illustration is provided for recipes dealing with the treatment of ear disorders, such as in an early thirteenth-century manuscript from southern Italy.[246] Alexander of Tralles (525–605) was sceptical about a great number of apparent cures for impaired hearing and for profound deafness. He remarked that some physicians had attempted to cure deaf and deaf-mute persons by using acoustic instruments and hearing aids, and also by making the patient perform hearing exercises; but in his time these 'experiments' were now discontinued[247] (presumably due to lack of success). A number of medieval Arabic and Western physicians distinguished between congenital and acquired deafness, and most regarded congenital deafness as incurable, for example Mesue (John Damascene, d. 1015).[248] A Salernitan text of the twelfth century also regarded congenital deafness as incurable, and acquired deafness or impaired hearing could not be cured if the disorder was older than two or three years.[249] The surgeon Lanfranc of Milan (d. 1306) did try cures for hearing impediments again. In the later thirteenth century he had written two surgical texts, *Chirurgia parva* (1270) and *Chirurgia magna*. In the latter work he discussed diseases of the ear and their treatments. With regards to impaired hearing (*diminutio auditus*) he remarked that one should awaken the hearing with a quiet voice,[250] a suggestion that Lanfranc returned to the practice of hearing exercises.[251] This may have helped in cases of hearing impediments, but profound deafness eluded therapies by physicians and surgeons. A fifteenth-century Middle English translation of Gilbertus Anglicus (originally writing around 1240), after discussing various types of so-called 'deafness', simply states the physician should understand that old sicknesses of the ears, and especially deafness, are incurable.[252] Guy de Chauliac in the mid-fourteenth century, following Avicenna, differentiated two types of deafness, 'kindly' and 'unkindly', the latter being chronic deafness of both ears which was incurable in his opinion.[253] But for actual, profound deafness no treatment is suggested beyond the religio-magical sphere. So as a cure for deafness Hildegard of Bingen, in the twelfth century, suggests that cutting off a lion's right ear and holding it over the patient's own affected ear just long enough to warm it, and to say 'Hear *adimacus* by the living God and the keen virtue of a lion's hearing', a process then to be repeated many times, is a way of restoring hearing.[254]

Moving further down the body in the scheme of treatments from head to toe, deformities of the nose and mouth will be considered next. One finds a rare incidence of 'cosmetic' surgery from the late medieval period. One Heinrich von Pfolspeundt, a member of the Order of Teutonic Knights, wrote a treatise of *Bündth-Erznei* ('Wundarznei'[255]) in 1460 where he mentioned a procedure for rhinoplasty. He described attempts to restore a lost or mutilated nose by using flesh from other parts of the face or from the upper arm of the patient. Apparently, in this he copied from Italian surgical techniques which had been developed in the earlier fifteenth century,[256] which in turn seemed to be derived from a description of the procedure for rhinoplasty in the *Surgery* of Albucasis (b. 1013–d. 1106).[257] Incidentally, Pfolspeundt also mentioned the use of anaesthetics, derived from opiates, in surgical procedures, so one may assume that his proposed treatment for rhinoplasty was not the ordeal for the patient it appeared to be at first. Knowledge of anaesthetics was not limited to the post-medieval period, as so many historians of medicine too readily assume: there is evidence from as early as the fourth century pointing to the knowledge and use of anaesthetics in surgical procedures. Hilary of Poitiers (d. 367), in his tract *De Trinitate*, already proposed that '...when through some grave necessity part of the body must be cut away, the soul can be lulled to sleep by drugs, which overcome the pain and produce in the mind a death-like forgetfulness of its power of sense. Then limbs can be cut off without pain: the flesh is dead to all feeling, and does not heed the deep thrust of the knife, because the soul within it is asleep.'[258]

Bald's *Leechbook* mentions a rather intriguing recipe, and a good example of the 'scientific' rationale behind Anglo-Saxon medical practice, for the correction of a congenital defect, namely a surgical treatment for harelip. 'For harelip: pound mastic very fine, add white of an egg and mix as you do vermilion, cut with a knife, sew securely with silk, then anoint with the salve outside and inside before the silk rot. If it pulls together, arrange it with the hand, anoint again immediately.'[259] Explained in modern medical parlance this would entail the adjoining surfaces of the harelip being cut so that they might grow together as a single tissue. The salve contains mastic (an antiseptic agent) and egg white (a binding agent necessary for proper adhesion to the wound). Possibly the text demonstrated an awareness of the Hippocratic observation that a sutured wound is likely to open if suppuration takes place; this awareness should not be taken necessarily as evidence that Anglo-Saxon medical authors had knowledge of Hippocratic medicine, since the observation could just as easily have been made empirically and independently. A salve that prevents 'rot' was therefore important. If it was necessary to handle the wound, then in such a case the text cautions the application of the antiseptic salve again immediately afterwards;[260] here also it is not paramount to have knowledge of the exact transmission of infections, or even the nature of bacteria, but an empirical observation suffices to make it apparent that wounds left untreated with the (antiseptic) salve do not heal so well as those treated with it. This procedure raises interesting questions: was this surgery performed on infants, for example. Infants with harelip find it very difficult to suckle, and since we are dealing with an age prior to the advent of bottle-feeding, let alone drip-feeding, the survival chances of babies born with harelip may well have been pretty minimal. If that is the case, how *do* infants with harelip survive to grow into the adults on whom, presumably, this surgery was performed? Are we to think, then, that perhaps this surgical technique was intended specifically for infants, as they would otherwise starve? As an aside, the mention of silk as the material to be used for the suture in this recipe[261] points to the availability of silk in Anglo-Saxon England; elsewhere even more specifically mention is made of the yellow 'good silk'[262] which would only be available from China (Chinese raw silk is yellow, whereas Coan silk is a pale creamy white).[263] Harelip treatment was also mentioned by the Flemish surgeon Jan Yperman (1295–1351), who described how to heal a harelip incision using freshened edges and special sutures.[264]

Speech disorders and their treatments were occasionally alluded to in the sources I have studied. From Anglo-Saxon England stems the case of a healing achieved through the application of a 'rational speech therapy'.[265] Bishop John of Hexham (d. 721), later to become St John of Beverley, gradually gets a young man who was speech impaired to speak, first by making the sign of the cross on his tongue, then asking the man to say 'yes', then getting him to vocalise the letters of the alphabet in turn, then syllables, then whole words, and finally the man was able to speak entire sentences.[266] However, Anglo-Saxon therapies for speech disorders could also be of a more 'magical' nature. From the text known as *Lacnunga* stems the following advice for dealing with speech impediments: 'For a woman suddenly going dumb: Take pulegium [pennyroyal], and grind to dust and wrap up in wool. Lay it under the woman. Soon will she be better.'[267] It seems that weaving and the association with woven materials was seen to have a loosening effect, so that here wool was believed to have the ability to 'loosen' the tongue.

Injuries to the head and/or neck were another area where difficulties ensuing from such wounds could lead to permanent impairments, something that did not elude one medieval surgeon. William of Saliceto (Guglielmo da Saliceto, 1210–76/80) wrote practical treatises on surgery, such as his *Chirurgia* (1268, and 1275 or 1276, as it is available in two versions) and also a work on hygiene and therapy, *Summa conservationis et curationis*.[268] In his texts he made the point that wounds sustained to the head or the neck could result in paralysis if the spinal cord or the brain were injured, but he hastened to add that such paralysis need not necessarily be either permanent or fatal to the patient, recommending a thick compress to prevent air entering the head, which he regarded as detrimental.[269] He gave three examples of such cases. First, a man who had received a sword wound to the head became paralysed and incontinent three days later, but 'thanks to the healing power of nature and William's treatment, however, he ultimately recovered completely and lived another twenty years'.[270] Second, a patient who had been wounded by an arrow in the neck also became paralysed and incontinent, and as a result of his impairment additionally became deeply depressed; he also made a partial recovery under William's treatment so that he survived for another ten years but could only walk with the aid of crutches.[271] And thirdly, a less fortunate patient whose arrow wound within less than a month's time resulted in rigour, fever and subsequent death – but it is interesting to note that this man had been attended to by another rival surgeon prior to being seen by William of Saliceto, who blamed the failings of the other medic for the patient's demise.[272]

Therapeutic measures to prevent orthopaedic impairments, that is impairments affecting the use of a person's arms or legs, were among the most commonly discussed themes in medical texts. Galen (*c*.130–200), commenting on earlier texts from the Hippocratic corpus, had already proposed treatment methods for club foot or inwardly twisted feet. His therapeutic measure was to be the realignment of the affected bones, which could be achieved in small children, due to the malleability of the infantile bones, by using soft linen bandages. These bandages were to be applied without too much pressure, and they were to be held together with wax and resin.[273] Following Hippocrates, Galen also suggested attaching a (shoe) sole made of lead or leather to the finished bandage.[274] Galen also cited the case of a child with a deformed chest which he treated – presumably successfully. The child's thorax deviated strongly from normal appearance, so he had the child wear a broad belt around its lower body, without, however, restricting the child. He also had the child carry out arm exercises and speech practices, whereby the child had to hold its breath. The inhaled air was to be held in the lungs while the chest was pressed in from around on all sides. With a further intake of breath the chest was in this way stretched and widened due to increased internal pressure. The speech exercises were intended to aid the organs located within the thorax. Galen reckoned that in still developing bodies, such as in children, this therapy helped to better a badly developed body.[275]

In Anglo-Saxon medicine *Leechbook II* advised that a broken limb was to be covered with a salve and with elm bark, then a splint was to be applied; or the broken limb was to be bathed, then stretched and subsequently a splint applied. This kind of advice could not generally have been very successful in dealing with fractures. 'All in all, treatment of broken bones did not do much to assure a sound limb after healing'.[276] The implication of this lack of effective medical procedure for dealing with fractures is that many people may have been wandering around with badly healed limbs, which could potentially have caused impairing conditions. Nevertheless, it appears that the authors of Anglo-Saxon medical texts at least recognised the possibility of ensuing complications in fractures, even if they could not do much to prevent them. For example, if the thigh bone is fractured, the muscles frequently go into strong spasm with the danger that then the fractured bone ends override (due to the tension of the muscles) and consequently the thigh bone knits together in a foreshortened manner, causing the fractured leg to be shorter than the other and therefore also causing a limping gait. The *Leechbook*[277] recommended that 'in the case of many a man where his feet shrink up to his thighs [i.e. the limb is shortening due to muscle spasm] give baths ... when they [the limbs] are in a sweat, then let the patient arrange the bones as well as he can and apply a splint ...'.[278] Bathing in hot water eases the muscle tension and allows for the bones to be set straight, without overriding ends, therefore at least potentially permitting a healing of the fracture without complications or deformity. Bathing as a form of therapy for chronic disorders was also advocated in later periods of the Middle Ages. For example, Peter of Eboli wrote around 1250 in his didactic poems on bathing, *De balneis*: 'The long standing burden of gout can be shed, and joints can be given repose' through bathing.[279] In law-codes of the Anglo-Saxon period, too, there was some recognition of the potential for complications ensuing from fractures. In the laws of King Alfred it was specified that 'if a man break another man's ribs within the whole skin, let 10 shillings be paid as *bót*: if the skin be broken and the bone be taken out, let 15 shillings be paid as *bót*.'[280] There was here the realisation that a compound fracture might not heal as well as a simple fracture, and the larger compensation fee reflected the degree of resulting complication and potential impairment. In the case of dislocated shoulders, again salves from a number of herbs were the preferred Anglo-Saxon treatments – no mention of using traction to reduce the dislocation was made in the medical texts of the period. A modern historian has commented that '... except for cases of spontaneous reduction, there was little hope of a successful outcome, and consequently deformity and loss of function could be expected'[281] in the affected arm.

An example of an intended cure that did successfully reduce dislocation nevertheless exists from after the Anglo-Saxon period, in the twelfth-century 'miracle' healing of a monk of Revesby whose dislocated shoulder was cured when he wielded a staff given to him by Ailred;[282] apparently the rotary movement the monk made when wielding the staff acted as a kind of physiotherapy. Another interesting case from twelfth-century England also exemplified successful healing of an impairment through a combination of the expectation of miracle healing and unwittingly performed physiotherapy. A man from Dunwich, Suffolk, named Adwyn, who was a carpenter by trade, had badly crippled hands and feet – it is not mentioned how or why he acquired his condition. He was taken by boat to London, from the Thames dockside to St Bartholomew's shrine at the eponymous hospital in Smithfield. There he was apparently expected to earn some of his own keep in addition to receiving charitable support while he awaited a cure. As time passed by he started making simple wooden objects, such as distaffs and loom weights. As he became stronger, he turned to heavier tasks like cutting wood. Eventually Adwyn achieved a complete recovery, and in gratitude he voluntarily worked some carpentry for free for several London churches.[283] It has been suggested that Adwyn suffered from 'a classic case of chronic contractures caused by a fixed posture during prolonged illness'.[284] His gradual healing may have been achieved through a form of physiotherapeutical exercises and occupational therapy, to put it in modern medical parlance.

In the case of paralysis, Anglo-Saxon medical texts acknowledged that not a lot could be done in treatment, but 'various heroic measures'[285] were attempted. An interesting assumption has been made by S. Rubin with regards to the regular occurrence of mentions of paralytic conditions in texts of the Anglo-Saxon period:

> in view of the frequency with which paralysed youths appear in the literature, as well as those suffering from weakness of their limbs, it is not impossible that some infectious and paralysing disease such as poliomyelitis was responsible. Despite the unhistoricity of Ingulf's *History of Croyland Abbey*, it does contain a detailed description of a disease which could be considered typical of poliomyelitis.... The sequence of pain, paralysis and muscle wasting with deformity is very characteristic of this most infectious disease.[286]

The episode related by Ingulf concerns an 'epidemic' at the council of Kingesbyry in 851, where many people appeared to have a disease 'like paralysis' which was wearing away the whole of England, with men, women and children all afflicted 'with a sudden and severe chill' and intolerable pain in their diseased members, hands and arms being the main areas which were 'withered or disabled' by the affliction. There was no remedy, at least not until Ceolnoth, archbishop of Canterbury, became the first to be cured by the relics of St Guthlac, thereafter hundreds of people were daily cured of the 'paralysis'.[287] If one accepts the suggestion that this was an outbreak of poliomyelitis of epidemic proportions then that still leaves the problem of a mass cure for incurable symptoms of a mass paralysis, unless one were to acknowledge that it is part of the function of miracle stories that incurable diseases are cured, or that such cures take place on a massive scale.

A disease similar to paralysis could be the 'half-dead disease' (*healf-deád ádl*) of the Anglo-Saxon medical texts, which has been identified as a kind of hemiplegia, a one-sided paralysis. Section 59 of the *Leechbook* described it as arising 'on the right half of the body or on the left, where the sinews are paralysed and are [afflicted] with a viscid and thick humour ... when the disease first comes on a man, then open his mouth, look at his tongue: then it is whiter on that side on which the disease is about to be'.[288] Treatment was suggested to be in the form of applying heat to the afflicted side.[289] Considering that modern therapeutic methods utilise heat, in the form of infrared lamps or ultrasound, to alleviate palsy and joint problems, it is likely that this Anglo-Saxon remedy may actually have had some effect. This was not always the case with remedies suggested by later writers. So Albertus Magnus in the thirteenth century stated that a diet of lion's flesh was said to benefit paralytics,[290] due to the properties ascribed to certain parts of the lion (and other animals), apparently basing his material concerning the lion on a discussion of that animal in Pliny, and on a compilation in the work of Thomas of Cantimpré. A similar animal-based remedy was suggested by John of Gaddesden in his *Rosa Anglica*, written around 1314, where he advised sufferers to bathe in water 'wherein an entire fox is boiled until its flesh separate from the bones; with rue and flagflower and caraway and peony and vervain'.[291] Bathing may have relieved some of the symptoms, or at least made the afflicted person feel better, as would have John's advice for follow-up treatment, namely to massage and wrap up the paralysed limb – but in fox's skin!

In the Anglo-Saxon text, the incidence of 'true' hemiplegia was linked to the age of a person, afflicting the middle-aged and elderly, while symptoms of hemiplegia in younger people were regarded as indicating a different disease:

Truly, the disease comes on a person after forty or fifty years; if he is of a cold temperament then it comes after forty, otherwise it comes after fifty years of his age. If it happens to a younger person then it is easier to cure and is not the same disease, although ignorant physicians think that it is the same halfdead disease. How can a similar disease befall one in youth on any limb as the halfdead disease does in old age? It is not the halfdead disease, but some other harmful humour has flooded the limb which it settles, but it is easier to cure. But the real halfdead disease comes after fifty years.[292]

Here, then, a humoral explanation is given for the disease, in that since the colder humours were believed to dominate in old age, older people were more likely to be afflicted by a disease that numbs and paralyses their limbs, and makes the affected limb feel cold. Lastly, the name for the disease warrants a brief discussion. 'Halfdead' disease is a very interesting term, as it conjures up associations with liminality. People who suffer from the 'halfdead' disease could be seen to be half dead themselves, they would be neither truly 'alive' nor truly 'dead', but halfway in between the two categories. Similarly, the impaired person is occupying an in-between state, as my discussion of anthropological theory demonstrated, so that impairment and 'halfdead' disease both place the sufferer in a liminal position, between the states of health and illness, dead or alive.

One of the main causes of acquired (as opposed to congenital) orthopaedic impairment will have been due to dislocations and fractures of bones that subsequently did not heal properly, and left the injured person with a permanent impairment. It is therefore useful to take a closer look at what medieval medical and surgical texts had to say about the treatment of dislocations and fractures, especially with a view of how to prevent such permanent physical damage. Here the bulk of my evidence stems from surgical texts. Even the accompanying illustrations to surgical texts are more likely to depict impaired people than 'regular' medical texts; an example is a manuscript made at Bruges in 1482, which shows three patients with orthopaedic disorders arriving to consult a surgeon.[293] Medieval surgery, more or less successfully, dealt with broken limbs, sprains, dislocations, burns, scalds, cuts, bites, bruises, swellings, but also bone setting, bandaging and suturing. In the early fourteenth century, the surgeon Henri de Mondeville delineated the sphere of activity for his 'craft': surgeons deal with those disorders which appear on the surface of the body, as well as with 'external afflictions of the head, arms, thighs and lower down, whose location can be determined, even if they do not appear on the surface, such as arthritis, short-sightedness, deafness, pain in the hands',[294] and so on. From the twelfth to the fifteenth century surgical literature, both in Latin and in vernacular languages, underwent a complex evolution, which was parallel to and therefore cannot be separated from the history of strictly medical writing of the period. The developments in later medieval surgical techniques were only possible in the contexts of a successfully transmitted tradition of the 'craft' of surgery (i.e. surgery as a non-academic profession) and due to the widespread social demand for surgery and appreciation of its benefits.[295]

Generally, one can find in the medical and/or surgical texts a recognition that fractures which are improperly treated, or just too difficult to treat, can lead to lasting damage, to what we would now call impairment. The texts I have studied either advocate specific types of treatment, or, conversely, caution against certain other types of treatment, which were regarded as making matters worse. In eleventh-century Arabic medicine, Albucasis (1013–1106), whose work was later made known to the West[296] and became one of the leading textbooks on surgery, already cautioned against too much medical intervention in the case of complex fractures:

> On the treatment of fractured bones when they mend crooked and are inhibited from their proper functioning.
>
> When a limb that has been set has some distortion after healing, or the bone that was broken has some prominence or callosity, so that the limb is deformed, but there is nevertheless no limitation of its natural movement, then you should not listen to those who think that the bone should be broken again.[297]

Greek medical writers also mentioned potentially impairing conditions. Dislocations in new-born children were discussed by Michael Psellos (1018–78), in his *Letter concerning all kinds of curiosities*, who mentioned using a kind of hook as part of one treatment, and alluded to a second method involving a substance which shone at night, derived from a plant he called *gorgoneion* (the meaning of this is unclear: it could be a magical plant rather than an actual botanical specimen).[298]

In the West, the association of fractures with the potential crippling of a person was made by William of Saliceto in the 1270s, who records the link between what he termed *crepitus* with trauma due to broken bones (*sonitus ossis fracti*).[299] Moving on to more general aspects of surgical procedures and the treatment of potentially impairing conditions, we encounter Roger of Salerno, who in his *Surgery* (*Chirurgia*) around 1180 wrote about precise indications for the reduction of dislocations.[300] Raimon of Avignon, who made a vernacular verse adaptation of Roger's text before 1209, mentioned that dislocations of the shoulder were often caused by knights falling off their horses, and advised that such injuries should be treated straight away 'while the bone has just recently been displaced.'[301] Treatment methods, in both Roger and Raimon's texts, were based on ancient (Hippocratic) methods, and involved applying pressure or tension to the affected bone with the help of assistants. A French manuscript, dating from the early fourteenth century, of Roger's *Chirurgia* illustrates the kind of treatment recommended for reducing a dislocated shoulder: two assistants hold the patient suspended over a padded pole, while the surgeon pulls down on the affected arm.[302] More material can be found in surgical manuals of the thirteenth and fourteenth centuries. Gilbertus Anglicus was the author of the *Compendium medicinae*, written about 1240, which dealt mainly with internal medicine, although, unusually for a physician, some coverage was given to wounds and fractures (such as fractures of arms and ribs, dislocations of jaw, shoulder and elbows), in other words those areas falling within the surgeon's sphere of competence.[303] In his chapter *De vulneribus cruris et tybie*, Gilbertus noted that separation of the sacrum (he called it *vertebrum*) from the ilium (*scia*), either by accident or from a corrosion of humours, left the patient permanently lame, although suitable fomentations and inunctions might produce some improvements.[304] Fractures of the femur which occurred within three inches of the hips or knee were regarded as particularly dangerous for the patient by Gilbertus.[305]

Some of the most extensive discussion of fractures, their potentially impairing effect, and their treatment can be exemplified from the work of the Italian surgeon Theoderic (Theoderico Borgognoni, 1205–98). Around 1267 he had completed his *Cyrurgia*, which dealt with fractures and dislocations. Theoderic displayed an extensive knowledge of fracture treatment, and associated problems and complications. Theoderic stated that 'the first objective is the treatment and correct reduction or realignment of the broken or separated bones.'[306] Traction was used by him to stretch the muscles, which allowed the bones to return to their proper position. On this subject he advised the following. 'Sometimes a fracture which occurs in the large limbs does not submit to setting without violent stretching, and sometimes to correct the shortening [of a limb], strong traction is necessary.'[307] He wrote that compound fractures of the humerus could on occasion lead to mobility impairments. 'The humerus between the shoulder and the elbow is sometimes broken in such a way that the muscle and the bone are equally damaged by a sword or some other like weapon striking it, and the hand hangs limp.'[308] Theoderic then continued by describing how a suture of the flesh wound, and the proper dressing and splinting of the upper arm should be carried out. 'With such a bandage the forearm will be included with the humerus in such a comfortable relationship that the fractured parts will be kept well united and cannot be distracted.'[309] Presumably the assumption was that this type of treatment would prevent lasting impairment in the form of paralysis or motor impairment of the affected limb. Some types of fracture or dislocation were regarded as having more adverse effects than others. So Theoderic thought that a particularly bad dislocation 'is the type in which the condyles of the bone are split or broken and can rarely be restored to normalcy. This occurs at the end of the femur, secondly at the end of the humerus and of the two bones of the lower leg near the heel.'[310]

He was aware of the difficulties a patient could encounter even after a fracture had healed. So, to overcome stiffness in a healed joint, Theoderic suggested to 'soak the part in the bath, and massage it gently until it move freely. And if you wish, apply melted ram's fat with butter, moderately warm, using it both before the bath and after.'[311] However, fractures in joints or limbs did not always heal properly, leading to deformed bones or impairing the affected limbs. His observations that sometimes 'after a fracture has healed the limb becomes thin and weak, and that is because the union has not been strong'[312] might be in reference to atrophy in the limbs. Concerning the 'mal-union' of limbs, where the bone has not healed with proper alignment, Theoderic advised on the causes and possible remedies. 'Sometimes a bone is not restored as it ought to be, indeed, the part stays misshapen; and the cause of this is either the ignorance of the physician, or a fault in removing the splints, or haste in removing them before the fracture is strong, or excessive motion during sleep.'[313] Theoderic mentioned that the ancient physicians sometimes advised to break the bone again, but that Albucasis had spoken out against this practice, 'saying that it is ruinous to rebreak a fracture which is badly healed.'[314] Theoderic himself was against the old method, on the one hand, because the ancient doctors did not actually describe the procedure – in other words, he was critical of the lack of practical recommendation – and on the other hand, because the procedure entailed risk 'and sometimes the part is completely ruined.'[315]

Following the standard medieval layout for a medical text, I will now discuss Theoderic's surgical advice on fractures and dislocations by commencing with the top of the body (the head) and working downwards towards the feet. Theoderic even had a few words to say about fractures to the head and face. He described how to repair a fractured lower mandible using gold or silver wire, or silk, to tie the broken bits together.[316] He was also concerned about the aesthetic implications fractures of the nose might have: 'When a fracture occurs in the upper part of the nose, and it is broken and not cared for, it leads to disfigurement, for sometimes it hardens and remains crooked, and later is not susceptible to realignment.'[317]

Fractures of the ulna were regarded as particularly tricky to deal with. 'Its fracture is calamitous and its healing is difficult, because the ulna supports the forearm . . .',[318] while dislocation of the elbow is 'more troublesome than all the others, and its reduction is more difficult.'[319] A dislocation of the elbow was a serious injury if had been dislocated posteriorly, because the reduction was deemed to be exceedingly difficult, and it might never grow sound.[320] The reduction of a broken clavicle, not surprisingly, was also regarded as a very difficult matter.[321]

With regards to spinal injuries in particular, Theoderic noted that complications could ensue, and could lead to the patient's impairment. He was aware of the neurological problems that lesions of the vertebrae could cause. He advised that to make a prognosis in cases involving trauma to the vertebrae of the neck, the surgeon must examine a patient's hands: if they were limp, senseless and immobile, then the situation was serious (i.e. a full recovery was unlikely, and the patient would be impaired).[322] In cases of damage to the lumbar vertebrae, similar signs of mobility loss should be looked for in a patient's feet,[323] while the symptoms of faecal incontinence, a distended abdomen and the inability to control urination were caused by damage to the spinal medulla, and indicated that the disorder was fatal.[324] The passage on spinal injuries is worth citing in full:

> The cervical vertebrae are often contused, less commonly fractured; the meninges may be damaged, and sometimes the spinal cord itself. If you wish to know whether the patient is recovering, examine his hands to see if they are flaccid and numbed and deadened, and if the patient cannot move them nor flex them, and if there is no feeling in them when they are pressed, then you should know that something awful has happened. But if he moves them and feels the pressure of your fingers, then you may know that the spinal cord is safe. If something similar happens to the lumbar vertebrae, examine the feet and make your decision in similar fashion. If rectal incontinence and distention occur when he lies on his back, and if he is not able to urinate when

he wishes, then without doubt it is a mortal injury. Otherwise, let it be cared for and set with all the physician's ingenuity. And if there should be any bone fragments to be removed which require excision, let that be done smoothly.[325]

Theoderic also discussed dislocation of the cervical vertebrae,[326] and dislocation of the vertebrae of the back,[327] which he regarded as especially dangerous and generally fatal conditions. An illustration of what kind of treatment was performed in the eleventh century for dislocated vertebrae, based on a commentary by Apollonius of Citium on the Hippocratic *De articulis*,[328] demonstrates this: the patient was suspended upside down in an attempt to reduce the dislocation. If there was a posterior dislocation of the vertebrae of the back, which Theoderic called gibbous, that had been around since childhood, it could not be cured at all, in his opinion.[329] Guy de Chauliac also believed in the difficulty of treatment for compound dislocations, and old dislocations, which were 'impossible to be cured' so that they should be treated as soon as possible.[330]

Theoderic warned with regard to hip fractures that the patient was liable to be impaired by a limp: 'Avicenna says that one whose hip or thigh has been fractured is very likely to limp. On this account one should summon up the greatest zeal and ingenuity in applying bandages.'[331] The surgeon is therefore to try the best that can be done for the patient. Lower leg, that is tibia and fibula fractures were regarded as similar to fractures of the lower arm, though Theoderic reckoned that tibia fractures were more difficult to heal.[332] With ankle fractures, Theoderic also noted the potential impairment that might be caused by complications: 'When the ankle is healed, walking about on it is painful; and when it is not restored as it ought to be, its usefulness is lost.'[333]

Theoderic appears to have delivered his verdicts on the prognosis of a patient's injuries and his advice on their treatment from a position of practical experience. He was not just citing previous medical texts, and cobbling together a textbook based on any earlier material he may have been familiar with, but was very much what would now be termed an empiricist. His dismissal of antique methods of re-breaking badly healed fractures, due to the lack of practical advice on how to actually do it, should be seen in this light. He said, by way of a conclusion to his book on surgery, that he was not willing to include anything that he had not tested himself, nor had he wished his book to contain more text in it by other writers (i.e. earlier medical authors and 'authorities'). 'For it would seem superfluous and vain to turn out a new book, if what we write could be found equally well or better in the books of other men.'[334]

Besides Theoderic, several other thirteenth- and fourteenth-century surgeons discussed fractures and their treatment. Lanfranc of Milan (*c*.1245–d. before 1306) wrote his *Chirurgia magna* in 1296, the fourth chapter of which concerned fractures and dislocations. He described the symptoms of and therapy for different kinds of fractures of the various limbs and other bones, including fracture of the skull.[335] He specifically excluded a discussion of fractures of the vertebrae, apparently because they just distorted and did not fracture as such.[336] He was the first medical professional to describe an ingenious method for tightening multiple splints by means of two or three wooden tubes, to allow the retention of tension in cords which in turn held the splints in place; this sophisticated method was later also used by Guy de Chauliac and others.[337] Since fractures take a relatively long time to heal (compared with flesh wounds) and it is important to keep the affected limb immobilised, a method for keeping patients still while not making them suffer through long periods of confinement to a bed is as important nowadays as it was in the Middle Ages. Bernard de Gordon addressed this issue in his *Lilium medicine*, which he commenced around 1303. In the section on broken limbs he had the following to say:

> Let the leg or arm be placed in a ship-like vessel and bound up so that it cannot be broken again by sudden movement, since this happens sometimes in sleep: hang a rope over the bed so that when the patient wants to move some part of his body he can lift himself up: and let there be a hole in the bed so that he can relieve himself, otherwise it might be dangerous if he had to lie there for forty days or more.[338]

Guy de Chauliac in the mid-fourteenth century provided further developments for the use of traction in the treatment of fractures to prevent impairment of the affected limb. He was in his sixties when he wrote his *Chirurgia magna* in 1363, of which book five dealt with fractures and dislocations. Concerning a fracture of the shaft of the femur, Guy rejected the earlier technique of Albucasis (d. 1106), whereby the leg was bent at the knee and was firmly tied against the back of the upper leg by way of a splint. (It is a matter of pure speculation, but since I have observed the frequent depiction of crippled pilgrims, beggars and others in medieval art, which show the crippled person with their impaired leg bent at the knee in a ninety degree angle, I could not fail to wonder whether it may not have been due to this 'old' method of treating leg fractures, advocated by Albucasis, that people's legs ended up in this characteristic position. Two examples from medieval iconography may illustrate this leg position: a miniature from around 1130, shows a man on the far right with his leg in just such a posture,[339] and again in a miniature from the fifteenth century.[340]) Instead, for femoral fractures Guy proposed to immobilise the broken leg in an extended position by means of splints. He also used a form of continuous traction by means of a leaden weight, suspended from a pulley, and fastened to the patient's foot.[341] It is described thus: 'After the application of splints attach to the foot a mass of lead as a weight, taking care to pass the cord which supports the weight over a small pulley in such a manner that it shall pull on the leg in a horizontal direction.'[342] Like Bernard de Gordon, who had already described a similar traction procedure, Guy de Chauliac also recommended suspending a rope over the patient's bed, so that it facilitated changes of position for the patient. As one modern medical historian noted, Guy de Chauliac worked according to the maxim that no cause furthered the malformation of a broken limb more than too tight a bandage, or an inadequate positioning of the fractured limb could lead to complications.[343] The correct repositioning of a fractured limb was therefore important for healing that did not result in impairments.

It is unfortunate that the *Chirurgie* of Henri de Mondeville (b. *c.*1260–d. *c.*1320), one of the greatest of medieval surgeons, was never completed in its entirety. Mondeville had planned to write five treatises,[344] of which most were written between 1306 and 1313, but those sections dealing with fractures and dislocations are missing since Mondeville never finished his work before he died. It is therefore exactly those areas of surgery that would deal with preventative measures as far as impairments are concerned which now cannot be discussed in relation to Henri of Modeville's important text.

'Surgery' in the modern sense, as in operations on patients, or amputations, was sometimes carried out successfully. The German emperor, Frederick III (1415–93), had to have his left foot and part of his lower left leg amputated, when he was already in his seventies. The operation took place at Linz on the Danube, on 8 June 1493. An illustration of this exists as a miniature, made by a contemporary Austrian master.[345] Two physicians were present to advise the emperor, three surgeons held down the emperor, while two more surgeons, master Hans Seyff of Göppingen and Hilarius of Passau, cut off his foot with a saw, so carefully that the emperor hardly felt any pain.[346] After six weeks the emperor's remaining leg began to heal up, and after a further four weeks the healing process was practically complete. Ironically, Frederick III died later that same year of a stroke brought on by fasting, not due to any adverse effects of the amputation.[347] Surgical procedures for amputations of limbs which had become ischemic or otherwise diseased due to wounds, blows or fractures had already been described in Anglo-Saxon texts, but, according to Cameron, 'we cannot be sure that the operation of amputation as given in the *Leechbook* was ever carried out in Anglo-Saxon England.'[348] Chapter 35 of book I of Bald's *Leechbook* described a procedure for removing 'blackened and deadened body',[349] which seems to have been a close translation of a Latin original. The operation involved cutting away all of a livid body which was so deadened that the patient had no feeling in it, admonishing the surgeon to ensure that the amputation was made right up to the first parts of healthy tissue;[350] the text, however, did not give any advice on how to control bleeding during the procedure, which is why Cameron believes it may not actually have been carried out in practice.

Finally, in the context of surgery it is worth pointing out that not all therapies involved the application of mechanical techniques that the learned masters, such as a Lanfranc of Milan or a Guy de Chauliac, wrote about. At the level of lay practitioners, alternatives to the setting of bones by means of splinting, traction or surgery were sometimes employed, which involved the application of various salves, unguents, poultices and other such substances. A thirteenth-century rhymed Anglo-Norman text known as *La Novele Cirurgerie*, which despite the title is actually a compendium of recipes for potions, ointments and poultices, contains one piece of advice dealing with fractured bones. The title of the recipe indicates that it is 'for fractured bones, splinting and a potion',[351] but after briefly mentioning that broken legs and arms ought to be splinted, continues by providing purely medicinal recipes, for potions and poultices. This vernacular text was presumably intended for use by a non-learned practitioner.[352] Similarly, two late medieval manuscript collections, one now at Salzburg, the other from the former Benedictine monastery of Farfa in Latium, together list 38 remedies, of which only one mentions a form of manual traction to straighten a fractured leg.[353] These methods of treating fractures formed another, independent thaumaturgic process besides the surgery of the educated professionals.

4.4   Social and 'alternative' medicine

Specific occupations, or specific tasks associated with work, could lead to lasting physiological damage – and still do in the modern world. Already in late antiquity Paul of Aegina (fl. early seventh century) recognised the existence of what we would now term 'occupational disorders'. He mentioned the calcification of the lungs and the coughing of blood – symptoms of phthisis – found among people working with dust, that is people working with stone or metal or mineworkers who were liable to inhale dusty particles.[354] Writing in the 1290s, Arnald of Villanova observed in his *Speculum medicinae* that not only smiths, but also glaziers, sweepers, gilders and other artisans were quite often made ill by their trade. The connection between metalworking and specific diseases was also made by a lesser-known figure, one Ulrich Ellenbog (b.1430s–d. 1499), who was employed as a civic physician by the city of Augsburg. Ellenbog wrote a popular pamphlet or flier, intended for an audience comprised of goldsmiths and other metalworkers, which would show them how they could protect themselves against the detrimental effects of fumes associated with their work. This pamphlet, *Von den giftigen besen* [*bösen*] *Temppfen Reuchen der Metal* (On the poisonous and noxious vapours and fumes of metals) had originally been written in 1473, but was not printed until 1524, and has been called the 'first publication in the world's literature that deals specifically with industrial hygiene'.[355]

Less dangerous occupations, however, were also deemed to be detrimental to health. Arnald of Villanova, in connection with his observations on artisans affected by their work, noted that even people in apparently harmless occupations, such as notaries, who may sit in poor light while reading and writing all day long, risk a progressive loss of sight; notaries additionally might suffer from kidney and bladder problems 'since the press of business forces them to go for long periods without relieving themselves.'[356] Arnald was perhaps picking up on the well-established topos of the occupational hazards of writing. The popular litany of the physical pains of writing occurred as a variation on a theme dating back as far as Roman times, and was often repeated by medieval scribes.[357] For example, an anonymous scribe put this conclusion to a twelfth-century text of the Silos Beatus: writing '... makes the eyes misty, bows the back, crushes the ribs and belly, brings pain to the kidneys, and makes the body ache all over'.[358] Visual impairments brought about by such work may not have been all that infrequent.[359] Another occupation with associated health hazards was textile working. Spinning and weaving were done in areas of high humidity, for reasons connected with the processes of textile manufacture, conditions which were around even as late as the 1960s. In such damp work areas there was a strong possibility of developing respiratory diseases and joint problems, which could become chronic, and in the case of joint problems, lead to impairments. Chrétien de Troyes in the twelfth century mentioned the complaint of the spinsters about damp working conditions (he also mentioned more general complaints by female textile workers regarding malnutrition, low wages and sufferance of many illnesses).[360] There is some evidence that in the later medieval period, at least, attempts were made to alleviate the working conditions of textile workers. In the guild house referred to as the Weaver's House in Constance one may find a fourteenth-century mural depicting a warming room, which shows a female textile worker reclining on a bed in front of a typical southern German tiled stove (*Kachelofen*).[361]

Further evidence both for the presence of occupationally caused impairments, and for medieval awareness of such conditions can be gleaned from an entirely different type of source: the patronage of certain saints with responsibility for specific ailments. St Andrew, as the patron saint of fishermen, was said to heal rheumatism and gout, because fishermen, through their damp working environment, were exposed to such diseases; similarly, St Nicholas of Bari (d. 324) was the patron of sailors and boatmen, who were prone to chills and colds, and St Nicholas, too, healed gout and rheumatism.[362] St Guimerra (d. 932) became patron saint of leatherworkers who easily got eye disorders, and healed blindness and other visual impediments.[363] Finally, St Walstan (d. 1016) was patron saint of mowers, and healed lameness, because mowers apparently easily got lame arms through their work.[364]

Mining and metal working were, and still are, two occupations that, if performed in the long-term, could have quite dramatic effects on a person's health. In the case of coal-mining one only has to think of the typical 'miner's lung', the phthisis caused by breathing in coal dust over prolonged periods, and ore mining also had its specific health hazards. For example, a discussion of palaeopathological symptoms found on the eleventh- or twelfth-century skeleton of a 40- to 50-year-old man, from northern Germany, led to the conclusions that he had apparently worked in the metal-working industry.[365] In central Europe ore mining was an important economic activity, such as at Goslar in the Harz region where silver had been mined since the tenth century, further the exploitation of ores in the Erzgebirge between 1100 and 1300, and the opening up of Bohemian silver mines from the thirteenth century onwards. One would therefore expect some medical literature on the diseases of mining. Instead, according to a study by George Rosen,[366] throughout the medieval period one can not find any textual reference to such occupational diseases. It is only since the early sixteenth century that these issues were being written about, with the publication of Paracelsus' *Von der Bergsucht und anderen Bergkrankheiten* in 1533–4, and sections in Agricola's *De re metallica*, published 1556. The development of new technical skills in mining and the greater commercial exploitation of mining by the end of the fifteenth century meant that the driving of deeper mines brought with it an increase in health risks,[367] so that only at that period, it has been suggested, the health of miners became an issue to people other than the miners themselves. Nevertheless, Rosen has argued that the conditions these two authors describe in the sixteenth century are likely to have been valid for the earlier (medieval) periods also.[368] Common problems, apart from catastrophic events like the collapse of tunnels, were inadequate ventilation, the foul air bringing about breathing problems, headaches and suffocation for the miners, conditions recognised by Agricola,[369] though, as Rosen points out, 'it is worthy of note that the conception of an occupational disease, that is, a specific disease characteristic of a specific occupational group, is still unknown to Agricola'.[370] Agricola divides illnesses affecting miners into categories such as those that attack the joints, those that attack the lungs, the eyes of miners and fatal diseases; he also mentions diseases resulting from the dust in the air of the mines,[371] intoxication by various other substances found in the mines,[372] and fractures with the possibility of consequent disability resulting from falling rocks and/or breakages of ladders in the mine shafts.[373] Paracelsus focuses on what he calls 'Bergsucht', which to him is a disease of the lungs,[374] and furthermore a disease about which, so he claims, he has not found anything in any of the earlier writers, not even in the sources from antiquity.[375] One need not, however, assume that until the publication of either Paracelsus's or Agricola's works nothing was known about miners' specific illnesses, nor that no form of help was available to impaired miners. There is some evidence that miners organised themselves in self-help groups; miners in the German empire emerged from feudal ties to have free status,[376] and the earliest free miners working in Germany around the fourteenth century got together in *Gewerkschaften*, while self-help organisations dealing specifically with issues of illness and funeral costs date from mainly the thirteenth century, although the Goslar miners already received a charter for that purpose as early as 1188.[377]

Connected with the theme of occupational impairment is the development of what one might term 'public health', that is, the provision of medical treatment, often free of charge, for those who needed it by municipal authorities. In the first instance, it seems such health care provision stemmed from the need to treat soldiers wounded in the course of military campaigns on behalf of a city, although in the North Italian cities free medical treatment was extended to poor citizens as well. Soldiers themselves, one could argue, were another group of 'workers' very much subject to occupational impairments,[378] and surgical techniques perfected on the battlefield were often groundbreaking advances that were later taken up by surgeons practising in a civilian environment. Because of the interconnectedness of free healthcare provisions with military matters, both seemingly disparate themes will be explored alongside each other, as two sides of the same coin.

In Florence doctors were hired by the community to treat those who had been wounded in battle at public expense. The *Book of Montaperti*, an official contemporary account of the 1260 campaign between Florence and Siena, first offers an extended description of doctors being on hire to the commune. The sick and wounded were often transported to the nearest town for treatment, or carried home to their native city, presumably depending on how serious their wounds were and how far they could travel. The government of the city either paid doctors directly for the treatment of injured soldiers, or the soldiers were later reimbursed for the costs of their treatment. The kind of surgery required for the treatment of battle wounds and broken bones was highly developed in late medieval Italy,[379] and one wonders whether this reflected the frequent conflicts between city-states which necessitated expertise in the treatment of such injuries.

The provision of (free) public healthcare in the North Italian cities had its first recorded instance at Bologna in 1214, when the physician Ugo of Lucca was contracted by the city to provide 'free treatment for the army, and for all injured residents of the city and for those of the countryside who have been brought to the city'.[380] Ugo could impose a differential scale of fees '... if he treats an inhabitant of the countryside for severe wounds, fractures or sprains',[381] whereby the poor, however, were still treated for free. Other cities during the thirteenth century followed the example set by Bologna, so that by the mid-fifteenth century there was a 'system of medical hiring almost universal through-out urban Italy'.[382] For example, in Florence during the later fourteenth century there were plenty of doctors. This comparative oversupply of trained medical practitioners together with public and private notions of charity had led to concern for how the poor could be treated (one could also surmise a less altruistic motive, namely that after the Black Death there was greater concern about public health, and the untreated poor could be seen as posing a health risk for the commune as a whole). Most doctors hired by the city of Florence tended to be surgical specialists, usually bone doctors, 'presumably because dislocations and fractures were common and easy to treat'[383]. There are records of communal bone doctors at Florence from 1336, who were to treat the poor free of charge and have the expense of their salary met by the city. By the later fourteenth century (well-off?) doctors were treating the poor for free anyway of their own accord, so after 1380 there was no longer a public doctor in the employ of the city.[384]

Tied in with the development of health care provided by a municipality for its citizens was the provision of healthcare for those injured on military campaigns. As Linda Paterson asks, 'If wounds were not immediately mortal what was the likely fate of the injured man? One possibility was that he would be treated by a surgeon.'[385] Already during the twelfth and thirteenth centuries some surgeons followed various armies, and the above mentioned Ugo of Lucca was obliged, bound by his contract of 1214 with the city of Bologna, to follow the Bolognese army when it went to war. During the fourteenth and fifteenth centuries it became common for rulers and campaign leaders to include surgeons among their entourage. For example, during the campaign culminating in the battle of Agincourt in 1415, Henry V had on his staff one Thomas Morestede as well as 12 other surgeons.[386] An idealised depiction of the kind of surgical treatment available on the battlefield exists, where a fashionably dressed officer or nobleman is having his wounded leg treated by a surgeon, in a miniature of 1465.[387] This presence, of course, need not imply that such surgeons were at hand to treat the ordinary soldier, they could have been accompanying an army just for the treatment of the officers and members of the nobility. Prior to the regular presence of surgical staff during a campaign, successful treatment for battle injuries was presumably erratic and a matter of luck. One modern historian of medicine, who tried to find evidence for what kind of arrangements (if any) were made during the Middle Ages for the sick and wounded on campaign, could not find much material at all, save the isolated case of the provisions made during the last years of Edward I's reign for a certain Harvey de Cornubia, a valet of the king's napery, who was wounded by the Scots during action in Galway; he was given his expenses to pay for his return to England, plus additional expenses to pay for the necessary medical treatment.[388] One may guess that this service was presumably not available to the ordinary foot soldier. However, there is circumstantial evidence from chroniclers of the first crusade, which indicates the presence of surgeons and other medical staff among the crusading armies. These medical personnel, according to one scholar who has examined such chronicles, were not named as individuals in the texts, but simply referred to as *medici* or *cirurgici*.[389] In England, a letter addressed to Ralph, bishop of Chichester, and written before 1230, mentions that the presence of a Master Thomas is useful to the royal army, because 'in the siege of castles, medics are necessary, and especially ones who know how to cure wounds.'[390]

One professional Latin surgical text, the *Chirurgia* of Roger of Salerno (written around 1180) was adapted into an Occitan verse form by Raimon of Avignon before 1209. The use of the vernacular and the verse form, which lends itself to better memorisation than prose, could indicate that Raimon's adaptation was intended for a lay audience, or for a less well-educated surgeon. Moreover, Raimon's adaptation placed greater emphasis on describing the kinds of trauma that would have been specific to soldiers, and provided practical advice on how to deal with such injuries. 'His version therefore reveals ... some of the wounds and treatments inflicted specifically upon late twelfth-century knights and sergeants, and in some cases how injuries were occasioned by defective equipment.'[391] Concrete evidence in France for the organised presence of medical personnel on campaigns does not appear until the early fourteenth century, when the Count of Savoy, Amédée V, hired approximately a half-dozen surgeons for various military engagements; thereafter some surgeons appear in fifteenth-century accounts.[392] Surgeons, or 'doctors' in general, are, however, mentioned in literary texts, which Linda Paterson has examined. The Occitan *Song of the Albigensian Crusade* (composed around 1230) mentions the presence of medical people on three occasions connected with sieges or battles.[393]

Whether professional surgeons or physicians were present on campaign, and whether they treated all ranks or just some of the injured combatants, is debatable and varies both geographically and chronologically. Nevertheless, one type of medical personnel available to wounded soldiers on the battlefield may have been what Nancy Siraisi termed 'amateur surgeons'.[394] Since not all armies, during all times of the medieval period, had professional surgeons with them, the assumption is made that knights, for example, would have had to learn some basic surgical techniques to help themselves and each other – similar to modern non-medical people taking a first aid course nowadays, one might imagine. There is some evidence for this theory in the sources. The surgeon Guy de Chauliac mentioned various categories of people who practised surgery, and in his list he included the German knights who treat battle wounds:

> The ferste secte is nerehande of alle kny3tes of Saxoun and of men followynge batailles, þe whiche procuren or helen alle woundes wiþ coniurisouns and drynkes and with oyle and wolle and a cole leef, foundynge ham þerfore vppon þat, þat God putte his vertu in herbes, wordes and stones.[395]

Prior examples can be found indirectly in early thirteenth-century romance literature. In Wolfram von Eschenbach's *Parzival*, the hero Gawan, 'who was no fool in the matter of wounds' (*er was zer wunden niht ein tôr*),[396] performed an operation for the drainage of blood from a chest wound. Gawan was called by a distraught lady to help a wounded knight, whose wound he immediately recognised as not being fatal, since the blood was only pressing on his heart. Gawan then grabbed the branch of a lime tree and removed the bark, so that it formed a tube, which he inserted into the knight's wound. Then he asked the lady to suck until blood was drawn up the tube,[397] thereby saving the knight's life. It seems that Wolfram von Eschenbach at least had some rudimentary concepts, if not actual knowledge,[398] of medical or surgical techniques, irrespective of whether we would now believe in the efficacy of Gawan's treatment. At a later stage in the epic Gawan was mocked by a haughty lady for his knowledge of medical things: Gawan and his lady were riding through a meadow, when Gawan spotted a plant which he knew to have medicinal properties. When he dismounted to uproot the plant, the lady sarcastically commented that her companion was both physician and knight, and that if one sold boxes of medicine, one need not worry about one's income.[399] Perhaps this is a disguised social comment on the rapacity of physicians, perceived to be making lots of money through the sale of more or less effective pharmaceuticals.

One other area where knights could be injured is of course in tournaments. An illustration in the Manesse codex of the early fourteenth century depicts a wounded knight having his broken leg set by a medical practitioner.[400] It is not clear from the context whether this is an example of battlefield surgery, or whether treatment is taking place elsewhere, for example at a tournament, or even whether the medical person is a surgeon or another knight (the man in background wearing a white cap looks far more like surgeon, judging by the dress other contemporary surgeons wear, than the well-dressed man in the foreground).[401] The illustration nevertheless demonstrates the 'occupational hazards', including potential physical impairment, of being a medieval knight.

My discussion of medieval medical notions of impairment has so far focused primarily on the two groups who produced the bulk of the textual matter we possess nowadays: physicians and surgeons. As was evident in the case of knights and soldiers injured on campaign, who may have treated each other, physicians and surgeons were of course not the only medical practitioners to whom a sick person could turn. In the case of impairment, turning to medical practitioners who were not physicians or surgeons may even have been preferable for an individual, since 'regular' medicine could actually offer very little in the way of cures for impairments. Therefore a brief examination of what we would now perhaps call 'alternative therapies', or 'complementary' medicine, is in order. It seems to be a commonplace that when one type of therapy has failed, and alternatives are available, people will, sooner or later, pursue other avenues for the restoration of their health – there is no reason to suppose that medieval people behaved any differently from their modern counterparts in this respect. Furthermore, different types of therapy may have been used concurrently, in the same way that today patients might, for example in the case of chronic backache, consult both a general practitioner and a chiropractor. 'Alternative' practitioners in the Middle Ages could be, for example, wise-women, herbalists, apothecaries, barbers or astrologers.

One 'alternative' practice that fell within the realm of healing activities was 'magical' medicine.[402] From *Piers Ploughman* comes a very succinct example of why a person might turn to 'alternative' therapies. *Piers Ploughman* may be a literary text, and the passage in question may be satirising those people who sought out such therapies, but the text can nevertheless reflect to a degree social attitudes and realities. One of the characters had a fever 'lasting a whole year. And then I began to despise the Christian doctors, and resort to witches; and I say quite openly that no trained doctor, not even Christ himself, can cure diseases as well as the old cobbler-woman of Southwark, or Dame Emma of Shoreditch.'[403] It is therefore out of desperation at the lack of success of 'proper' medicine that someone is seen to turn to magical remedies. The astrologer, natural philosopher and sometime court physician to emperor Frederick II, Michael Scot (d. 1220) had also pointed out that people consulted 'alternative' therapists in similar situations. He in fact recommended that in certain cases, 'where medicine fails, the physician should advise the patient to go to diviners and enchantresses, although this way seem wrong (*inhonestum et nephas*) or contrary to the Christian faith, but true nevertheless.'[404]

One area of magical practice that appears to have been used in connection with therapies for impairments is 'transference' magic. Transference magic relied on the notion that an illness or impairment could be transferred from the afflicted person onto another thing, onto an animal (one is reminded of the 'scapegoat') or a plant, or passed into the earth.[405] An example of such a ritual in relation to impairment can be found in fifteenth-century Italy. A woman called Matteuccia Fransisci of Todi was tried for witchcraft in 1428 (she had used all sorts of 'illegitimate' magic, like love magic, contraceptive magic, using wax images etc.). But besides her ritual magic, she also tried to cure a client's lameness. This was done by making a potion out of thirty different herbs and then enhancing its power with an incantation, before throwing the potion out onto the street so that the lameness was transferred from her patient onto an unsuspecting passer-by.[406] Perhaps another type of transference ritual was acted out by adherents to the cult of St Guinefort, located in the Rhône and French Alps region in the mid-thirteenth century. The contemporary source, by the Dominican writer

Stephen of Bourbon, has been extensively discussed in a seminal study by Jean-Claude Schmitt,[407] and it is therefore superfluous to repeat his analysis here in detail. Suffice it to say that part of the cult concerned the transference by ritual or 'magical' means of a child's impairment. The thirteenth-century mothers in Stephen of Bourbon's narrative would take children whom they perceived as impaired to the site of the cult (a wooded grove), where nails were driven into the trees. Then the naked babies were passed between the trunks of two trees, presumably transferring their impairment onto the trees.[408]

Another area of 'alternative' medical practices concerned what I have termed 'preventative magic'. In particular, this involved the use of ritual, Christian or 'magical', to ensure that the outcome of a pregnancy was not a deformed or impaired child. An example of this can be found in the early eleventh-century *Lacnunga*, in the following charm:

> The woman who cannot nourish her child [in the womb]. Go to the grave of a dead person and then step three times over the grave and then say these words three times: 'This be a remedy for me for the loathsome late [slow] birth; this be a remedy for me for the grievous dismal birth; this be a remedy for me for the loathsome imperfect birth (laðan lambyrde)'.[409]

Performing the ritual was presumably believed to protect against some of the complications associated with pregnancy and birth, such as miscarriage (this may be the meaning of the lack of nourishment in the womb). Connected with notions of preventative magic is the belief in supernatural, especially demonic, causes of impairment. Wilfred Bonser suggested that the many charms found in Anglo-Saxon medical texts against 'nocturnal visitors' might allude to a belief in certain demons who were regarded as the cause of deformed and monstrous children; such belief could also relate to the origin of narratives surrounding incubi and succubi in later periods.[410]

Sometimes it is not possible to draw a dividing line between 'regular' medicine and 'magical' medicine – the two (modern) categories were not always seen as disparate entities in the Middle Ages. An example would be the late medieval recipe for curing a fractured leg, which involved wrapping the skin of a one-day old dog's whelp around the leg. The recipe is found in a collection of vernacular medical texts concerning the treatment of fractures, probably intended for use by lay practitioners, in a manuscript now at Salzburg.[411] This appears to be a case of sympathetic magic, where the analogy between the skin of the whelp, which encloses and protects the dog, and the closure and protection of the fractured leg is part of the therapy.[412]

4.5   Summary

Using the distinction made by modern theorists of disability studies between disability as a social construct and impairment as a physical phenomenon, this chapter investigated the description of physical impairment in medieval medical textbooks and texts relating to natural philosophy – what one might call medieval 'scientific' sources. To understand what differences there might be between modern and medieval notions of medicine, a brief discussion of medieval medical concepts was entered into. The main distinguishing factor of medieval medicine from its modern counterpart appeared to be the wider range of notions and activities that the medieval concept of medicine encompassed. Modern medicine was seen as a purely biomechanical model, while medieval medicine included what we would now classify as religious, metaphysical or supernatural elements. This was partly due to the strong association of medieval medicine with religious ideas about *Christus medicus*, Christ as healer.

The crucial point about medieval medicine to emerge has been that medieval medicine, similar to its modern counterpart, had, in fact, very little to offer the physically impaired. Physical impairment was essentially regarded as an incurable condition, and some medieval medical texts made it quite clear that the physician was not to 'waste' time or reputation with trying to cure the incurable, hence was to refrain from attempts to cure those conditions we now describe as impairments.

There were, however, several areas in which medical or 'scientific' theories and practices did concern themselves with physical impairments. These were found to be the realms of aetiology and prevention, that is, theoretical approaches to explain the causes behind (mainly congenital) impairments, and practical measures (mainly in surgery) to prevent a mundane physical injury or trauma from becoming a permanent impairment. Since medieval medicine derived to a great extent from older, especially from Galenic sources, a brief analysis of late antique and early medieval Greek medical aetiologies of impairments was made. One of the most important causalities of impairment in medieval medical thought was the influence of the humours on the functioning of the body. A variety of disorders that we would classify as impairing, such as paralysis, speech impairments, deafness and visual impairments, were ascribed to imbalanced or corrupted humours by the sources studied. Humoral imbalances could also be passed on from the parents to their child. Different medieval opinions circulated as to whether certain impairments were inheritable, or whether some, like missing limbs in a parent, were not transmitted to the children.

One of the key areas of medieval aetiologies of impairment related to ideas about the conception of children, and what impact various internal and external factors had on foetal development. Again, humoral reasons, which were seen to affect male sperm or female 'seed' at the time of conception, constituted the most important internal causality. Planetary, or what we would call astrological, influences were also regarded as crucial external causalities. Conception of a child during menstruation and conception by non-standard sexual positions were seen to almost certainly result in the birth of an impaired infant. However, in this context it was noted that such parental sexual activities perceived as sinful were not invariably reflected onto the child – medieval notions concerning sin, sexuality and congenital impairment were not uniform but displayed an ambiguous and diverse range of reactions.

Several other causes of congenital impairment were also mentioned in medieval aetiologies. One concerned the maternal imagination, whereby external influences upon the pregnant woman impacted on the development of her foetus. Similarly, the type of food eaten by a pregnant woman could also impinge on the physical or mental development of her child. Once a child was born, a frequent peri-natal cause of impairment ascribed by the sources was incorrect swaddling of the infant.

What we now term iatrogenic causes were briefly discussed in relation to medieval notions of impairment. The analysis centred on two aspects: physical damage done to adult patients by medical practitioners in the course of their treatment, and damage done to children (cutting the tongue string) in the belief that it would prevent or cure speech impediments.

This was followed by a discussion of what preventative measures medieval medical and surgical therapies could offer patients with potentially impairing afflictions. In my discussion, I followed a thematic structure, that is the head to toe scheme of disorders and their treatments that medieval medical and surgical texts themselves employed, rather than a chronological structure centred on the sources. Medical and surgical texts dealt with preventative measures in the case of head injuries, visual and aural disorders, facial deformities, speech disorders and spinal injury. The vast majority of therapies centred on the prevention or alleviation of orthopaedic impairments. Since fractures were a common cause of orthopaedic or mobility impairments, the bulk of my evidence in these cases derived from surgical (rather than medical) texts. Several medieval surgeons, such as Theoderic or Guy de Chauliac, were aware of the potentially impairing effect of certain treatment methods, and either criticised such (older) methods and/or tried to devise their own improvements.

Because textbook-derived medieval medicine, as was seen, did not have much to offer the physically impaired, it was found useful to turn to a discussion of social medicine and 'alternative' medical practices. In this context, the recognition by medieval sources of what we would now describe as occupational impairments was dealt with, as well as measures concerning 'public health'. Participants on military campaigns were identified as one particular group that would have been especially prone to 'occupational' impairment therefore medical provision on the battlefield was regarded as one important aspect of this theme. Under the rubric of 'alternative' medicine, practices we would refer to as magical medicine were briefly discussed, insofar as they related to physical impairment.

In conclusion, what we would now term 'regular' medicine, that is treatments such as those described in the learned texts of a Gilbertus Anglicus or a Guy de Chauliac, may have had little to offer the impaired person in the Middle Ages. That does not mean that impaired people received no care whatsoever, but that instead care will have been primarily in the form of what we might now call 'palliative', concentrating on sustaining physical needs such as food, clothing and shelter through charity. As Faye Getz observes:

> When historians remark that there was little in medieval England that medicine actually could do for sick people, what they really mean is that medieval doctors had little in common with modern scientific practitioners.

A very important point that is often forgotten applies to care for people living on the margins of society. There was quite a lot that medieval society could do for the hungry, the homeless, the crippled, the unwed mother, the aged, and the orphaned.[413]

'Social medicine' and 'social security' through charitable actions could then be regarded as alternatives to effective medical therapies for impairment. The main form of 'alternative' therapy, however, that medieval people would have turned to when regular medicine failed to bring about the desired results, was of course seeking cures through miracle healing. Therapeutic miracles and their surrounding narratives therefore constitute the subject of Chapter 5.

5   Medieval miracles and impairment

5.1   The context of saints, miracles and healing

Medieval sainthood, the miraculous in general, and accounts of healing in particular, have been studied repeatedly by modern scholars. For example, Raymond Van Dam[1] has examined the cult of saints in late antique Gaul with particular reference to the healing miracles of various saints in the writings of Gregory of Tours, while André Vauchez[2] has contextualised sainthood and the realm of miracle in the later medieval period. The everyday aspect of later medieval life as reflected in miracles of rescue and salvation in saints' cults of the fourteenth century has been discussed by Michael Goodich.[3] More generally, Benedicta Ward[4] has tried to discover what the concept of the miraculous meant to people of the high Middle Ages. Of more direct relevance to my own interests in miracles as curative processes has been the work of Ronald Finucane.[5] The illnesses in general, not impairments in particular, which afflicted children and their cures by five English saints have been studied by Eleanora Gordon,[6] and in a more recent book by Ronald Finucane[7] the general rescue, cure or resuscitation of children is described.

Yet none of these studies have been explicitly concerned with disability and miracle. 'Disability' has never been treated as a separate, distinct condition from 'illness' by any of these authors. Indeed, most of these modern scholars (Raymond Van Dam being the exception) have employed interchangeably the terms 'illness', 'sickness' and 'disability', regarding them as transferable and, presumably, as one and the same phenomenon. Even in such thorough and impressive a study as Finucane's, 'disability' is shunted into the epistemological realm of 'unqualified illness'[8] and is thereby marginalised. Finucane regards descriptions of illness in the sources as vague or 'unqualified' if they purely refer to the pilgrim being 'bed-ridden and disabled, or simply "paralysed" without further qualification or "paralysed" on one side'.[9] In his view, then, 'disability' is a problematic term, one that cannot be pinned down to a specific disease aetiology. He further blurs those distinctions, which modern disability theorists would make, between 'disability' and 'illness' by referring to the very group of cures which revolve around impairments as 'illnesses':

> Another group of cures (or illnesses) involved impaired locomotion or articulation of the limbs, hands or fingers, those paralysed in *specific* areas, 'cripples' and the lame, deformed or contorted such as the woman, *contracta*, who was unable to move, raise her head or look at her own feet.[10]

He states that it would be pointless trying to establish what medical conditions such pilgrims had, but then tries to position the medieval descriptions of impairments within a medical discourse again, by suggesting it may have been due to 'anything from arthritis to hysterical paralysis'.[11] As demonstrated in Chapter 2.2, making distinctions between 'disability' and 'illness' is one of the cornerstones of disability theories. Re-reading medieval miracle narratives from the perspective of how disability – more accurately: physical impairment – features as the subject of the miraculous, as I propose to do in this chapter, is therefore a completely new approach to the topic.

To study and understand the interplay between impairment and miracle healing I have taken an emic approach, trying to explain the types of impairments presenting at the tombs and shrines of saints and their (apparent) cures by locating these phenomena within the context of medieval notions of miracle, cure and the transcendence of what was deemed natural. Using such an approach permits, to a degree, the avoidance of some modern tendencies which dismiss any possibility of veracity in the medieval accounts of miracle, to the extent that even the impairments, never mind the cures, presenting at the sites of pilgrimage are regarded as figments of the medieval imagination.[12] Moreover, I have followed the methodological approach taken originally by Ronald Finucane, in that I have tried not to impose modern medical diagnoses onto the conditions which presented at shrines. As Finucane put it: 'We will follow the clues given by the registrars and pilgrims and classify ailments not by what we think they "really" were, but according to the symptoms and signs as given in the miracle collections even if this only conveys a vague idea of the events going on at the shrine.'[13] Some registrars in Finucane's study did categorise curative miracles by the type of ailment, but the problematic tension between medieval and modern medical terminologies makes precise, exact diagnosis or comparisons practically impossible.[14]

With regard to the nature of miracle stories as historical sources, Benedicta Ward has pointed out that collections of miracle narratives surrounding a particular saint or the events at a specific shrine are biased sources, in the sense that they already take the possibility of miraculous events for granted, a priori, and instead function as eloquent advertisements for that saint or shrine.[15] But precisely for that reason, namely that these texts advertise successful cures and other miracles, these sources provide a wealth of information about the condition, both physiological and spiritual, of impaired people – information and description which is for the most part omitted in other types of source material. If a miracle collection describes the physical condition of the supplicants at the saint's shrine or tomb in great detail, mentions the effort they underwent to reach the site of pilgrimage, and finally narrates a spectacular cure, then that makes for wonderful advertising for the powers of that saint. Because of the detail these sources go into, it is possible to extract incidental information about the lived experience of impaired persons, such as what mobility aids they had available to them, or how they made their living. As Finucane remarked with regard to healing miracles revolving around medieval children, 'while the "miraculous" core may be unbelievable, the incidental or circumstantial details – the *nonessentials* [*sic*], as far as most witnesses and shrine-keepers and parents were concerned when reporting these cases – are of primary importance'[16] to historians interested in cultural and social attitudes. These are details which, again, other types of sources rarely, if ever, inform upon. Notable exceptions are the depictions of impaired people in art, such as illuminated manuscripts, wall paintings and so on, which are, however, beyond the scope of this work. Equally beyond the present scope are further investigations into the textual form of these miracle narratives, full linguistic analyses, studies concerning the dissemination of these texts, or questions of gender imbalance in attendances at healing shrines – all of which would provide fascinating studies in their own right, but do not help in providing immediate answers to questions concerned with concepts of medieval impairment.

Records from canonisation processes in particular constitute very interesting sources, because of the standardised fashion in which information was obtained. Canonisation enquiries tended to follow a set of very specific questions, which included asking personal details of the person who reported a miracle, such as their age, place of origin, what affliction they suffered, how long they had the condition for and interviewing witnesses for the 'before and after' condition of the person who had allegedly experienced a thaumaturgic miracle.[17] Although one can make a formal, textual distinction between hagiographical material,[18] such as *Lives* of saints, or collections of miracles worked at shrines, on the one hand and records of canonisation processes on the other hand, both categories of source material contain valuable information about the lived experience of impaired people. For the purposes of my argument, therefore, I have grouped together both the canonisation protocols of St Elisabeth, and the miracle narratives surrounding the other saints which I have studied, under the rubric 'miracula'.

Medieval accounts of saints and the miracles ascribed to them very often involve themselves with the healing of illnesses in general and the cure of impairments in particular. Certain saints are associated with specific ailments, body parts or even medical practice. Sts Cosmas and Damian are probably the best-known example of 'medical' saints, in the sense that they were associated with the art of medicine, and especially with surgery. Cosmas and Damian, twin brothers,[19] were believed to have lived in Arabia during the third century, becoming famous for their cures of both animals and people, their most remarkable cure being the legendary surgical graft of a dead black man's leg onto the body of a living but cancerous white man, who had lost his leg – a popular topic for medical illustration in later medieval art.[20] The growth of their cult during the Middle Ages was phenomenal. It originated in Byzantium, spreading from there to Sicily (where it continues strongly in modern times), was present in the rest of Italy in the fifth and sixth centuries, finally arriving in the Rhineland by the ninth century, after which it dispersed widely to other regions of western Europe.[21] An anecdotal story relates that St Louis of France founded the College of Sts Cosmas and Damian in Paris for surgeons in the thirteenth century, showing how important they were deemed to be as patron saints for this occupation.[22]

Many saints became the patron saints of specific ailments and bodily afflictions.[23] Not all those saints were equally popular for the same illnesses at all times in all locations of medieval Europe, but one can make some generalisations. Most important, in the context of impairment, was St Giles as the patron saint of cripples, lepers and nursing mothers. Giles was a hermit who died around 710, and who had founded a monastery at what is now known as Saint-Gilles in Provence, which centuries after his death turned out to be strategically placed along the pilgrim route to Compostela, therefore attracting many pilgrims as well as being a shrine popular in its own right.[24] In one of the legends surrounding St Giles he was shot by an arrow during a hunt. He refused to let himself be healed, believing virtue was perfected in infirmity, so that he remained chronically ill, and in some versions of the legend he became lame.[25] In England, Gilbert of Sempringham (*c*.1083–1189) was also associated with patronage of the crippled, perhaps because Gilbert had himself been physically impaired since birth.[26] Also in England, St Osmund (d. 1099), bishop of Salisbury, was invoked to aid cases of paralysis.[27] Other saints particularly relevant to impairment were St Aurelianus, believed to have lived during the first century, who became the patron saint of deafness, and the seventh-century St Meriadocus, who restored hearing to the deaf with his bell or through the sound of its ringing.[28] Saints associated with diseases of the eyes were Sts Bridget (Brigid, Bride, of Ireland, sixth century), Triduana (of Scotland, perhaps fourth century) and Lucia (Lucy, martyred in Sicily in 304), each the favoured saint for such ailments in a different region.[29] Associated with blindness in particular were Sts Dunstan and Thomas the Apostle, as well as the archangel Raphael,[30] the latter invoked because of his part in the healing of blind Tobit.[31] Saints associated with other illnesses were Sts Dymphna (for insanity), Avertin (vertigo and epilepsy), Fiacre (haemorrhoids and fistula), Roch (plague), and Sebastian and Cyprian (also associated with plague); while saints with particular concern for specific body parts were Sts Blaise (or Blasius, for the throat), Bernardine (lungs), Apollonia (teeth), Lawrence (back), and Erasmus (abdomen).[32] In addition, many lesser-known saints were associated with eye disorders and blindness, dropsy and lameness, paralysis and crippled limbs, either through healings performed by them or their relics, or through having themselves suffered from such conditions.[33]

One can infer from the sheer number of saints who were linked with patronage of impairments and diseases how important this aspect of the wider function of a saint will have been to medieval people. Healing, if not the most important function of a saint, certainly played the greatest part in the accounts of miracles recorded at saints' shrines, and in the acts of the processes of canonisation, during the high Middle Ages, as a study by André Vauchez demonstrates. 'In the majority of accounts of miracles linked to the cult of the saints, however, the latter appear primarily as miracle-workers, to whom one appealed to recover one's health.'[34] Vauchez' statistical analysis of the types of miracles recorded in the process of canonisation for eight saints in the century between 1201 and 1300 reveals that just over 90 per cent of all miracles could be categorised as therapeutic.[35]

These miracles include resurrections, and the healing of contagious and organic diseases, paralysis, motor problems (people referred to as *contracti*), wounds, fractures, blindness, deafness, muteness and mental illnesses, and also help in difficult births or sterility (Table 1). In fact, here we encounter just the kinds of afflictions we would now classify as 'impairments', together with conditions that we would now term 'illnesses' (the problems of distinguishing between impairment and illness had been discussed in Chapter 2.2). Amongst these miracle cures, the healing of paralysis and motor problems alone account for nearly 29 per cent of all miracles, non-therapeutic ones (categories 8–10 in Vauchez' table) included. Furthermore, the *contracti* or 'cripples' occupied the largest single group of all recorded miracles. In the following century, 1301 to 1417, the picture changed dramatically. Of ten processes of canonisation in that period analysed by Vauchez, now only 79 per cent of miracles refer to therapeutic cases, and more interestingly, the number of *contracti* cured has fallen from nearly 29 to 12.5 per cent, with a somewhat less marked fall in the number of blind, deaf and mute cures (from 12.4 to 11.7 per cent); only resurrections increased over the thirteenth-century miracles, from 2.2 to 10.2 per cent. During the fourteenth century, it seems, non-therapeutic miracles, such as miracles of deliverance and protection, and religious miracles, gained at the expense of healing miracles, with resurrections forming the one exception in this set of examples.

More statistics are provided in an article by Pierre-André Sigal on the miracles of St Gibrien at Reims.[36] Sigal, as also Marcus Bull in his discussion of the Rocamadour miracles, initially argues that medieval miracle narratives follow literary stereotypes in their concentration on the themes of curing the sick and disabled, resurrecting the dead, freeing prisoners and so on. In the narratives, a particular saint cures 'difficult

Table 1 Development in the typology of miracles recorded in canonisation processes

Types of miracles	% of total miracle numbers	
	1201–1300	*1301–1417*
1. Resurrections	2.2	10.2
2. Contagious and organic illnesses	28.6	31.2
3. Paralysis, motor problems (*contracti*)	28.8	12.5
4. Wounds, fractures, non-fatal accidents	5.2	5.6
5. Blind, deaf, mute	12.4	11.7
6. Mental illnesses (possession, epilepsy, mad)	10.7	5.1
7. Difficult births, sterility	1.2	3.3
8. Deliverance and protection	3.2	11.8
9. Religious miracles[a]	3.8	5.0
10. Miscellaneous	3.9	3.6
Therapeutic miracles (categories 1–7)	90.2	79.3
Other miracles (categories 8–10)	9.8	20.7

Source: Adapted from table 31, in Vauchez, *Sainthood in the Later Middle Ages*, p. 468.

Note

a That is, punishments for blasphemy or broken vows, visions and apparitions, sacramental miracles.

cases' that other saints and shrines have been unable to achieve to prove that saint's superiority over the others,[37] and hence to increase the flow of pilgrims and revenue to that particular shrine. However, Sigal admits that many miracles deal with healing activity, and this allows us, to a degree, to examine certain aspects of medieval morbidity.[38] Of St Gibrien's 102 miracles, a staggering 98 deal directly with healing, that is almost 97 per cent.[39] The miracles of St Vulfran at Saint-Wandrille[40] from the second half of the twelfth century reveal a somewhat smaller ratio, namely 75 per cent (of 89 miracles) are about healing people. Among the miracles recorded for St Gibrien, one category dominates, that concerning motor impairments, contractions and withering disorders (or as Sigal tries to rephrase it in modern medical terminology, disorders of the nervous system, especially paralytic disorders), with 49 cases, or 50 per cent of all Gibrien's healing miracles.[41] Possession or madness was cured in 8 cases, eye disorders in 16 cases, hunchbacks in 7 cases, lameness in 4 cases, muteness in 6 cases (1 deaf-mute), 3 people with fistulas, and 3 with ulcers or abscesses, 2 with St Anthony's fire, 2 cases of fractures, 1 burns case, 1 case of kidney disease, 3 cases of dropsy, 1 man with cancer, another man with an injured knee, and 2 resuscitations of infants.[42] With regard to the 49 motor impairments, Sigal believes that in some of these cases a more precise diagnostic can be made: 13 people were contracted or curved (*curvae*), 8 had a general paralysis, 7 suffered from hemiplegia, 8 from paraplegia, 7 had lost the use of an arm and 6 the use of a leg.[43]

Similar patterns can be found in other saints' miracles. Among the miracles of St Martin, recorded by Gregory of Tours in the sixth century, 75 cases of paralysis were among a total of 185 miracles. In ninth and tenth century Poitou 31 of 150 miracles related to paralysis; St Foy's miracles recorded 11 paralyses out of 70 miracles; St Vulfran at Saint-Wandrille in the eleventh century cured 16 paralytics out of 66 total healings; however, by the end of the fourteenth century the number of paralysis cases had dropped (a statistic also found by Vauchez, see above): at the canonisation process for cardinal Peter of Luxembourg only 11 cures of 145 healings dealt with paralysis.[44] Overall, though, the kinds of ailments with which pilgrims presented in general, and at the shrine of St Gibrien in particular, broadly follow along the pattern outlined by André Vauchez's study, in that healing miracles (up to the fourteenth century) account for the vast majority of types of miracles, and within the category of healing, conditions we would now classify as impairing – motor, visual, aural and oral impediments – become the main focus of attention for the miraculous.

My own studies (see Appendix) have analysed a series of miracle narratives, chosen especially for their chronological range, covering a span from the earlier medieval period (ninth-century texts relating to seventh-century saints) up to the thirteenth century, and also chosen for their geographical range, since I include miracles performed at shrines in the German and French regions as well as those by English saints. The sources I have used, in brief, constitute the following texts:

- *vitae* from manuscripts produced at the monastery of St Gall, including three *Lives* of St Gallus, one from the eighth, the other two from the ninth century; two ninth-century *vitae* of St Otmar; and a *Life* of St Wiboroda, mainly of tenth-century date with eleventh-century additions;

- miracles of St Foy recorded at her abbey church at Conques, and written up by Bernard of Angers in the early eleventh century, with additions by an anonymous author in the middle of that century;
- miracles of St Ithamar occurring at his shrine at Rochester during the twelfth century, extant in one manuscript from the late twelfth or early thirteenth century;
- miracles of St William observed at Norwich between 1144 and 1172, recorded and written up by Thomas of Monmouth during 1172–3;
- miracles of Our Lady of Rocamadour, collected and written between 1172 and 1173;
- miracles of the Hand of St James at Reading abbey, occurring during the later twelfth century, but recorded in a thirteenth-century manuscript;
- miracles of St Godric from the late twelfth century, collected by Reginald of Durham in the thirteenth century;
- and the canonisation protocols of St Elisabeth, covering the period from 1232 to 1234.

The original language all these sources were written in was, of course, medieval Latin, although I have had to rely, due to accessibility in some instances, on translations into English and German.[45] Some narratives are fairly long, covering more than two hundred miracle stories, in the cases of St Godric and St Elisabeth, while the collection for St Ithamar describes only a handful of miracles. Only those stories dealing with impairment have been fully quoted or paraphrased in the appendix, and been counted for statistical purposes here.

Among this group of *miracula* that I have studied in more detail a similar pattern of healing emerges to that discovered by Vauchez and Sigal. The vast majority of healing revolves around motor impairments, closely followed by eye disorders/ blindness. Different saints seem to have 'specialised' in different types of miracle, but in most of them impairments of the limbs and general immobility of the body appear to be the main reasons why people sought their aid. This is demonstrated in Table 2.

All the miracles studied amount to some 458[46] healings performed. Of these, 47.6 per cent relate to mobility impairments, 25.5 per cent to blindness, 7.6 per cent to deafness, 11.1 per cent to muteness, 3.7 per cent to insanity and 4.3 per cent to epilepsy. In some particular cases more than one miracle may occur to a single person, for example a man cured by St William was both mute and blind.[47] Such cures have been treated for statistical purposes as two different healings. In the cases of three saints, Our Lady of Rocamadour, St Elisabeth and St Godric, the vast majority of miracles deal with impairing conditions, so that in compiling the study I have been able to list every single miracle irrespective of what condition was being cured.[48]

What clearly emerges from the three sets of statistical data provided by André Vauchez, Pierre-André Sigal and myself is that an overwhelmingly large number of those saints' miracles concern themselves with the healing of conditions we would now refer to as impairing. In addition, Finucane, in his study of English

Table 2 Types of healing and frequency in miracles

Saint	Healing activity relating to					
	Mobility[a]	Blind	Deaf	Mute	Insanity	Epilepsy
James (Reading)	6	1	—	1	—	—
Ithamar	2	5	2	2	—	—
William (Norwich)	24	8	3	7	—	—
Godric (Finchale)	81	44	18	11	11	4
Foy	17	15	3	7	—	—
Elisabeth	61	24	2	6	4	14
Mary	15	16	3	12	2	2
St Gall *vitae*	12	4	4	5	—	—
Total in category	218	117	35	51	17	20
	(458 miracles in all categories)					

Note

a 'Mobility' covers impairments relating to total immobility of the entire body (irrespective of medical cause), 'infirmity' (the quasi-generic medieval term for 'impairment') which has caused immobility, crippling, contraction or withering of upper or lower limbs and paralysis of all the body or of the limbs, as well as the rather vague medieval term 'weakness' in cases where it is implied that the person affected was immobilised.

and European shrines between the twelfth and fifteenth centuries reckons that nine-tenths of all miracles reported there dealt with the cure of human illnesses.[49] Furthermore, when one breaks down the cures into more specific categories, the largest number of miracles deal with motor impairments, closely followed by visual impairments. It would be interesting to compare the incidence of these medieval impairments with incidences among modern, contemporary populations, which is beyond the scope of this book. Such a comparison, however, might in future establish whether perhaps motor impairments constitute the largest form of impairment in actuality; it might then be possible to shed more light on the debate as to whether medieval miracle narratives are simply literary stereotypes, speaking of healing the impaired because Christ set the example in the Gospels, or if they do in fact reflect a 'real' medical situation, and that 'real' impaired people turned to saints and their shrines in the hope of a cure because other avenues (medical cures) were closed to them.

The question of whether medieval miracles narratives are simply literary stereotypes, echoing Christ's Gospel miracles, or concerned 'real' medical conditions among medieval populations, seems to have fascinated scholars for some time.[50] Some 35 years ago Sigal had already tried to address this issue. Sigal had been struck by the predominance of impairing conditions presenting in the miracles, and had asked whether there really was a very strong proportion of people suffering from paralysis and eye disorders during the medieval period, or if these miracles were imitations based on the Gospel model, where the two typical New Testament miracles were exactly those concerning the blind and the lame.[51] He tried to answer his question by pointing to research done on Byzantine miracles,[52] where similar results appeared, but concluded that due to the state of research then (in 1969) it was too difficult to come up with a satisfying answer. More recently, in discussing the miracles of the Virgin Mary at Rocamadour, Marcus Bull[53] has made similar assumptions about the literary stereotyping of miracle narratives (i.e. that they are based on New Testament precedents). Perhaps instead of looking purely at medieval narratives, one should turn to investigate the apparent model the medieval stories imitate, namely the gospel miracles. This is precisely the approach I take, since examining the original 'model' for what it might tell us about notions concerning the cure of impairing conditions can tell us a lot more about the cultural assumptions that revolve around the concepts of impairment, miracle and cure.

Christ's miracles in the gospels have often been regarded, both by medieval writers and modern historians of the medieval period, as models for medieval miracles. In the New Testament, Christ and his apostles frequently healed impaired or sick people. For example, in the gospels alone there are some 35 instances of Jesus healing, among others, blind, deaf, dumb and lame people, people with disabled (withered/shrivelled) limbs and paralytics.[54] The Acts of the apostles contain further miracles of healing, this time performed by Paul. Many miracles one encounters in more than one gospel, such as the healing of the man with dropsy,[55] the healing of a man's withered hand[56] and the healing of a blind beggar,[57] while other miracles are recounted in only one gospel, for instance the cures at the pool of Bethesda,[58] or the healing of the man born blind.[59] Occasionally the healing is described as being an example of Jesus' compassion, but more often than not the miracle is treated as a sign of the presence of God's holy kingdom, so that there is, apparently, no discernible pattern to the kinds of people cured in the healing miracles of Christ.[60] For example, as was discussed in Chapter 3.1, whether the person to be healed by Christ had sinned explicitly, or not, was not always an issue. The underlying assumption of the New Testament, taken over from the Old Testament, seems to be that 'all affliction has sin (generically in the human race) as its ultimate cause',[61] but that says nothing more with regard to impairment other than that *all* the ills afflicting humanity are due to the primal sin of the Fall. Jesus sometimes explained impairment as the work of God alone, as in the miracle of the man born blind,[62] but at other times viewed illness as directly due to an individual's present sin.[63] The miracles in the gospels are conducted both with and without a concern for the moral condition of the person, as was shown in the discussion of sin and illness/impairment.

Medieval miracle healings sometimes echoed the view of the gospels that healing is quite possible without reference to a person's spiritual state. In his *Life* of St Anselm (d. 1109), Eadmer recounted the episode where Anselm was alone in a chapel after mass when a man 'guiding his footsteps with a stick'[64] approached and tried to burst in, disturbing the saint. Anselm's aide Alexander detained the man, but when Anselm heard the commotion, he made the sign of the cross three times with his thumb on the eyes of the blind man, praying: 'May the virtue of the Cross of Christ illuminate these eyes, and cast out all their infirmity, and restore them to perfect health.'[65] Alexander then told the man to come again the next day if the cure had not worked on the first attempt, but the man answered that there would be no need for a repeat of the action, as his blindness had gone away and he could see with perfect clarity. In this story there is no mention of sin in connection with the man's blindness, nor is there any mention of a need to absolve sins prior to a successful miracle healing, nor even do the words Anselm uttered reflect a link between spiritual and physical state – Anselm just blessed the man irrespective of his moral condition.

Returning to the gospels, one aspect of the miracle healings is strikingly consistent, namely the sense of a kind of transcendence of the natural order of things. The healing of impairments is mentioned in the same breath as the raising of the dead in Matthew and Luke: 'the blind receive their sight, and the lame walk, the lepers are cleansed, and the deaf hear, the dead are raised up'[66] and 'the blind see, the lame walk, the lepers are cleansed, the deaf hear, the dead are raised'.[67] These passages are commonly regarded as allusions to the prophecies made in Isaiah[68] on the deliverance of those redeemed, thereby prefiguring the advent of Christ, a time when God's power will manifest itself. The healing of lame, blind, deaf and dumb people, or of disabled people, as we would now say, is thereby positioned into a very special context. Essentially, it takes a miracle to heal such impairments in the gospels. To cure the disabled is likened to raising the dead, impossible for 'normal' human beings, and by implication therefore impossible for 'normal' therapeutic measures such as those practised by physicians.[69] One may find a further example of the analogous relationship between curing the impaired and raising the dead in the context of the raising of Lazarus; to overcome the scepticism some people have of Christ's powers, other bystanders say: 'Could not this man, which opened the eyes of the blind, have caused that even this man should not have died?'[70] Quite clearly, then, in the gospels the healing of impairments is regarded as on a par with bringing back to life the dead, and both actions are deemed miraculous in the sense that the performer of such miracles is acting above and beyond 'nature', transcending the boundaries of what normal human beings are capable of, in curing the incurable.

This notion of the miraculous, if not to say supernatural, aspect of curing the impaired is also evidenced in the reactions of bystanders and witnesses to Christ's miracles in the gospels. Several times 'great multitudes' approach Christ, bringing their blind, lame, mute, maimed and otherwise impaired people to be healed. Having seen the healing, the crowds are often described as being amazed, wondering or full of astonishment at what they regard as an impossible feat. On one occasion 'the multitude wondered (*turbae mirarentur*), when they saw the dumb to speak, the maimed to be whole, the lame to walk, and the blind to see';[71] on another occasion, the people 'were beyond measure astonished (*eo amplius admirabantur*), saying, he hath done all things well: he maketh both the deaf to hear, and the dumb to speak';[72] yet again, after curing a man of dumbness, 'the people wondered (*admiratae sunt turbae*)'.[73] The point here is that what makes the people witnessing the healing miracles be amazed are the *kind* of ailments being cured: had Christ cured something that would not have been beyond the capabilities of physicians, there would not be anything astonishing about the performance. Curing a person who has stubbed their toe is not particularly miraculous by any standard, whereas curing a crippled person is. One may argue that the healing miracles are purely literary devices to emphasise the power of Christ, and should not be seen as actual cures of the impaired, which may or may not be the case, but that still does not detract from the fact that as a prime example of Christ's powers, whether literary or not, the cure of impairments is paramount in the gospels.

For the authors/compilers of the gospels, as well as for the medieval hagiographers writing later, the cure of conditions we would now term physical impairments, and which they regarded as incurable by 'natural' or medical means through ordinary human beings, pertained to the realm of miracle. This notion that the healing of an incurable condition transcended the natural order of things, and was therefore a miracle, is expressed in one of the accounts from the miracle narratives I have studied in detail. A vision of St Elisabeth curing the monastic lay brother, who, while on milling duty, suffered what we might term an 'industrial accident', having had his hand crushed badly by the millstone. The bones of his hand were smashed to pieces and his nerves were ground up, and the remains of his mangled hand were crippled so that he could no longer stretch out his hand. After the miraculous cure had occurred, the miller, one of the witnesses, testified he thought it was impossible that the lay brother could ever have made use of his hand 'according to the course of nature'.[74] More dramatically, the restoration, attributed to St Foy, of both the eyes to a man who had them torn out in a brawl, is compared by the writer of the narrative to Christ's healing in the gospels of the man born blind,[75] except that this contemporary miracle is said to be 'much more marvellous by far'.[76] St Foy was also responsible for another such miracle, which the author terms 'contrary to nature',[77] namely the restoration of the eyes to a man who had had them gouged out by a local lord.

Healing miracles worked by medieval saints are sometimes referred to as 'divine medicine'[78] in the sources I have studied, or else the curative process is regarded as having been worked by the 'hand of the heavenly doctor',[79] as in the miracle stories of St Foy. St Godric is also described as working medicine in his miracles.[80] In a vision, St Ithamar touched the eyes of a blind priest with his hands 'like a physician'.[81] One of St Foy's miracles, where a 'little old woman'[82] with a severely curved spine was cured, is also likened to the cure of a similar condition performed by Christ[83] in the gospels. Earthly medicine is actually described as inferior in one text, where God restores a man back to health 'not by means of the trifles of physicians, but thanks to his Mother, Our Lady'.[84] To understand such statements, the tension between physical and spiritual medicine needs to be contextualised, by looking wider afield at other sources beyond the *miracula* I have studied.

The miracles ascribed to medieval saints are very much following the pattern set by the miracles of Christ and his apostles in the gospels, in that the medieval miracles, too, are described by contemporaries as having a transcendent quality about them, of God working above and beyond nature through the medium or conduit of the saint. Medieval writers themselves, from Augustine onwards, regarded miracles as transcending nature, as *super naturam* rather than *contra naturam*, acts of God which were not subject to nature or human actions in the usual way.[85] Already a figure as influential as the Venerable Bede, in the late seventh/early eighth century, had pointed out the astonishing and wonder-arousing aspects of the healing miracles of Christ and the apostles in the New Testament. Bede used the example of Peter and John's healing of the man born lame[86] to show that Christians and Jews were so moved by what they witnessed that they were thereby prompted to have faith; Bede also pointed out that this was the reaction of the uneducated crowd, while the scribes reacted differently, either denying the same wonder or trying to put a negative angle on it.[87] For Bede, of course, the gospel miracles had an importance going beyond the cure of the purely physical: 'In general the miracles of physical healing worked by Christ announce on the allegorical level his ability to cure the spiritual ailments that afflict humankind.'[88] Nevertheless, the sense of wonder inherent in a miracle remains, and, allegorical or not, miracles for Bede were a sign of the power of God over creation.

Miracles were also regarded as a sign demonstrating the divine power, and thereby strengthening the faith of believers, by Ælfric, abbot of Eynsham (*c*.955–1010). In his *Homilies* he had the following to say with regard to miracles and physical healing:

> We have the belief that Christ himself taught to his apostles, and they to all mankind; and that belief God has with many *wundrum* [miracles] confirmed and strengthened. First Christ by himself healed dumb and deaf, halt and blind, mad and leprous, and raised the dead to life. After, through his apostles and other holy men, he worked the same *wundra*. Now also in our time, wherever holy men rest, at their dead bones God works many *wundra*, because he wishes to confirm folks' belief with those *wundrum*.[89]

Ælfric's *Homilies* were also intended to be used as material for sermons, specifically to provide priests with access to basic sermon examples,[90] in other words, they were intended to be preached, so that they initiated a greater distribution of knowledge among late Saxon culture beyond just individual readers of a manuscript text.

The sentiments voiced by Ælfric regarding the similarity, in the powers of physical healing, between saints and Christ are echoed by Thomas of Celano in his *Life* of St Francis, written in 1228. Thomas writes about events at the shrine of St Francis:

> At his tomb new miracles are constantly occurring, and . . . great benefits for body and soul are sought at that same place. Sight is given to the blind, hearing is restored to the deaf, the ability to walk is given to the lame, the mute speak, he who has gout leaps, the leper is healed, he who has a swelling has it reduced . . . so that his dead body heals living bodies just as his living body had raised up dead souls.[91]

Of course there is a strong resemblance here to the miracles performed by Christ in the gospels, even in the wording,[92] but then, like Christ, St Francis cures the incurable and raised a person from the dead. Episodes from the miracles of

St Francis were illustrated early on, the images following the miracle stories quite precisely. An example can be seen in the work of Bonaventura Berlinghieri from 1235 at Pescia, where St Francis is depicted healing various crippled persons and a lame man.[93] St Godric, too, during his lifetime, is said to have cured the swollen feet and shins of a man by telling him to rise and walk in the name of Christ,[94] just as Christ himself did in the gospels.[95] So after a fashion, saints *are* imitators of Christ in their healing function. I argue that that imitation is precisely what distinguishes the saint from the 'ordinary' physician, who can only cure the mundane afflictions, but cannot perform 'miracles'. Medieval saints are therefore transcenders of nature, while the physician has to work with nature.

Finally, the notion of miracle is intrinsically bound up with the performance of healing physical ailments. A fourteenth-century Middle English text, not without some irony, demonstrates what the notion of a proper, 'true' miracle entails, by contrasting the miracles performed by God in church with the 'false' miracles attributed to the Devil. In this satirical homily, God's miracles are performed on the blind, who are made to see, the crooked who can walk again, the mad who are made sane, the dumb who are enabled to speak, the deaf enabled to hear and so on, while the Devil's miracles all relate to the setting of a tavern, which the sane, or rather, sober, man enters and emerges insane, or drunk:

> At cherche kan god his uirtues sseawy. and do his miracles. þe blynde: to li3te. þe crokede: to ri3te. yelde þe wyttes of þe wode [mad]. þe speche: to þe dombe. þe hierte: to þe dyaue. Ac þe dyeuel deþ al ayenward ine þe tauerne.[96]

The text continues by describing the false miracles the Devil performs in the tavern, which are an inversion of God's miracles performed in church: the glutton enters the tavern in an upright state, but when he exits he cannot support himself; when he enters a tavern he can see, hear and speak clearly, and has understanding, but when he leaves he has lost all those senses and has no reason or understanding left. Even in satirical reversal, this notion of miracle still revolves around the effect it has on the body.

A very unusual attitude to miracles, effectively contradicting the predominant notion of healing miracles as something supernatural, is taken in one specific text. In a tenth-century *Life* of Mary Magdalen, Magdalen is described as having a discussion with the famous physician Galen. Galen explains to her how Christ cured blind Bartholomew,[97] namely by using minerals, which, in fact, would be the method the historic Galen would have recommended for treating eye disorders (minerals as remedy for such ailments are found in Galenic texts)[98] – a 'medical' explanation for one of the gospel miracles performed by Christ is reiterated in a hagiographical text.

5.2   Medicine, transgression and miracle

One problem regarding the connection between medicine and miracle concerns modern misinterpretations of medieval healing miracles, by making the assumption that miracle narratives, because of their focus on conditions we would now term 'impairments', rather than a wider range of medical disorders, were not a reflection of the 'real' cases of ill-health medieval pilgrims to miracle-working shrines would have had. In the chapter on medieval medicine and natural philosophy, I have argued, basically, that medieval medicine, not unlike modern medicine, relegated impairment to the status of incurable, and was therefore not worthy of discussion by the medical profession. In modern medicine, too, disability issues are shunted into the specialised corner of 'rehabilitation' and are seen more as social work than 'proper' medicine. Medieval medical texts, as we have seen, barely said anything on curing impairment at all, only the surgical texts mentioned a little, in the sense that they tried to describe methods of preventing impairments arising from accident, trauma, or other injury. I will argue here that precisely because medicine, medieval as well as modern, had so little to offer to the physically impaired by way of cure, that people turned to miracles.

In discussing the twelfth-century miracle accounts of Rocamadour, Marcus Bull asserts that the terminology used in the *miracula* to describe the ailments (e.g. *surdus, mutus, caecus, paralyticus*) with which pilgrims presented at the shrine is nothing more than an allusion to, or echo of, the biblical language employed by the description of Christ's miracles in the gospels. In other words, Marcus Bull relegates the descriptions in the Rocamadour *miracula* to the status of a literary device, rather than according them historical validity. 'What these stories do not amount to, then, is a comprehensive catalogue of the medical conditions that afflicted medieval men and women, nor even a list of most of the symptoms that ill people would have presented.'[99] This statement does, however, miss the point somewhat. The medical conditions presenting at Rocamadour, and at the other shrines which I discuss, are only those conditions that medieval medicine, as practised by surgeons, physicians and a wide variety of other, more 'populist' healers, found difficult and even impossible to cure; many of the conditions described are difficult or impossible to cure by medical means even today, for example profound deafness or blindness. What the *miracula* of Rocamadour, and those of other shrines, are describing are in fact those very impairing conditions that are not dealt with in the medieval medical discourse, as was discussed in Chapter 4.1. Furthermore, Bull's assumptions that these miracles do not even represent a picture of *all* the varieties of symptoms that people may have had stems, perhaps, from the prevailing modern view that medieval medicine was so ineffective and dreadful that an impaired or sick person had solely miracles to resort to, rather than physical medicine. Again, it is only the difficult to treat or even incurable medical symptoms that we hear of in the *miracula*. Bull argues that this is the case because the discourse which the *miracula* present 'was not predicated on the need to address the full variety of human ailments'.[100] In my view, the *miracula* do not intend to address all human ailments, only those which are medically difficult or incurable ones, all the more so if the narratives of miracles are modelled on Christ's miracles in the gospels, as Bull had assumed himself.

When it comes to discussing the medical element that may exist in the miracles, Bull proceeds to state: 'In addition this discourse [of the *miracula*] was detached from – although not completely unaffected by – contemporary medical learning, diagnostics and practice.'[101] However, such detachment can also be due to the kind of cases presenting at the shrine, and need not be ascribed to a lack of interest in or knowledge of contemporary medical matters. Bull notes that the *miracula* are more concerned with describing the symptoms rather than the aetiologies[102] of the conditions presenting, which is not surprising: the conditions presenting are those that are difficult or impossible to treat medically, so one may wonder why the aetiology should be of concern to the medieval author. If it is not possible to cure something medically, the medieval reasoning may have been, why speculate on medical origins, especially if the author is a compiler of miracle narratives and not a medical professional? Essentially, the problem seems to stem from the fact that Marcus Bull does not differentiate between disease and/or illness on the one hand, and impairment and/or disability on the other hand, but treats them both as one and the same category, thereby doing precisely what modern disability studies have criticised the medical profession for doing. By not differentiating disease and disability, one may fail to notice that medieval medicine and miracle interplay and complement each other in the different areas (illness and impairment) that each tries to cure by its own means.

Evidence for this criticism can actually be found in the Rocamadour miracles themselves. The medieval perception of the incurability of impairment, and furthermore the relegation of cures for impairment to the realm of the miraculous, instead of to the medical domain, can be found in several of the miracles in the Rocamadour collection. In miracle I.48 of the collection, a knight with a lumpy growth (tumour?) in his throat is only cured at Rocamadour: 'The physicians said that they did not know what this was, and that it was incurable.'[103] Here we encounter precisely the situation of the miraculous cure of what was deemed medically incurable. This is a situation emphasised in the prologue to the *miracula*, where the notion is expressed that miracles deal with the wondrous and supernatural, with the inexplicable: 'Let them come and witness the amazing sights, and let them put their faith in things that are incredible.'[104] The cure of routine, mundane illnesses is not incredible, but the cure of impairments or disabilities is, and hence pertains to the realm of the miraculous. Other instances in the same collection of miracles can be found where the person cured miraculously first sought out the aid of physicians, and only when they could not help, turns to the shrine. For example, a woman who was stabbed in her pregnant belly was cured 'who could not be healed by doctors' medicines'.[105] A knight who had been run through with a lance up to his spine (a potentially impairing spinal injury, and spinal injuries often even now can be one of the main cause of mobility impairment) came to the shrine for a cure after medical practices failed to help him: 'Doctors sewed up his entrails, bound the wounds and applied poultices. But their skills were not enough to make the patient well... So when the doctors' attentions failed to heal the injured man, they became afraid of his friends [in case they, the doctors, did not succeed] and, declaring that he would be dead within three days, seized the first opportunity to run away.'[106] A mad woman could not be helped by the physicians' arts, so her relatives focused on the possibility of a healing at Rocamadour.[107] Even more noteworthy, because of the allusion to surgical measures, is the miracle of one Bernarda, who suffered from a tumour. On the advice of her doctor, who said she would not survive the opening up of the tumour, she was not 'placed under the surgeon's knife'.[108] Instead she went to Rocamadour. On her journey there, Bernarda met a grey-haired pilgrim, who turned out to be a messenger from the Virgin, who then performed the surgical procedure, 'perforated the tumour by means of an incision, and bloody matter bubbled out of her body like a spring rising up from deep below the ground. He applied poultices' and 'dressed the wound'[109] and she was cured. What is striking here is that the actual miracle relating to Bernarda is reminiscent of regular, non-supernatural surgical treatment. Perhaps Bernarda had simply met a superior surgeon on her travels, who could do what her first surgeon at home dared not to do, and her subsequent cure was handily ascribed to the Rocamadour miracles.

What all the examples demonstrate is that if the medical or surgical profession failed, then a person might turn toward the miraculous in the hope of a cure. The Rocamadour miracles seem not to have been unusual in this respect. It is probably an anachronistic image of the Middle Ages to assume that medicine, and physicians, were always held in far lesser esteem than religious cures, and that people therefore automatically went to a shrine for healing rather than to a medic. The people mentioned in other miracle accounts, this time of the thirteenth and fourteenth centuries, also sometimes looked to medical intervention for their illnesses and impairments before turning to a shrine, as André Vauchez has shown: 'Some witnesses admitted that they had only considered resorting to a celestial intercessor when all treatments had failed and they had been abandoned by the doctors to their unhappy fate.'[110] Other people did, of course, turn to aid by a saint straightaway, without ever consulting a physician. The important point is that both attitudes were present simultaneously in high and later medieval society. Therefore, what the *miracula* tell us about medieval medicine provides of necessity a distorted image, since only those cases where it was thought that medicine could not help, or was expected not to be of help, are the cases where people went on pilgrimage, so that the successful cases of medical intervention went unnoticed, not featuring in the miracle narrative.

One need not restrict oneself to the one set of miracle narratives from Rocamadour to find echoes of the attitude that medical treatment is more than likely to have preceded a recourse to the miraculous. In his *Life* of St Cuthbert, Bede related how in another monastery near to Lindisfarne a young monk was immobilised with paralysis; this monk's abbot knew that 'the Lindisfarne monastery housed some extremely skilful physicians' and the monk was carried there on a cart.[111] At Lindisfarne, the physicians 'applied every ounce of skill and knowledge they possessed' but the monk regressed until he could no longer move except to open his mouth and his doctors 'having so long exerted all their human skill in vain, gave up hope'.[112] It is only then, when the young monk is 'lying there despaired of'[113] that he turns to heavenly medicine and asks for a relic of

St Cuthbert, and is cured by the shoes of the saint. Miracles were far from routine events for Bede, it has been pointed out:

> Not even at Lindisfarne, where the power of Cuthbert should have been particularly effective, was there expectation of a miraculous cure. In the first instance at least, faith was placed, not in the relics of the saint, but in the skill of the physicians.[114]

The Bedean stance on miracles and medicine was, however, not the only viewpoint a medieval author could take. For an alternative attitude towards miracles and medicine, one need only turn to another writer from the earlier Middle Ages, Gregory of Tours. In a study of *vitae* and Merovingian healing shrines from sixth to eighth century France, Valerie Flint[115] has concentrated on the writings of Gregory to analyse the position of the two main early medieval healers – the physician and the saint. She argues that the early medieval 'medicus' was a figure positioned midway between the healing saint and the (non-Christian) enchanter. Nevertheless, even with such a critical initial view, healing was performed in the *vitae* by the saint *after* healing by the medicus had failed. Sometimes punishment by the saint might be elicited if healing by a physician was sought *in addition* to saintly healing. Such a story is told by Gregory: the archdeacon Leunast of Bourges had cataract in his eyes and went from physician to physician without being cured. Finally he was healed by fasting and praying at the church of St Martin. But thereafter he went in search of professional medical attention to reinforce his miracle healing, and he became blind again.[116] Gregory, in Flint's words, almost displayed *schadenfreude* in relating this story: the affront was not so much a case of seeking medical help over saintly help, but in trusting the medical help more than the heavenly. Additional prejudice in Gregory is evident in the fact that he saw it necessary to mention that the physician whom Leunast consulted after his miracle healing was a Jew.[117] Gregory complained that 'Leunast would have retained his health, if he had not sought the help of a Jew after he had received God's grace. ... Let this story be a warning to every Christian man, that when it has been granted to him to receive a cure from Heaven, he should not then seek earthly remedies'.[118] Flint has interpreted these kinds of stories as signifiers of competition between the saint and the physician.[119] Competition existed furthermore between the Christian Church and enchanters (who were presumably also in competition with physicians, although Flint does not press this point); the solution emerged by which the medicus and the saint in effect joined forces against the enchanter. Overall, the portrayal of medical aid in the *vitae* and in Gregory of Tours is not totally negative, it is just a more cautious and less enthusiastic stance than found in Bede. Even a critic of physicians and a proselytiser of spiritual medicine such as Gregory of Tours on occasion tried medical treatment first for his illnesses, before resorting to heavenly cures.[120] What is still apparent is that people sought *both* medical and spiritual aid for their afflictions, and did not turn exclusively to spiritual healing.

Turning to the sample of miracle stories that I have studied in detail, one too finds a number of instances in which the impaired pilgrim had tried physical medicine before resorting to the 'divine medicine' of saints, relics or shrines. In some cases previous treatment by physicians is only hinted at in the sources, whereas in other cases it is explicitly stated that the pilgrim had received (unsuccessful) medical treatment. A man who had been lame for over a year 'found no cure with others' and so went to the shrine of St Elisabeth.[121] The contracted hand of a woman who went to St Godric was 'incurable',[122] until healed through Godric's powers, of course. Also 'incurable'[123] was the weakened and tumorous knee of a woman, as was the incurable tumour in the feet and legs of a youth, 'whom no [efforts of] medicine could help or cure'.[124] A man who had broken his leg, knee and shin 'so that no doctor could cure him'[125] was healed by St Godric as well. St Elisabeth cured a woman of dropsy whose physicians declared her incurable,[126] and another woman with the same disorder whom an 'experienced physician'[127] had declared incurable; furthermore a woman with cancerous growth who could not be cured 'by any art'[128] was healed. The point is made even more strongly in another of St Elisabeth's miracles regarding the incurability of a condition, which may then lead to a visit to a shrine once the likelihood of a 'conventional' cure is seen as very slim: a man with pains in his legs for more than twenty years was cured, whose daughter testified that she had tried 'many medicines' on her father, while another witness said that he could not be helped by medicine, 'even though he had a very experienced physician'.[129] Cured by the hand of St James was one Gilbert, whose blindness was incurable by ointments or remedies.[130] One of St Foy's visitors was a man whose physicians could not agree on the diagnosis of his condition, whether it was dropsy or paralysis, though this man was partially cured by the 'constant care of doctors'[131] even before he made the pilgrimage. Two of St Ithamar's pilgrims had tried medical treatment first: an elderly blind monk[132] and a bishop with another eye disorder 'which his doctors could neither remove nor assuage'.[133] And a boy had to visit St William to be cured as the 'doctors who were consulted did him no good',[134] while Claricia's leg and kidney pains could not be cured by physicians even though she spent a lot of money on them.[135]

Mention of seeking the aid of physicians first before turning to the aid of a saint is most frequently made in the narratives of St Mary of Rocamadour. In addition to the cases already discussed above, there are further miracles relating more specifically to impairing conditions. Count Robert of Meulan was cured by his doctors after dislocating his shoulder, but after a second accident injuring the same body part and rendering his arm immobile 'doctors applied poultices which did absolutely no good … and nothing the doctors could do' would improve his condition.[136] A dropsical woman could not be cured by doctors' treatments.[137] A knight had his leg amputated at the knee, but the 'infernal burning' he suffered from returned to his other leg.[138] A squire who was both dumb and mad had physicians labour 'long and hard without success' in an attempt to cure him, and, interestingly, when 'they had exhausted all their means of healing they pronounced the squire incurable'.[139] A man diagnosed with dropsy had to make a vow to St Mary, 'for the attentions of physicians did nothing to cure him.'[140] And Guillelma, who was crippled by paralysis in the middle part of her body, could not be cured by anything 'anyone could think of, nor the treatments of doctors'.[141] In the harrowing tale of Stephana, the knight who rescued her also provided her with medical aid; she recovered somewhat 'thanks to the attention of doctors' but she felt that 'none of the doctors' medicines or poultices would make her well' completely.[142] An aspect of contemporary medical opinion is alluded to in the story of William Boarius, who became blind for six years. 'The skill and hard work of physicians did not work on him, failing to restore to him any degree of sight. They were astonished how it could be that only his sight was affected when the rest of his body was perfectly healthy.'[143] Again, the topos of a person going on pilgrimage only after unsuccessful medical treatment was tried is expressed in the case of a young man with epilepsy and paralysis, who was unable to find a doctor who could cure him so he decided to go to Rocamadour.[144] An explanation expressed in medieval medical or physiological terms is even provided in the story of Godfrey, who was so debilitated by an illness in his legs that he was confined to his room for a year: 'When one limb hurts, the others do so too because the parts of the body are joined in such a way that one part cannot be damaged without injury to all the others. ... Medical science was ineffective and quite useless because no remedy existed to make this sick youth better. His family had lost hope for his recovery, particularly because a long-lasting illness is said to be incurable.'[145]

Only in one miracle of the numerous narratives I have examined is the attitude to physicians so negative that the patient dies after recourse to secular medicine, and that is in the context of a cautionary, moralising tale: William the sacrist, already cured once by St William, was instructed by the saint that 'he will never henceforth take any medicine except this of mine', and recovered. But when his condition worsened again, his doctors 'kept advising him to take measures for his safety, and try some medicine' and 'he yielded to the advice of the doctors and sought refuge in the deceits of medicine'.[146] The crucial factor seems to be that he reneged on his 'deal' with the saint and broke the vow by which he had been bound.

The overall impression that emerges strongly from the analysis of these sources, varied over time as well as place of compilation, is that seeking the aid of saints was not invariably the first port of call for medieval impaired persons. In contrast to the assumptions of some modern scholars, 'normal', secular medicine appears to have been the norm, and visiting shrines or placing one's hopes in relics was actually a secondary thaumaturgic measure. Finucane's work on miracles and pilgrims reinforces my point, in that according to his estimates a substantial number of supplicants had already sought medical treatment: 'At the very least, ten out of every hundred recorded medieval English pilgrims who arrived at a shrine to seek or report a miraculous cure had already sought some sort of medical assistance.'[147] Medical treatment was resorted to in the first instance, and often the pronouncement of physicians that a disorder was incurable was the deciding factor that prompted the impaired individual to embark on a pilgrimage for curative purposes. In this context one can borrow a term from anthropology, and speak of a 'hierarchy of resort', that is the hierarchy in which people themselves sought aids or cures for illness.[148] It has often been remarked that the bias of the sources, namely the hagiographical texts and canonisation protocols, naturally had a vested interest in advertising or proving the powers of a saint over secular therapies.[149] To this one can one can add that secular medical texts themselves sometimes emphasised the incurability of impairments and shied away from discussing treatment methods for such conditions. Additionally, following Finucane, one may surmise that the description of the 'useless' medicine of physicians also reflected the 'natural disappointment felt by pilgrims who had consulted doctors whom they thought had failed them'.[150] Impairments due to punishment for transgressions are a separate category, discussed below, but even in those instances medical aid was sometimes sought first and foremost.

Occasionally, miracle and medicine were both used as attempts to cure. Bede relates the story of the miracle of Heribald, the future abbot of Tynemouth, who in his younger days had a riding accident while racing his horse. Heribald fell off his mount and hit his head on a stone, fracturing his skull and thereby becoming paralysed. He was carried home, speechless and vomiting blood all night. Bishop John (later St John) of Beverley stayed with Heribald in vigil and in prayer all through the night, blowing on his face while talking to him.[151] By the next day, Heribald was able to speak again – a miraculous cure effected through the actions of bishop John. However, as Bede says, when Heribald could already speak again, bishop John 'called the surgeon, and told him to close and bandage up the crack in [Heribald's] skull'.[152] There was still a place for the surgeon in the curative process, and Heribald did not rely on miracles alone. In fact, relying on miracles alone could be a lengthy and uncertain process in the quest for healing, as the following two narratives illustrate. William of Malmesbury related the story of a man named Wulfwin, blind for 17 years due to 'blood stagnating in his eyes', who visited 87 churches with their shrines in the hope of a cure, until he was finally treated by Edward the Confessor, by dipping his hands in water and placing them on Wulfwin.[153] And a paralysed priest from Melksham 'dragged his half-dead body round all the holy places in England'[154] before finally being cured at Worcester by the relics of St Wulfstan, as the thirteenth-century *Miracles* of the saint recount.

Frequently, though, aspiration to a miracle was seen as the preferred alternative to medical intervention. The risks associated with medical intervention, especially with surgery, may have been a factor influencing people's decision to visit shrines or seek healing at the hands of holy men and women instead. This is not to state categorically that medieval medical methods and standards would have been so primitive or appalling that people invariably chose the vagaries of 'faith healing' over medicine, but instead the sources reflect what appear to be medieval contemporaries' own fears regarding medicine and surgery. (This should not be surprising, as even today patients still fear surgery.) In the *Life* of St Otmar, a beggar who was sinistrally lamed was directed for a cure to St Gall in a dream, otherwise his foot would have to be amputated.[155] From an Icelandic source, the B version of the *Life* of bishop Gudmundr Arason of Hólar, written between 1315 and 1330 comes the anecdote of a man with frostbite in his feet which had become so bad that he required amputation at the ankles; he was spared the ordeal due to miraculous intervention by bishop Gudmundr's holy water.[156] In one of St Elisabeth's miracles the refusal to consult a physician apparently stemmed from a more general mistrust of the medical profession: a mother was admonished to call a physician after her son had broken his arm, but she refused, because she would only trust in the merits of the saint.[157] Physicians did sometimes make matters worse, too, as in the following case of iatrogenically caused illness, which necessitated a visit to St Foy. A young warrior had suffered a lance wound, which was treated:

> by the unskilled hands of physicians who erred in bandaging the wound too quickly. In so doing, they trapped putrefying, congealed bloody matter inside his body and it began to infect his internal organs. And since the confined fluid inside him had no outlet it raged on the inside and his body swelled up on the outside.[158]

The text does not actually criticise physicians *per se*, but only the unskilled ones, and it is interesting to note that the argument is very much formulated in medical language – more a case of one doctor criticising another's methods than a critique of medicine as a whole. One of the Rocamadour miracles tells of a youth from Montpellier who was 'gravely stricken by paralysis and, on the advice of his physicians, was carried to the baths. Whereas only part of his body had been withered up till then, when he was brought back from the baths his whole body was now desiccated and crippled'.[159] However, this story is told neutrally and no criticism is vented at physicians for apparently making matters worse through their treatment.

Because physicians (purveyors of secular medicine) had a rather ambiguous status as healers in relation to saints (purveyors of divine medicine), and the question of whether one should turn to earthly or heavenly medicine has been addressed, in this context it is worth taking a closer look at the issues of transgression and punishment in the miracle narratives. Not all healing miracles were straightforward cures, enacted after the supplicant had implored God, the relevant saint, or made a pilgrimage or an offering, and was cured without further ado. In some cases the miracle cure is attached to a cautionary tale, or moralising story. Such cases often involve a protagonist who receives their impairment (or illness) initially as a kind of punishment for some mundane or spiritual transgression. Once the protagonist has seen the error of his or her ways, a miraculous cure for their affliction ensues. Thereafter they are fully healed both in body and soul. Sometimes there are even a series of punishments and cures, when particularly stubborn, or stupid, protagonists relapse (an example would be the story of Guibert in the St Foy miracles[160]) and repeatedly need to go through the process of transgression, punishment and cure. What is interesting is that specific collections of miracle narratives are more keen than others to relate stories of transgression, physical punishment and subsequent redemption – that is in relation to impairment, there may be other forms of punishment inflicted on a sinner. The narratives surrounding St Foy and St Mary of Rocamadour are particularly eager to expound such moral tales, whereas the miracles of St James, St Godric and St William each only relate one story of illness or impairment as punishment, and the St Gall *vitae*, St Ithamar and St Elisabeth do not punish anyone physically. One may surmise that different saints had different 'characters', reflected in the kinds of miracles they performed, and that the authors/compilers of the *miraculae* worked these into their texts.

In one of the St James's miracles one finds the story of Gilbert, a keeper of hounds, who was overly fond of hunting, and was punished by blindness for hunting on the saint's feast day;[161] after visiting other shrines unsuccessfully, he was eventually cured by the relic of the hand of St James. St William punished a man, also called William, who was sacrist at his shrine in Norwich, for breaking the vow he had made to the saint.[162] And St Godric had to cure a youth who was struck blind in one eye in punishment for working in the fields on a Sunday.[163] In the works of Gregory of Tours one already encounters the theme of punishment for transgressions, especially for violation of the sabbath.[164] Similarly, other sacrilegious actions are punished, as in the story of abbot Leofstan of Bury St Edmunds. To verify for himself if the decapitated head and body of king Edmund had actually miraculously joined again in the martyr's tomb, abbot Leofstan tried to pull the body of the relic apart. He held onto the head of the saintly body, while another monk, Thurstan, pulled at the feet. In this unseemly tug-of-war, the saint's body, head still firmly connected, and the monk Thurstan were pulled towards Leofstan, who was struck with paralysis for his impiety. Leofstan's hands were distorted and palsied, and he became blind and dumb. After healing of his sight and speech by Baldwin, physician to king Edward the Confessor, he could nonetheless never recover the use of his hands, since his hands had been implicated in the impious act.[165] From another source comes the story of Richard de Belmeis, bishop of London 1108–27, who was hit by a paralytic stroke on the same day that he gave orders for the confiscation of the lands of St Osyth's minster – a neat and convenient accident disguising a politically motivated story here, of a Norman bishop attempting to grasp formerly Saxon ecclesiastical landholdings. Richard repented, and founded an abbey to the glory of St Osyth,[166] and one assumes he was of course cured.

St Foy and St Mary of Rocamadour have already been mentioned as being particularly keen on punishing transgressors, and their miracle narratives will now be discussed in more detail. St Foy had to cure a man who had to spend the night out in the open keeping watch over some horses. He was exhausted and 'gave in to sleep',[167] and found next morning that he had become blind overnight. The author states that the man knew that he deserved his blindness. In another of St Foy's narratives, blindness is meted out as a 'precautionary' punishment, a case of using the impairment as a way of reminding the protagonist not to err in his ways: the previously secular Gerbert had been cured of loss of his eyes, became a devout man living in the monastery, but then, 'to prevent the happenstance that he might be corrupted by arrogance or by the seductive counsel of those near him – and might wish to return to the secular life, through divine will the sight of his left eye began to disappear almost completely afterwards'.[168] Robert, the lord of a castle, tried to attack one of St Foy's monks, and was not only struck blind, but also his entire body was stricken and his mouth wrenched back towards one ear; he was cured after repenting.[169] A crippled girl was initially cured, but when she refused to stand up and leave her work during a procession in the saint's honour, she

> began to be made pathetically deformed throughout her whole body. She became so misshapen that it was just as if she had never been healed but had remained bent and crooked, wholly deprived of the function of her muscles. Her body was completely drawn together and she didn't have the strength to let go of the tools of her loom – the very shuttle was held fast in her clenched hand. ... [she] could speak only hoarsely because her condition greatly restricted her voice (though she had been able to speak normally before).[170]

After being carried in procession, and keeping vigil for several nights – suitable acts of repentance, in other words – she was 'transformed a second time from a cripple to a person who could stand upright'.[171] The lengthiest cycle of healing and punishment is found in the story of the servant Guibert, who had his eyes torn out by his master. He had his sight restored after staying at Conques for a year, where the abbot put him in charge of selling wax to the pilgrims. Then Guibert took up with an 'unchaste woman'[172] and was blinded in one eye, which was cured once he repented, only to lapse a second time, be blinded again, and cured again on repentance. Apparently this 'tit-for-tat' continued for some time until Guibert became blind in the other eye, which made him reconsider and decide to become a monk, whereupon he regained his sight.[173] Cycles of cure, punishment for transgression and repeated cure seem to be a hallmark of the St Foy narratives.

The miracles of St Mary at Rocamadour also contain the theme of punishment following transgression. So robbers who assaulted a pilgrim had their hands paralysed and shrivelled, but when the frightened robbers prayed to the Virgin, they were cured.[174] A man whose fellow-pilgrims had entrusted him with their money for offerings kept some of the money for himself and therefore lost his speech. Pleas from his companions and the revelation where he had hidden the money brought about a cure.[175] Vow-breaking is also punished by St Mary, as it was by St William: a woman who had vowed to go to Rocamadour if her blindness was cured fails to fulfil her vow, and in punishment had a sharp bone from some meat she was eating block her throat.[176] Also, a young knight who had been a gambler, irreverent and blasphemous, was punished by epilepsy. He was cured at Rocamadour after vowing not to commit those sorts of crimes anymore, but after returning home he eventually broke his vow and his disorder returned; he had to return to Rocamadour a penitent and was completely cured.[177] A squire who had insulted the Virgin was punished by losing all his bodily strength and becoming both dumb and mad, but after visiting her shrine he was healed.[178] As in other miracle narratives, working on a saint's day is also punished as transgressive: a woman from Burgundy who worked on the feast day of St Anthony had her hand suddenly seize up and wither.[179] Curiously enough, mistreatment of animals seems to warrant a harsher treatment, in that no cure was forthcoming: a guardian of the church threw a stone at a sparrow that was trying to fly into the basilica at Rocamadour; he 'lost the strength in his arm, and it remained withered for the rest of his life'.[180] Lastly, a knight who had gone on pilgrimage to other shrines criticised the presence of votive offerings in wax he found at Rocamadour. In a very sceptical, almost 'modern' way, he stated that they had been placed there fraudulently by the monks and not by visiting pilgrims who had actually been cured, since apparently at the other shrines he had been to, he had not seen this sort of thing. For this he became paralysed in all his limbs, but again was cured in due course after suitable repentance.[181] A similar punishment of unbelief is found in one of the child healing miracles Finucane cites, except here the perpetrator is punished by proxy, so to speak: a Welsh mother was disapointed because St Wulfstan had not healed her blind daughter, even though they had waited for three days at the shrine, so she complained that if 'the things they say about Wulfstan were true, he would have cured her'.[182] Since no cure occurred, the mother said she would never believe in the saint again, and in punishment, another of her children was struck with an eye affliction.

The theme of thaumaturgic miracles that reverse an affliction originally sustained in punishment has been addressed by a scholar of late antiquity. Raymond Van Dam,[183] in his discussion of miracles in the texts of Gregory of Tours, has proposed to explain such miracles as the cure of 'social illnesses'. He regards illnesses and impairments that afflicted people who themselves thought, and admitted to it, that they had transgressed as social illnesses, whose cure re-integrates the transgressive person into society. Significantly for Van Dam, the illness or impairment strikes parts of the body that acted transgressively in the first instance, that is, people who work on Sundays are rendered paralysed or crippled in those limbs with which they performed the forbidden activity,[184] an observation which also seems valid for the punishment miracles of the high medieval period which I have studied. However, punishment miracles are not that numerous in the sources I have examined, comprising only some 20 miracles out of over 400, whereas in Gregory of Tours' writings, their incidence appears to have been far more frequent. One should therefore assume a shift in attitudes to transgression and physical impairment as punishment between the late antique (or early medieval) period and the high Middle Ages.

For all the physical impairments (and other afflictions) placed in punishment upon transgressive individuals, there are equally a number of cases where the texts quite clearly state that the physical condition of the protagonist was caused purely by chance or accident, with no moralistic overtones or edifying religious sentiment attached to the narrative. In these cases one can distinguish, to a degree, between 'chance' and 'accident' as causes, since the texts themselves make such a differentiation. 'Chance' tends to refer to the presence of congenital impairment, an impairment present and observable 'from birth', as the sources phrase it (though sometimes such congenital impairment is referred to as an 'accident of nature'). 'Accident' more often than not refers to, quite literally, an 'accident', as in an injury sustained while performing some activity or other. The theological importance of regarding impairment as caused by chance or accident lies in the fact that thereby the issue of sin as the cause of impairment becomes negated: if it is recognised that someone accidentally, or 'by chance', became impaired, their moral status becomes irrelevant.[185] Whether or not they have sinned in any way is therefore not important, and their healing can take place without any reference to personal sin.

One of the lengthiest miracle accounts in the narratives of St Godric discussed just that issue of sin and chance.[186] There, a man had been born congenitally blind, which the text says was brought about by chance and not by merit of his sins.[187] Furthermore, as the text puts it, 'perhaps neither he himself nor his parents had sinned'.[188] Interestingly, the theme of sin and chance which this miracle addresses echoes the same sentiments evident in a miracle Christ performed in the gospels, the miracle of the man born blind.[189] Although the St Godric text makes no direct reference to the biblical passage, presumably the allusion would be familiar enough to the medieval reader. Besides such a direct discussion of sin and chance, some of the *miraculae* mention instances where the protagonist of the miracle was impaired purely accidentally, sometimes even employing the actual term 'accidental'. A 5-year-old boy had been placed on a horse and had fallen off, breaking his arm, so that he was impaired for six weeks until his miracle cure happened.[190] A man fell hard (it is not mentioned why) and broke the bone of one leg, his knee and shin.[191] And a woman named Gilliva lost her vision through an (unspecified) 'accident', becoming blind for three years.[192]

Some of the accidental causes of impairment which the texts speak of could be regarded as what we would now term 'industrial accidents', in other words, injuries leading to impairment that were sustained by the individual while performing their work. Five such cases alone occur in the miracle protocols of St Elisabeth, where the cause of impairment is most definitely 'accidental', and no mention whatsoever is made of the individual having sustained their accident through their sinful state. A man had got a hernia after leaping from a cart during harvest time (perhaps he was some kind of farm labourer?). He had become unconscious and had also lost the ability to speak.[193] Another man had fallen from a tower and fractured his spine in three places, as well as his sternum and one of his shins[194] – this may well have been a building site accident, a type which even now is one of the most frequent causes of industrial injury. A third man, aged about 30, injured his knee with an axe.[195] A 30-year-old woman had been injured in the knee so badly by a pig that she was bedridden for 11 weeks, and even after the wound had healed she could still only walk with the aid of crutches due to her lamed leg; while she was impaired she was sustained by the alms of her master (*Dienstherrn*).[196] One may speculate that the woman in question was employed by her master to look after the pig(s). A monastic lay brother, while on milling duty, had his hand caught accidentally (*zufällig*) by the millstone and severely crushed.[197] A very clear example of an industrial accident can be found in the miracles of St Foy: Hugh the master mason had been working on the church when his lower legs were crushed by a cart which was carrying stones from the quarry.[198] And another building accident is mentioned in the miracles of St Godric, where it is actually stated that a youth was injured on a building site, breaking his spine in three places.[199] In his study on miracles and pilgrims, Finucane, as usual without providing practical traceable references, lists a series of accidents involving children and adults, and also refers to 'industrial accidents' on construction sites.[200]

Not all impairments that required a cure at the shrines of saints were attributed to punishment in the texts I have studied. In fact, only two sources in particular, the miracles of the Virgin at Rocamadour and the miracles of St Foy, are keen to emphasise physical impairment as punishment for transgressions, while the other texts are less concerned about such issues. As was demonstrated above, impairment as punishment was linked to specific transgressions which the texts themselves emphasise. In contrast, in some cases the texts state explicitly that impairment was caused by chance or accident. The vast majority of impairments, however, were described without attribution of either punishment or chance/accident. One can conclude from this that the medieval writers of these *miraculae* of the central and high Middle Ages[201] were far less concerned about whether sin caused impairment or not than some modern commentators, who ascribe to the entire medieval period an unsubstantiated obsession with sin and physical punishment. Ronald Finucane has reinforced this point of view, emphasising that in the miracle accounts he has studied, 'sin is nearly as rare as a *stated* cause of illness'[202] as illness caused by demonic influence; where it was expressed, sin was most frequently linked with leprosy, and therefore not with physical impairments as defined in Chapter 1.2.

Loosely connected with the theme of impairment, punishment and cure is the reverse situation: where the impaired protagonists are cured reluctantly, as if their cure were in fact the punishment. A rather curious story was narrated by Jacques de Vitry (d. 1240), in his *Exempla*,[203] whereby the cure that the impaired protagonists received was apparently not entirely welcome to them. The two people in question, one blind, the other crippled, had to be almost forcibly cured in the end. Lame and other 'deformed' persons were assembling for healing at the tomb of a saint, and refused to leave when they had not been cured yet after two days there. The local priest, in a strange psychological healing experiment, eventually told them that 'he who is most disabled amongst you must be burned' and his ashes would be scattered over the others to heal them (perhaps in a perversion of the usual application of saintly relics as curative measure?). Every one of the impaired persons became afraid, and each one forced themselves to such an extent that they all ran away together from the shrine: 'fear added wings to feet!'[204] This narrative can be interpreted in various ways: on one level there is the assumption that maybe the protagonists were not 'really' impaired, hence their 'cure' when they ran away. As such we would be dealing with a cautionary tale for those people who feign impairment, so that they avoid 'proper' work and make a living begging at shrines.

None of the sources I have studied in detail mention fraudulent cures or supplicants who feigned their impairments, for obvious reasons, in that these texts are concerned about promoting the status and powers of their saint. However, some of the additional material consulted by Finucane in his study of miracles and pilgrims does occasionally mention 'fake' impairments, fraudulent cures and a thirteenth-century scheme of what sounds reminiscent of 'organised crime'. A Scottish lady cared for an apparently paralysed man until he was discovered to be a 'fake' and she threw him out; a boy who made out to be speech-impaired was challenged by someone who had already witnessed his 'cure'; a blind man already 'cured' by St Thomas Becket around 1290 was later recognised attempting a 'cure' at St Cantilupe's tomb;[205] and the 'organised crime' was evident at Oxford, where a con man suggested to some Franciscan friars that they could make money from the tomb of a recently deceased friar by having miracles worked there, and he, the con man, had 24 people all over England under his control who were prepared to experience miracles anytime anywhere.[206]

On another level we are dealing with an example of the immense healing power of the saint's relics, whereby even those people who are reluctant to be healed are cured. The saint 'sees through' the deception of the fake impaired people and forcibly 'cures' them, perhaps. We encounter yet another level in the possibility that medieval priests may have known more about psychology than modern historians normally credit them for. Whether the 'healing' actually took place historically is less relevant than that we are told how it took place: through instilling fear in people. Jacques de Vitry appears to have been concerned with the moral of the story, that hell fire (punishment for lying about and feigning impairment) was the real object of fear, not the threat of earthly fire the priest uses, and may therefore have been less concerned with his story as an example of a rather unorthodox miracle healing.[207]

It may sometimes happen that it is not the supplicants who are reluctant to be cured, but that it is the saint who is reluctant to perform a cure, as was the case with three grudgingly performed miracles of St Anselm. Though these miracles do not, strictly speaking, revolve around the cure of impairments, they are worth mentioning here in the context of miracles performed reluctantly. In his *Life* of Anselm, Eadmer normally passes over examples of Anselm's healing powers for the sake of brevity – the implication being that these are too numerous to mention – though he hints at the kind of miracles Anselm performed in his lifetime: 'We have also decided to pass over in silence the countless cases of men cured of divers diseases, and especially fevers, by water in which he had washed his hands and by morsels of his food surreptitiously removed from his plate.'[208] However, Eadmer does cite three examples of healing miracles in which Anselm, a very modest saint, either unwittingly or reluctantly heals the protagonists. Seeing as crumbs from his food were 'misappropriated' for curative purposes, Anselm refused to let two knights suffering from a fever have these crumbs; instead, they could eat the actual food but not the leftovers. 'Anselm would do nothing in this matter which could be ascribed to a miracle,'[209] offering his own food so that the knights would not have access to the apparently miraculous power of the crumbs, not out of meanness but out of modesty. Another time a man was cured of fever and belly-ache, but Anselm 'affirmed that no credit for this belonged to him, but that it must be ascribed to the man's own faith and to the merits of the blessed martyr to whom he had resorted'.[210] Finally, Anselm refused at first to cure a madwoman on the grounds that 'on no account would he attempt anything so extraordinary',[211] although he relented and cured her by making the sign of the cross. One may deduce from this that not only was Anselm rather modest with regard to his healing powers, but also that he regarded some 'cases' to be more difficult than others, with the cure eventually due to manifestations of divine grace (i.e. through the sign of the cross and the protagonist's faith) and not Anselm's own status.

5.3   Narratives of impairment in medieval miracles

This book has been primarily concerned with theoretical approaches to impairment. I shall now turn to the actual miracle stories as they are described in the sources, and critically examined in the secondary literature. These accounts of miracle cures at shrines or by living saints display a wealth of information about how the impaired were treated, in both the medical and social sense of 'treatment'. Attitudes towards impairment become apparent through such narratives, with regard to various cultural assumptions about impairment and constructions of 'disability'. In this sub-chapter I will explore some of the themes one can identify in the miracle narratives that relate to attitudes and reactions to physical impairment, starting with descriptions in the *miracula* of impairment as a physical defect, deviating from the perceived norm. Next I will address the 'liminality' of impaired protagonists, one of the key criteria in connection with physical impairment (as was discussed in Chapter 2.2 in the context of anthropological theories of impairment). Having so far preferred to refer to 'impaired' people in the Middle Ages, rather than to 'disabled' persons, I will also address the question of how far these medieval sources perceived of the impaired as disabled, by looking at the topics of the inability of impaired pilgrims, their perception as a burden or object of mockery, and the connection with poverty and charity.

Although mainly concerned with theories and cultural attitudes, I cannot ignore the evidence presented in the *miracula* that sheds light on more practical aspects: the issue of personal mobility for the physically impaired. I will therefore also discuss examples of how impaired pilgrims managed to travel to sites of saintly healing, and how they got around in their daily lives. In connection with mobility I also examine different methods of obtaining cures which need not require the personal presence of an impaired supplicant at a shrine, that is votive offerings and cures by proxy. Lastly, a speculative note on the question of the veracity of miracle cures concludes this chapter.

Some of the most detailed descriptions of the conditions from which the impaired people seeking cures suffered can be found in the miracle protocols of St Elisabeth (this may be due to the fact that these cases were recorded for an 'official' purpose – canonisation – and greater importance was placed in such detail than in the more 'fictional' narratives of the *vitae*). The worse the impairment, the more merit due to the saint in healing such a condition, so even the most horrific ailments are described in relentless detail. The detailed description does not of itself mark out the impaired person as 'defective', and I have therefore not discussed all such cases, but only those where a value judgement is made implicitly or explicitly which positions the impaired person in opposition to 'normal' notions of physical appearance.

In the miracles associated with St Elisabeth this implicit notion of 'deficiency' is found sometimes, as when a girl with multiple impairments is described as 'disfigured'[212] by the growth of her lip, or a boy with multiple orthopaedic impairments is also portrayed as 'dreadfully and horribly'[213] disfigured by the witnesses. In other instances the pilgrims seeking cures are more explicitly referred to as 'defective'. A young boy was impaired by a hunched back, contorted neck, twisted feet and lame hands, and his father is said to have 'shrunk back as if from some monster' when he saw his son; in addition the boy had parts of his mouth 'twisted inhumanly'.[214] Another little boy had a hump growing out of his back and a growth on his chest, plus his legs had contracted, forcing him to lie for a year and three weeks 'like a monster'.[215] A woman suffering from nasal polyps was in so awful a condition that 'she appeared deformed' and even her own son became reluctant to share a house with her since she 'insulted people's senses of sight and smell'.[216] Similarly, a boy who was lame additionally suffered from a discharge of pus from the skin of his belly and his legs, so that the smell was 'hardly bearable'.[217] At Rocamadour, a woman called Stephana was cured who had been attacked by wolves, and mauled such 'that it was scarcely possible to recognize in her a human form ... She was terrifying to behold'. Stephana was abandoned by her community because the 'people decided that this deformed member had to be removed from the body as something useless and putrid'.[218] It is worth emphasising in the language of the story the imagery of surgical amputation, and also the analogy between society and the body (Stephana as the diseased member that needs to be removed from the body of the village community).

Other narratives also focus on the notion of a 'defect'. In the St James miracles, John the clerk's speech impairment is referred to as a 'defect of nature'[219] which required a cure by the 'creator of nature', and William, a boy from Reading, suffered from congenital impairment so that 'from his birth nature had so punished him by the awful laws of her indignation, that, with both legs shrunken, he was regarded as a spastic'.[220] Furthermore, concerning a girl from Suffolk, 'nature had so condemned this girl from birth'[221] that she appeared to have no firm bones in her legs. It is interesting to note that all three cases from the St James collection are described in terms of natural defects, whereby nature is to be seen in opposition to divine will or punishment: in other words, none of these people were impaired through any fault of their own, but solely due to the caprices of 'nature'. Analogous notions of 'nature' are also expressed in a story of St William: Huelina of Rochesburch had her heels adhering to her back by a 'vice of nature'[222] – in contrast to an impairment sustained by divine will. Also cured at Norwich was a woman called Matilda who had been afflicted since her youth by a 'sorrowful debility' whereby she had such an immense curvature of her spine that she was completely doubled up.[223]

St Foy cured a deaf-mute man named Stephen 'on whom nature herself had inflicted his defects while he was still in his mother's womb'[224] – again a view of impairment that does not imply some kind of justified divine intervention. In the same miracle story, a girl with multiple impairments is also described in terms of having sustained these due to 'nature': she had been 'thrust out of her mother's womb into the light blind, deaf and mute'[225] by nature, and in addition her hands were perpetually closed into fists. While her condition was caused by 'nature', her healing involved reshaping of her hands by the 'highest Craftsman'. However, in another of St Foy's miracle narratives, the congenital impairment of the protagonist is blamed on the mother. A man called Humbert was partially paralysed: 'His mother's livid nature had sent him forth from her womb in a condition in which his lower body, from the kidneys down, lay lifeless.'[226] This could be a reflection of the different views of the different authors of St Foy's miracles, since the first two cases mentioned occur in the second book, written by a named individual, Bernard of Angers, in the early eleventh century, while this latter case occurs in the fourth book, written by an anonymous author half a century later. In the narratives surrounding St Ithamar, a lengthy discussion is devoted to the miraculous cure of a woman who had been hearing impaired and completely mute since birth. Here, too, her affliction is described in terms of her being 'badly deformed by nature',[227] but the writer then embarks on an extensive justification of her cure. People might doubt such a miracle, the author surmises, because it might be impossible for a woman who had never uttered a word in her life to suddenly start speaking (an action which could be seen as 'contrary to nature'). Such potential doubters are referred to an analogy with the miracle of Balaam's ass[228] which spoke suddenly in a human voice; similarly, the mute woman could speak suddenly, because for God nothing is difficult, and nothing against nature is impossible to do for the author of nature.[229] Miracles then, after a fashion, are contrary to nature, but since God, as the 'author' of nature, can transcend nature, God or his saints can work such 'contrary' wonders.

Connected with notions of the 'defectiveness' of impaired people in the miracle narratives is the idea of liminality. The topos of liminality has already been discussed in the analysis of modern disability theories, where the liminal status of impaired people has been identified, first and foremost, by scholars working in the disciplines of anthropology and ethnography. I proposed elsewhere[230] that medieval impaired persons, too, could hold a liminal position, especially with regard to the incurability of their conditions; this means that impaired people were liminal in the sense that they occupied neither the category of being 'well' nor the category of being 'sick'. In general, liminality can be identified in spiritual terms in many cultures, whereby people, objects or places that occupy the territory between the boundaries of this world and the supernatural (or other world, or the next world, but always a metaphysical space) hold a liminal status. So in tribal religions a shaman or witch doctor might be an example of a liminal figure. The very word 'liminal' is derived from the Latin *limes*, meaning a boundary or border, as in the boundary of a temple or sacred site. By inference, liminality could also relate less metaphysically to being in-between, as in occupying a space between two different states of being, dead or alive, for example. It is this aspect of liminality that has been proposed for impaired people. As discussed in Chapter 3 on theory, impaired persons are neither sick nor healthy, their condition is not an illness that either disappears again, or gets worse and kills the individual, but a permanent, incurable state between the two categories of health and illness. In some of the medieval miracle narratives I have examined, precisely these notions of liminality may be encountered, whereby the protagonist falls between the two categories of alive and dead, of healthy and sick, and occupies a liminal position.

St Foy cured a man who was terribly injured in the face, whereby he lost the faculty of speech, and his wound was regarded as incurable. His condition was described as that of being 'half-alive'[231] for almost three months. St William partially healed a boy who had been unable to take a single step, and could not even move or turn himself, so that his condition was likened to that of one 'almost dead'.[232] Among the Rocamadour miracles one finds the story of a knight punished with epilepsy and paralysis for his transgressive behaviour. His condition is described in detail:

> Up until that moment this man seemed to be soaring through the clouds and considered himself second to no mortal being. But now he lies frothing at the mouth in agony. He gnashes his teeth, he contorts his mouth, and his eyes stare terrifyingly. He clenches his fists, and there is no use in his limbs *as if they were dead.* [my emphasis][233]

This is the man whose case was already discussed above in connection with transgression and punishment; he was cured, only to fall back into his immoral lifestyle again, and his affliction returned.

> In full view of the many people who were there he began to foam at the mouth and collapsed onto the ground, falling more heavily than he had done before. His right arm and right hand – the one he used to throw dice – became withered, as did the middle part of his body, which became paralysed. ... The man screamed that he would be fortunate if he departed this life, in that he had become *scorned by men and despised by the people.*[234] He said that he would have been better off if he had never drawn breath: better that than be afflicted by a destructive illness and daily die a hateful death.[235]

In another of the Rocamadour stories a youth suffers from a similar condition, only this time not in punishment. His whole body was desiccated and crippled. 'He was immobile, like a statue, and he could not feel anything. His eyes were permanently closed, his mouth was twisted back, and he could not do anything with his hands: he appeared to be dead yet did not die.'[236] He was just about breathing and 'was not properly alive', until his relatives made a life-size wax effigy of him to send to Rocamadour, which worked, because '[a]s soon as this was done, the youth came back to life'.[237] Further, a man called Gerald was immobilised by dropsy, to such an extent that 'Contrary to nature, or rather exceeding the bounds of what is natural, his bodily substance came to resemble soil, and he lay like a lopped tree. He was dead yet unable to die'.[238] These three narratives form as clear an expression as any of the liminality of an impaired person: they are alive yet daily die a death, they are dead yet do not die. In the miracles of St Godric one also finds such descriptions of the impaired as liminal figures. A boy with a general 'weakness' is described as being 'half-dead',[239] as is a girl whose body is swollen is in such a bad state that she is 'half-dead',[240] while a woman suffering from a tumour is also in the same state.[241] The liminality of impairment may also be expressed in other texts besides the miracle narratives I studied in detail. Finucane cites a case where doctors declared a patient to be dead who had lost his reason, sight, hearing, speech and breath.[242] Extreme cases of illness or injury, which need not necessarily have led to impairment, might also position the protagonist within a liminal category. In the Rocamadour miracles, for example, one Siger was run through the chest by a lance, resulting in a deep wound from which he suffered for almost a year. Siger barely remained alive 'if indeed this was alive, in that the loss of one's very nature may more properly be called death rather than life'[243] and even his friends eagerly awaited his death. Long-lasting, serious illness was therefore regarded in a similar fashion to chronic illness or impairment, and all these disorders could place the sufferer in a liminal state, somewhere between life and death.

As in the descriptions of impairments as 'defects', not all the writers of the miracle narratives share the same views, and similar physical conditions are not all described or labelled in similar fashion. So one might expect some of the severely impairing conditions detailed in the St Elisabeth accounts to be also regarded as liminal, but there the writer makes no mention of such a state. Nevertheless, those miracle narratives that do touch on the liminality of the impaired make the point very strongly, and such evidence permits the conclusion that modern anthropological/ethnographical theories of liminality may be transposed to discussions of medieval notions on the impaired as liminal figures.[244]

Next I will address the issue of the impaired as disabled, by looking at narratives of inability in the *miraculae*. In the chapter on modern and medieval theories of the body and of disability, I had emphasised the difference between 'impairment' and 'disability', pointing out that impairment is a physical condition, whereas disability is a socio-economic state. One of the questions my research raises is to enquire whether one can actually refer to medieval people with impairments as 'disabled' persons. To that extent I had examined and criticised the theories of a modern disability studies scholar, Brendan Gleeson, who had claimed that for socio-economic reasons, impaired people would not have been 'disabled' in the modern sense – the medieval economic system, and pre-industrial, pre-capitalist societies in general, Gleeson had claimed, allowed greater scope for impaired people that did not render them 'disabled'. It is striking, then, to find just such modern notions of 'disability', whereby the inability to fully function physically, or to perform tasks related to work,[245] are the criteria for labelling an individual 'disabled', in some of the medieval *miraculae*, even though, of course, these sources do not employ the actual word 'disabled'.

In the St Gall *vitae*[246] a crippled man (*paraliticus*) was so contracted together that he could no longer walk by his own means: the implication being that this man had to rely on (unspecified) mobility aids or on the help of other people to get around. A miracle of St Foy describes the case of a girl who was unable to work properly due to her impairment. 'Her body was completely drawn together and she didn't have the strength to let go of the tools of her loom – the very shuttle was held fast in her clenched hand.'[247] Another girl also had contracted hands which prior to her miracle cure had been 'inflexible and not suited for work'.[248] And in the Rocamadour narratives, Godfrey the son of Count Hartman in Germany had an illness in his legs for over a year which so debilitated him that he was confined to his room.[249] Two of St Ithamar's cases were victims of a weakening illness, which appears to have confined them to their sickbed.[250] Similarly, a woman cured at Reading was confined to her bed for two years because she was bent up and shrunken (*curva et contracta*).[251] Another Reading case revolved around a monk with a withered hand which he 'could neither raise...nor keep hold of anything he might grasp'.[252] St William's miracles mention a woman whose swollen knees meant she could no longer walk,[253] and a boy who was weak in all his body so that he was 'deprived of the use of his limbs'.[254] Finucane mentions a miracle recorded in 1282 at the canonisation process of Louis IX, where a girl was cured who had not walked until the age of four and a half (when her father took her to the tomb of Louis IX) even when she was given crutches by her father: she fell over 'like a lump of wood' as soon as her father left her unsupported, although he tried this 'more than a thousand times'.[255]

More implicit inability is mentioned in the miracle accounts of St Godric and St Elisabeth. St Godric, while still alive, cured one of the monastic brothers of a swollen foot which had affected the monk so badly he could barely get up out of his bed,[256] and Godric himself became afflicted in his old age by a condition that meant he had to use a 'triple stick' (*baculo tripes*) to get in and out of his oratory, but also relying on the hands of others to lay him down and carry him.[257] St Godric's relics cured a cleric of pains in the legs which had rendered him unable to walk,[258] and a man with contracted knees who had been deprived of the use of all his members,[259] while in two other cases the loss of function of a limb is mentioned.[260] A woman's hands were so contracted from birth that she could not move any object,[261] while another woman was both unable to use her hands and unable to walk.[262] St Elisabeth's pilgrims were also described as implicitly having lost the ability to make use of their limbs. A girl's hand was so swollen she could barely make any use of it,[263] another girl's legs and feet were swollen so that she could not walk,[264] yet a third girl's limbs were so weak she could no longer stand on her feet,[265] and a boy was lame in all limbs below the liver, so that wherever he was laid down he remained unless he was able to crawl with his hands.[266] Lastly, a man was so crippled he could not sit properly, and could not move about at all unless with the aid of crutches.[267]

What may be regarded as more explicit reference to the inability of the impaired person is, however, also a theme in the miracle narratives. Several of the sources I have studied make such references, though it is predominantly the

St Godric and St Elisabeth accounts that provide the greatest detail. St Godric's miracles, even in their short textual forms, refer to the two main aspects of 'disability' that the medieval sources emphasise again and again: the inability to work, and the dependency on help for mobility provided by other people. For example, he cured a woman who could do no work for three years because of her paralysis,[268] and a woman with an impairment in her feet who could not go anywhere, apart from with the help of other people.[269] Another woman, who was incapable of moving her arms, legs and entire body for five years, was unable to move herself without the aid of others.[270] Inability both of motion and of capacity to work come together in a woman who lost her ability to walk, nor was she able to move or could do any work properly.[271] A man with an incurable ulcer in his thigh was also unable to work or to move without aid from other people.[272]

Similar themes are found in the miracles of St Elisabeth. The inability to move unaided is expressed in several accounts, as is the dependency on others for help. A little boy was lame so that he could neither crawl nor walk, nor move himself,[273] while a little girl had lame legs and feet, so that from wherever she was placed she was unable to move herself, neither walking nor crawling,[274] and the son of a knight was completely immobilised due to a withering of his legs, consequently wherever he had been carried to he remained, unable to move.[275] A 13-year-old boy had been lame since birth, so that he could not walk at all and could barely sit with the help of a support, and additionally his hands and arms trembled so much that he could hardly eat and drink by himself, and even his eyes trembled.[276] A woman is described as bedridden due to 'weakness' which meant that she needed help from others if she had to move out of the bed,[277] and a 16-year-old girl who had lame arms and legs had to be moved, laid down and carried by other people.[278] A man aged about 40 had a withered leg, and could not move himself in any way; he is described as lying 'like [a piece of] wood'.[279] The inability to do work is also mentioned. A girl had lame legs and one lame arm due to some lumpy growths, and she could not keep her head upright any more, so that she could neither walk, nor stand nor sit; after four visits to the saint's tomb she could control her head movements again and use her limbs so that now she could walk, spin and do other work.[280] And a 40-year-old woman suffered from a 'weakness' in her hands, causing them to swell up and tremble constantly, so that when she was eating she could move her hands to her mouth only slowly and with difficulty; for four years she could do no work whatsoever. After the first two years of her impairment she was also afflicted by a second ailment, in that she completely lost her ability to walk and had to be carried by others.[281] Additionally, a youth had a 'weakness' in his legs and in his entire body, so that he could do no work and could walk only with difficulty, supported by crutches.[282] In one case of what we would term severe disability, the protocol writers do not even touch upon the issue of whether the protagonist can work or not, but simply describe the effects of physical impairment. A 12-year-old boy with severe multiple impairments had some mobility in a restricted fashion, but only by crawling along on his hands, and his ability to 'make use of' his limbs, as the sources often phrase it, was limited to using his mouth to carry objects.[283] Interestingly, it is only in the St Elisabeth narratives that one of the miracle stories details the loss of faculties and consequent inabilities for the visually impaired: a girl had such weakened eyesight that during a waning moon she could not see anything, and during a waxing moon she could see but a little; in addition, she could not follow the path she was meant to walk along.[284]

Some of the other *miraculae* also refer to the 'disabled' aspect of an impaired person. One of St Foy's miracles cures an old man who was very decrepit. This story provides more detail than most about the man's personal and economic circumstances as a result of his impairment, and is worth citing at length:

> From his youth he had been unable to use his arms and legs. In addition he suffered from a condition that had developed at the same time, namely that his limbs were stiff and unbending; he could neither move them to walk nor sit with any comfort. Since he suffered from such a physical impairment and had to struggle with it every day, he lacked any means of support and patiently joined the ranks of poor beggars.[285]

Here is a very explicit reference to the 'struggle' that physical impairment could bring with it, and the economic disadvantages. According to the modern theoretical criteria discussed above, this old man would be regarded as 'disabled' and not just as impaired. One of the St William miracles refers to an 8-year-old girl who from birth had suffered severely from 'gout' (*podagre ciragreque*) in her hands and feet, and a twisted neck. She was

> unable to raise herself or even to turn from one side to the other without assistance. To make matters worse, the sinews in her neck were contracted and her left cheek adhered so firmly to her left shoulder that you saw the one imbedded in the other, and the neck could not be bent in any direction whatever without bending the shoulder. All these afflictions therefore she suffered: walk she could not with her gouty feet, nor touch anything with her contracted hands, while the adherence of her head to the shoulder deprived her of the wonted power of seeing, standing, turning, nay, eating: for when she had to take food, it was cut up on the ground or on a trencher, and she lay down and fed like a beast, able only to eat what her tongue or teeth caught hold of. In this absolutely helpless state she was turned, raised, and moved about by others' help.[286]

Her story exemplifies another aspect of 'disability', namely the dependency on extraneous aids to fulfil 'normal' physical functions – whether such aid be in the form of other people providing help (as mainly the case in the medieval period) or in the form of technical aids (as in modern times). For the impaired person, 'disability' is then an issue when such aids are not available, insufficient, or, in the case of other people providing the help, unreliable or grudgingly given. The dependency on other's help is also emphasised in another of St William's miracles. A woman's sinews were all contracted so that her whole body was in a weakened state, and for many days she was unable to feed herself with her hands, nor walk on her feet.[287] The psychological or emotional problems that might be associated with 'disability' due to dependency on other people are hinted at in the text, when her condition before the miracle cure is contrasted with her 'able' state after the successful cure: 'And so, she who had come sad and in need of others' help, went away in joy trusting to her own feet'.[288]

Less dramatically, another case cured by St William mentions that a young boy was unable to make a single step, and for a long time had been incapable of moving or turning himself,[289] until after the miracle he could turn about unaided – again the dependency on extraneous help is emphasised. Similarly, a woman had been afflicted by gout so badly that she could only go to the tomb of the saint with difficulty and with the help of others, whereas after her cure she was able to go away alone.[290] Relating to the inability to work as well as to loss of motion is the case of a woman who suffered from an illness where her limbs were racked with pain, and she could not make a step without using a stick nor do any sort of work using her hands.[291] The impaired person as 'disabled' due to their 'uselessness' and as the object of pity for others is a theme encountered in one of the St James miracles. A girl had

> disabled her body and lost her agility. In fact, her left side from the sole of her foot to her shoulder had withered and lost all living movement. Her hand was shrunken and paralysed and hung motionless from her side close to her back. Her foot was bent round and, incapable of acting as a foot, was so twisted that (?her main foot bones took the place of her heel, her toes were in the place of the bones, and the nails of her shoe were where her toes should have been[292]). And the girl, being thus made useless to herself and pitiable to others, was harassed by her stepmother with many insults and taunted with abuse of various kinds.[293]

The 'evil'[294] stepmother sent the girl off to various shrines for unsuccessful cures, until the girl had a vision to go to Reading. The writer of the miracle narrative has the girl protest that she cannot go there because she is 'crippled and weak, ignorant of the way and penniless'[295] – in other words the girl's position as object of pity and dependency is highlighted. Needless to say, she was cured successfully in a spectacular fashion after finally getting to Reading.

One may conclude, then, that at least some of the more detailed miracle narratives describe the impaired person who is seeking a cure in such a way as to reflect notions that come close to our modern notion of 'disability'. The inability to possess the mobility needed for functions (such as feeding oneself, turning one's body around, sitting upright) that the able-bodied take for granted is recognised by some of these medieval texts to 'disable' the protagonist. So too is the (complete) inability to do any form of physical work – though one may wonder how this would have been described with regard to those classes of people (such as the nobility, or wealthy merchants) who did not have to rely on their own physical labour to make a living.

The notion of the impaired person as 'disabled' because they are incapable of doing something is closely linked in the sources with the idea that that person is a burden. However, it needs to be emphasised that the notion of the impaired person as burdensome is only reported by the sources, and is not actually endorsed by the writers of the miracle narratives. In fact, only four of the narratives studied even hint at the notion of the impaired person as a 'burden'.[296] It is, after all, an element of Christian charity to help the needy, and to an extent the miracle narratives function as texts exemplary of proper moral behaviour.

The miracles of St Foy relate the case of one Raymond, presumably a member of the nobility, since he had vassals, who had been injured terribly by a sword wound. He was carried home by his friends and vassals and watched over by them for almost three months. 'Because Raymond had sustained an incurable wound, his life was more of a loathsome burden than a pleasure to his friends.'[297] He did manage to get his friends to take him to Conques, however, where he was cured.

One of St Godric's miracles also mentions that the impaired person was a 'burden': a boy who was lame and mute appeared to be burdensome for his parents and all his friends.[298] And in the miracles of St James one finds the story of Gilbert, a keeper of hounds who was punished by sudden blindness for hunting on the saint's feast day.

> he began to become a burden to those among whom he had previously been very popular [*cepit fieri onerosus quibus prius fuerat gratiosus*]. In his adversity he found few friends, in his poverty very few, and in his blindness scarcely any physicians [*Raros enim amicos repperit adversitas, paucissimos paupertas, fere nullos medicantium cecitas*], as in the saying, 'when you are successful you will number many friends; in bad times you will be alone'. Bound by poverty and grief he sat in darkness[299]

His wife did not abandon him, and guided Gilbert around various shrines until he was cured at Reading. From another source there is also evidence for the perception of the impaired person as a 'burden' on their family or friends. Cured at the shrine of St Frideswide at Oxford, during mass, was one Mathilda, a girl of 17, who had lost her sight in both eyes for six years, and had been spurned by her relatives and friends.[300]

On occasion the impaired pilgrim regards himself as a burden or object of derision, as in the case of a young knightly man called William who became afflicted by contracted limbs. He toured the shrines of saints accompanied by two servants in the hope of finding a cure. 'Or, if he was not to be cured, he wanted to hasten his death through the hardships of travel. For it is said that members of the nobility deliberately prefer to exile themselves and leave home rather than to be viewed with disdain by their kin.'[301] It seems that his servants, too, had begun to regard William as a burden, because after having visited the Frankish, Germanic, Celtic, Belgic and Ligurian regions, they abandoned William on the way back from the shrine of St James (at Compostella). The suicidal tendency that is hinted at in this story – William travels to 'hasten his death' – is encountered in a few of the other narratives as well. In those stories no express mention is made of the perception of the impaired person as a 'burden' by others, but it is the impaired person who apparently feels that way. In the St Foy narratives is the case of another young noble, Rigaud, who was wounded severely and his arm was paralysed and numb. He became depressed and wanted to die 'rather than to drag out a disgusting and useless life with his body in such a shameful state'.[302] It appears that in the St Foy stories it is members of the knightly class who had most to lose by being physically impaired, since no mention is made of feelings of being a burden or wanting to die with regard to other groups of people in the St Foy collection.

That it may have been especially members of the upper classes who were (self-) conscious of the loss of physical ability through impairment is borne out by Ronald Finucane's research into miracle healings. Finucane noted that upper-class pilgrims were more likely to report miracles of a non-healing kind at the shrines they visited, rather than the cure of impairments or diseases; he surmised that this tendency of the nobility may have been associated with feelings of shame concerning their physical condition.[303] In the second edition of his work, Finucane briefly indicated that feelings of shame or embarrassment concerning physical impairment, illness or defect were also found among some urban popu-lations in central Italy, not just among the wealthiest, upper classes or nobility.[304] Also, a German scholar, Rudolf Hiestand, has pointed out that reactions to illness and impairment differed according to social status: the illnesses and impairments of rulers such as emperors and kings, and of the higher nobility, were concealed and marginalised by their contemporaries, whilst the lower classes, especially the peasantry, demonstrated no such reservations in acknowledging the phenomena of ill-health.[305]

However, among my sources, it is again a knight who expresses a death wish in another miracle collection, in a story from Rocamadour. The case of the young knight who was struck with epilepsy and paralysis has already been analysed twice, once in the context of impairment as punishment, and again in the limi-nality of impairment, but has yet a third facet to offer here. After his affliction returned, the man 'screamed that he would be fortunate if he departed this life, in that he had become *scorned by men and despised by the people* [Psalms 21:7]. He said that he would have been better off if he had never drawn breath: better that than be afflicted by a destructive illness and daily die a hateful death'.[306]

Perceptions of the impaired as a burden are therefore comparatively rare in the sources studied. Equally rare is the notion that the impaired person is an object of mockery, a figure to be made fun of by the able-bodied. Only four such instances were found in the narratives analysed by me. One case relates to a visually impaired man aged about 40 – he had developed spots (*macula*) over his eyes so that he could see only very little – who was cured by St Elisabeth. He is described as often straying off the path and wandering through the fields, for which he was laughed at by others going along the path.[307] In a miracle related to the Virgin, an elderly knight (he was about 60) who had four of his front teeth knocked out during a battle had them restored at Rocamadour. He was afraid of being made a mockery of for not being able to speak properly anymore: 'To prevent himself from becoming an incoherent-sounding object of universal derision, he eagerly prayed to the glorious Mother of God for the teeth to be restored.'[308] Speech and hearing impairments appear to have been especially problematic for the impaired individual concerned. In another instance, a woman who had been growing deaf with the passage of years was afraid of the social implications, as she perceived them, of her hearing impediment. In the miracle stories of St William, Alditha had been getting deaf over the years 'to such an extent that you could only make yourself heard by putting your lips close to her ear... She was consequently afraid to go out, and only talked to her own family, fearing lest the reproach of her deafness should be detected by others, and bring derision upon her'.[309]

It seems that the physical deteriorations of old age were in themselves something to be perceived of as derisory,[310] as the following story from St Foy's miracles shows. A 'little old woman' who had been afflicted in all her body by rheumatism was finally cured during a procession in honour of St Foy, after she at first had to endure the mockery of some young monks:

> The old woman had been carried down to the procession in a shabby litter, for she was poor and completely without means. She was lying there in the midst of the crowds violently pushing forward to converge on the statue [of Sainte Foy]. Although all around her people were rejoicing as they received the gift of health, she obtained no healing at all. She was simply an obstacle to the swarms of people. Finally some mischievous young men who belonged to the community of monks, most of whom knew her, came over to this poor, wretched woman and ridiculed her:
>
>> What are you doing here, stupid old woman? Why are you taking up space? Do you think that when boys and girls have been left behind, useful people of our age, Sainte Foy might heal a decrepit and useless old woman like you? Besides, what sort of health could be granted to you? You and your wrinkled, ugly skin and your feeble, grating voice would completely terrify a madman! Clear out of here now, you foolish woman. Don't spend the whole day deliriously cooing like a pigeon. You are already falling apart. You're in your final dotage, which is the most unhappy kind of disease – it's incurable, and now you ask to be cured![311]

Needless to say, after being denounced by the young monks, the woman miraculously leapt up from her litter and was able to walk again. The writer of the miracle narrative made full use of this story for moralistic and edifying purposes, comparing the cure of the old woman to some of Christ's cures,[312] and pointing out to the reader that partly the purpose of this miracle was to teach a lesson to those people mocking the old woman: 'But now the Compassionate One looked on her and He wanted at least to confound those who were deriding her, so He helped her on her bed of sorrow' [Psalms 40:4 (41:3)].[313] It is interesting to note that the writer also touched on the question of whether the old woman had become impaired due to a sin of hers, or whether her condition had come about so that divine 'works might be shown in her'[314] – a rhetorical question the writer left unanswered.

If the impaired were (sometimes) regarded as a 'burden', and part of the condition of physical impairment encompassed bodily and/or socio-economic inability, as has already been discussed, it should not be surprising to find that the sources make some mention of the poverty of the impaired supplicant. Overall, the poverty of an impaired pilgrim is not mentioned too frequently – only about 18 cases out of the total of more than 400 studied – so one should not assume that *all* impaired people seeking a cure at shrines were *automatically* flung into poverty and dependence by their physical condition. Too often modern scholars, especially those from the discipline of the history of medicine, have simply equated physical impairment with poverty during the Middle Ages, and modern textbooks on the whole dismiss the medieval 'disabled' person as economically impaired as well: all physically impaired people were apparently beggars, in this view. Other factors, such as support from family or friends, or independent economic and financial means, which are occasionally mentioned in the texts (see also later in the section on charity), would have prevented poverty in most cases. Where the pauper status of a pilgrim is mentioned, it is therefore useful to look at that individual's full story, if the text goes into that much detail, to analyse the circumstances, such as type of physical impairment, age, or life history, that led to the person's poverty.

Mobility problems and orthopaedic impairments were the most common impairments cured at saints' shrines, so one would expect to find a mention of large numbers of crippled beggars. However, the material condition of a mobility-impaired person as 'poor' or being a beggar is not alluded to very often in the sources. One example concerns a man who had been unable to use his arms and legs since his youth, and who additionally had stiff and unbending limbs; this man, however, is also described as 'very decrepit and extremely aged'.[315] He was impaired to such an extent that he could not walk or sit with comfort, and the text in this instance draws a link between the man's physical condition and his poverty: 'Since he suffered from such a physical impairment and had to struggle with it every day, he lacked any means of support and patiently joined the ranks of poor beggars.'[316] Another mobility impaired man mentioned in the sources was also afflicted from an early stage on in his life. This man, in fact had been born severely contracted, with one foot going backwards and the other foot curved back and bandaged to his thigh,[317] softened bone in his shins, and a deformed hand. In the miracles of St Godric, this man is described as crawling on hand-trestles ('two stools': *scamnis duobus*) and begging for a living for many years.[318] Congenital orthopaedic impairment also was an issue in the case of a boy from Norwich, who from infancy had been contracted. The narrative of St William states that the boy had lived there for many years and begged at many houses there, 'kneeling on his knees and getting about by trestles which he held in his hands: for the power of walking was denied him, inasmuch as his sinews were dried up, his knees contracted, and his calves wasted away'.[319] While it seems, then, that congenital impairment may have been more likely than impairment sustained later in life to lead to poverty and dependence on alms, the severity of an impairment, irrespective of when acquired, was another factor. In the protocols relating to St Elisabeth we encounter a hunch-backed man from Frankfurt who had also been crippled for a year in such a fashion that he could not move unless he pulled himself forwards on his hands, dragging his legs behind him which were bent backwards and totally lame. This man is described as a beggar who had nothing, and openly begged for alms of the faithful in the church.[320] Three of the witnesses in the protocol referred to this man as a servant (*Diener*) whom they saw begging for necessities within the church – was he a metaphoric 'servant of God', or a domestic servant who had become unemployable for the duration of his impairment?

Continuing the topic of severe impairment, it seems that sensory, as opposed to motor, impairments were regarded as such severe cases, and their descriptions are often more detailed than those of the orthopaedic cases. One of the St Gall vitae mentions a multiply impaired man – he was both deaf and mute (*surdus et mutus*) – who begged for his sustenance by rattling with two wax tablets which he always carried about with him.[321] Regrettably, this source is silent on one of the most intriguing aspects of the story: the use of wax tablets. Is it possible that this man possessed wax tablets for the purposes of communicating with other people, to draw or even write things? Why did the man not simply rattle two plain pieces of wood, if that was all the tablets were used for? The double affliction of hearing and speech impairments is also a factor in the story of a woman in the miracles of St Ithamar. This woman is described as being 'poor in material things but rich in faith...young but badly deformed by nature',[322] due to her complete inability to speak and partial deafness. Poverty, as in the need to beg for sustenance, is also mentioned in the case of another speech and hearing-impaired woman in the Rocamadour miracles.

> For a long time Polilia, who was deaf and dumb and came from Périgueux, lived in the village of Rocamadour with a poor woman called Juliana. When she wanted to get food, whatever she could come by, she used to stand outside the doors of the villagers' dwellings, tapping on the doorposts or the doors themselves and not stopping until the inhabitants were moved by her wretchedness to take pity on her.[323]

An interesting aspect of the communication problems for the speech impaired is also mentioned in this story, in that able-bodied people can verbalise their wishes and vows to a saint, whereas Polilia has to sigh in the direction of the shrine: 'it was with weeping and moaning that she expressed herself because she could not speak'.[324] The special problems posed for the hearing- or speech-impaired are mentioned elsewhere as well. In a narrative of St Foy, a man called Gozmar who was mute is described as asking for alms 'by moving his lips',[325] the implication being that he was unable to make any sound. A late thirteenth-century mute boy who had to beg is also mentioned by Finucane in his study of child healing miracles: this boy called John had to push food down his throat with two of his fingers since he lacked a tongue. He apparently 'grew up knowing nothing about his parents', so one may presume he was forced to beg primarily because of his familial situation and not necessarily due to his impairment.[326]

With regard to blindness as a contributory factor to the poverty of the supplicant, one example is found in the miracles of St James. Gilbert who had been a keeper of hounds was punished with blindness for a transgression, and his blindness is described as an 'adversity' in which he 'found few friends, in his poverty very few, and in his blindness scarcely any physicians'.[327] Not only was Gilbert poor, but the potential support of his friends did not materialise either, so that '[b]ound by poverty and grief he sat in darkness'.[328] In other cases, the impaired person was luckier, in that they had a support network to rely on. Such support could come from individuals, from family, friends or compassionate strangers, or from an institution like a monastery or hospital. An example of private support may be encountered in one of the miracles of St William. There one finds the account of Gurwan the tanner, who in the days of famine and pestilence had in his house a blind man, along with other poor persons.[329] The blind man is classed as one of the poor people, and while the condition of the other paupers is not specified, they appear not to have been physically impaired, since the text goes on to relate solely the healing of the blind man, and not that of the other lodgers in Gurwan's house.

Support, in the widest sense, from the village community might be the case, as in the story of a 9-year-old girl with a hunch back and swellings in her legs, who had to wander around the village begging for alms.[330] An example of some basic measures of public support is found in the miracles of St Foy. Though physical impairment need not invariably have caused poverty, it does seem to have been the case that those of the impaired who were destitute often relied on direct support by pilgrims and indirect support by the clergy, as happened at Conques. A little boy of almost 5 years of age was the victim of a feud, set upon in an act of vendetta by the relatives of a man the boy's fugitive father had killed. In this attack the pupils of his eyes were pierced with pointed sticks and he was left for dead by his assailants. Other villagers rescued the boy, and took him to the door of St Foy's church, where he was instructed 'that with the others who were sick or injured he should beg alms from the people coming to pray. For several months he sought contributions there'.[331] The narrative just briefly states that after his miraculous cure, the boy lived from monastic support for the rest of his life. What is noteworthy in this story, is that the boy's physical impairment alone may not have been the crucial factor for his dependence on the charity of others: the story mentioned that his father was a fugitive, so the boy's family would have lacked one of its main income providers, even before the little boy became impaired. In another case, a paralysed man named Humbert was brought to Conques by his parents, and then apparently deliberately left there by them, to rely on pilgrim and monastic support, spending many years at the shrine supported by alms.[332] At other shrines, too, destitute impaired people could be supported by alms from pilgrims. This happened at Rocamadour, where one Gerbert of Creysse, who was crippled and had had himself carried to the shrine in a basket, begged for food from other pilgrims.[333] Support of the impaired and charitable actions towards them are also mentioned in other sources besides the miracle narratives I have studied in detail. Ronald Finucane cites a family who put up 20 of Thomas Becket's pilgrims, a Canterbury baker who cared for impoverished and sick pilgrims, citizens of Lincoln who supported poor pilgrims, and, more specifically in relation to impairment, one Samson of Old Sarum who cared for a paralysed man for a year.[334] However, such charitable actions could be limited according to the resources and the attitude of the benefactor: Samson had to abandon the paralysed man at the city gate (where the ill usually lay, as Finucane states) after he was no longer financially able to support the man.[335]

After being cured, the economic circumstances of the supplicant might be improved, as in the case of the rheumatic 'little old woman' who was already mentioned above, in the context of an example of a derisory figure. After she was healed, she became a servant in the house of a respectable widow, since now 'she had ample strength to do her work'.[336] From the St Elisabeth miracles comes the case of a man who had been lame in his limbs (arms and legs) for over a year; after he had been healed, he no longer begged as before, but provided for himself through the work of his hands.[337]

Poverty and dependence on charitable support could also come about completely accidentally, not necessarily related to physical impairment, in other words. A paralysed girl should have been brought to the shrine of St Foy, but she was abandoned by those people who were meant to take her there – it is not made clear in the text why she was abandoned, and it would be an unsubstantiated assumption to think it was due to her impairment. She had to beg alms off passers-by for many days, until some members of the monastic community ordered that she be carried to the monastery. Like the small boy earlier, she seems to have begged alms outside the abbey church from visitors to St Foy's shrine.[338]

Apart from receiving direct material support, in the sense of sustenance and shelter, the impaired were sometimes singled out as the recipients of 'charity' in the wider sense. Charity, as one of the theological virtues, was of course part of every Christian's duty, and charitable acts towards the impaired, not surprisingly, therefore figure in the miracle stories. Several of the narratives emphasise the charity shown towards the impaired in the help provided them by friends, neighbours or even total strangers in actually getting to a shrine. A completely blind woman who had no one who would lead her to the shrine of St Elisabeth by chance found three women who did lead her there;[339] two blind people living in the same village were taken to the Virgin's shrine at Rocamadour by their neighbours;[340] and a warrior in the St Foy stories appeared to be particularly concerned about helping the speech-impaired: on three separate occasions he helped two mute men and a mute boy get to the saint's shrine.[341] Day-to-day help provided for impaired people could also be regarded as charitable, such as in the case of a woman mentioned in the St Elisabeth protocols. She had accidentally been lamed in one leg, and was often helped by one of the witnesses for the protocol (a male relative, friend or neighbour?) to the table of her master (*Dienstherrn*) by whose alms she was sustained.[342]

The gruesome story of Stephana, already encountered in the Rocamadour miracles, includes the charitable act of a knight who took in the injured Stephana and ensured she received medical treatment.[343] And in the St William narratives the text itself speaks of the *caritas* shown towards a severely mobility-impaired woman by one Peter, the priest of a village called Langham: he had 'long housed her by way of charity, and supplied her with food and clothing'.[344]

Other charitable acts could be provided by the saints themselves during their lifetimes. St Elisabeth, most notably, was famous for her concern for the sick, poor and destitute. An image on one of the decorated panels of St Elisabeth's shrine, dating from the mid-thirteenth century, depicts St Elisabeth distributing alms to the needy, who include an orthopaedically impaired man shown in the bottom left.[345] St Wiborada in her youth cared for and nursed the sick and the impaired (*aegrotos ac debiles*).[346]

Connected to the themes of charity, poverty and aid provided by other people, as already discussed, is the issue of transportation: how did impaired persons actually manage the often long and difficult pilgrimage to the site of a saint's cult? More often than not, if the sources mention modes of transport at all, travel by impaired people was heavily reliant on help given by other people, either in the form of financial support (paying for the impaired person's travel) or active support in mobility (carrying the mobility impaired, for example). Modes of transport to a shrine also shed some light on how impaired people may have travelled on other (unrelated) occasions, and it is for this reason as well that the sometimes detailed descriptions of how people travelled to a shrine are important. Details on transport seem to be provided by the texts mainly in unusual circumstances, in other words, when the mode of transport is interesting enough for the writer to warrant a special mention. The 'normal' method for a pilgrim to reach a shrine appears to be on foot, by walking, for reasons in part connected with the spiritual state of the pilgrim and religious convention, symbolising the humility of the pilgrim when approaching the saint for help. Finucane, who devotes but a single paragraph to issues of mobility and transportation in his entire earlier work on miracles, points out that even rich pilgrims who could afford horses 'usually dismounted to walk the last few miles of their journey, as an act of piety'.[347] So of course in those cases where pilgrims were unable to walk, the writers sometimes mention whichever alternative form of transport (such as handcart, horse or basket) was made used of. The emphasis placed on walking as the 'correct' way for a pilgrim to reach a shrine becomes apparent when one reads of those miracles where the impaired protagonist is singled out for praise by the writers for the effort they have undergone in walking, crawling or otherwise moving themselves by their own ability on their journey to the shrine. Examples are the cases of a woman called Matilda who struggled to reach Norwich and the shrine of St William on foot,[348] or the 16-year-old boy who set out for the tomb of St Elisabeth on crutches, who 'suffered constantly' and could therefore barely manage the ten miles from his home to the tomb in eight days.[349]

In the case of mobility or orthopaedically impaired people, the most frequent form of transport to a shrine was constituted by actually being carried there by other, able-bodied people. Most of the time, the sources purely mention that the protagonist was 'brought'[350] to the shrine without providing further information. However, on those occasions when more details are mentioned, the texts speak of the impaired person being 'carried' to the site, as in the case of a young woman at the shrine of St Elisabeth,[351] or a 9-year-old boy who was carried to the same site,[352] or a 'poor girl who had been crippled in all her joints and had been carried to Ste Foy's monastery'.[353] Interestingly, it was not always just the mobility-impaired who were carried: from the St Gall *vitae* comes a case of a girl who was blind from birth, who was carried to the monastery by her mother.[354] How exactly people were 'carried' is sometimes detailed a bit further: a 9-year-old girl was carried by her father in a basket on his back to St Elisabeth's shrine.[355] Another girl taken to the same shrine on two occasions was first carried in a small box or chest 'since she could not be transported any other way',[356] and then a year later, presumably because she had grown larger, she was carried in a different contraption 'which the porters of diverse goods use'.[357] An old woman was carried to a procession in honour of St Foy in a 'shabby litter, for she was poor and completely without means',[358] while in another case the monks of that saint ordered that an abandoned paralysed girl be carried to the monastery on a pallet.[359] At Rocamadour, one Gerbert of Creysse arrived after having himself carried there in a basket.[360] Finucane also draws attention to the use of litters by impaired people, stating that at Hereford around 1290 one could have observed several litters on the floor of the cathedral, which pilgrims could have hired for a penny or more to be carried from nearby villages.[361] An illustration of transport by litter can be seen in the depiction of the admission of a sick man to the Hôtel Dieu at Paris;[362] a similar litter is also depicted in a miniature illustrating the healing of a paralytic by Christ.[363]

Transport could also be carried out by animals. An old man who had been mobility-impaired since his youth was helped to a procession in honour of St Foy by some young people who 'prepared a beast of burden to transport him, placed him on it, and conducted him to the town of Talizat'.[364] A lame boy who additionally suffered from severe trembling was taken to the tomb of St Elisabeth tied to the saddle of a horse.[365] A woman called Matilda who suffered from severe curvature of the spine used to be 'laid like a sack across a horse'[366] whenever she desired to visit a shrine. Finucane cites the example of a woman who was lifted by her family onto a special feather-cushioned saddle.[367] One of St Godric's pilgrims was a boy, unable to walk, who was brought on horseback.[368] A woman who became contracted was set on a horse with the help of her husband and some others, and brought to St William's shrine.[369]

Several instances of vehicular transport of the impaired are mentioned in the miracle protocols of St Elisabeth. A woman impaired by 'weakness' was carried to the shrine in a carriage, which broke down en route, but by this stage she was recovering already so that she could continue her pilgrimage using two crutches.[370] Another woman suffering from 'weakness' was also taken to that shrine in a vehicle, and carried the last stage from the vehicle to the tomb itself,[371] as was the case for a young man, who was taken by his brother in a vehicle drawn by two horses (*Zweigespann*) up to the portal of the basilica, from where he was carried to the actual tomb.[372] A severely mobility-impaired young man was placed in a wagon for the outward journey, and because he was only partially cured, he had to return home in a two-wheeled carriage.[373] Two crippled boys from the same village were placed in a cart and taken to the tomb.[374] In the miracle narratives of other saints, further details of transport can also be found. In the St Gall *vitae*, a man who had become blind and deaf was brought to the tomb in a cart,[375] and a lame and crippled boy from Orléans travelled with his father on a small push-cart (*Schiebkarren*) first to Rome and subsequently to St Gall, where he was healed in 864.[376] Another case of a pilgrim being brought to the shrine in a contraption like a wheelbarrow comes from the St William narratives. There, a 10-year-old boy with curved spine and a humped back was brought to Norwich in a hand-barrow (*manuali uehitur uehiculo*).[377] Finucane mentions two instances from the miracles of St Thomas Cantilupe where supplicants were brought to the shrine in a wheelbarrow: a person from London was pushed all the way to Evesham in a barrow 'with one wheel and two feet', and around 1300 a person was transported by wheelbarrow from London to Hereford.[378] An illustration of using a wheelbarrow to transport an impaired man can be found, most famously, in the Luttrell psalter, dating from the early fourteenth century.[379] The daughter of a peasant was carried by her father to the shrine of St Foy on a horse-drawn pallet.[380] A supplicant to St Godric was a woman who was unable to walk; she was brought in a cart with a driver.[381] Furthermore, an impaired girl was brought to Norwich by her father 'in a wheeled vehicle of the kind called a litter (*civière*)',[382] and on the same day her miracle cure occurred, a lame boy was brought by his father 'also in a litter with wheels'.[383] From the Hand of St James miracles we hear of the case of a woman from the Oxford area who had been bent and contracted (*curva et contracta*), so that she was bedridden; she was set in a two-wheeled carriage by her brother and sent to Reading.[384] On the way there she was cured and arrived at Reading on foot. This miracle seems to exemplify the notion, discussed above, of the special circumstances requiring a supplicant to have need of some form of transport other than their own feet (or foot): a proper pilgrim should ideally make the journey by walking.

An example of the effort undergone by the supplicant when they do attempt the pilgrimage by walking, despite their impairment, can be found in the story of Matilda in the miracles of St William. She had a severe spinal curvature, and had been taken to other shrines, unsuccessfully, on horseback, without obtaining a cure. She finally decided to make the journey to St William's shrine at Norwich, setting out with her stick as mobility aid. 'Each step was hardly a finger's length, and there was considerable delay between them, so that one watching her progress would judge her to be slower than any tortoise.'[385] When she finally got to the cathedral, she felt the soles of her feet 'pricked as if by thorns',[386] and then in front of the shrine she was racked by pain, so that she writhed and rolled on the ground, after which she managed to get up, and still feeble, made her way along the screen of the shrine by clinging to the shafts, until she reached the tomb itself.[387] Perhaps the fact that she was cured after making the last pilgrimage on foot, with great effort, is significant: the moral of her miracle story could be that being taken to a shrine on horseback is 'too easy' and she may not have deserved a cure until making a suitable effort herself.

The survey of modes of transport used by the impaired to travel to a shrine demonstrates the widely differing types of mobility experienced by the supplicants. Undoubtedly social status and economic position was reflected in the mode of transport used, so that those lower down the social and financial scale were more likely to use the 'cheaper' alternative of being carried by a relative or friend, while those with more material means had access to horse-drawn vehicles.[388] The wide variety of modes of transport also shows how people tried to make do according to their circumstances. In a period such as the Middle Ages, before the invention of the wheelchair, mobility of the impaired was not necessarily curtailed or restricted, but relied on improvisation, making the most use of already existing transportation methods – the carts, baskets and handbarrows mentioned in the sources – and adapting them for the specific needs of the impaired person.

Having discussed the question of how impaired people made the often long journeys to the shrines and tombs of the saints whose aid they sought, it is worthwhile to examine the day-to-day, personal mobility of those same supplicants. The sources sometimes mention how impaired people moved (or could not move, as the case might be) in their home environment, prior to receiving their miraculous cure. These texts allow us to gain some understanding, therefore, of how mobile, for example, an orthopaedically impaired person was, or of how visually impaired people managed to negotiate their surroundings. Mobility is one of the key issues in modern disability politics, since access, or lack thereof, to public buildings and spaces constitutes one form of restriction imposed on the modern disabled person. Examining the issue of personal mobility is therefore an important aspect of gaining some understanding of the overall lived experience of medieval impaired persons.

Personal mobility with regard to orthopaedic impairments is most frequently mentioned by the sources, not surprisingly, since the overwhelming majority of conditions pilgrims were described as having can be classified as mobility impairments (see Table 2 on p. 133). Crutches, either described as such, or simply referred to as 'sticks', were the most frequently utilised method of mobility aid for the orthopaedically impaired. Finucane, in his study of miracles and pilgrims, briefly mentions the use of walking-sticks and crutches by supplicants, including a pair of padded crutches presented to an impaired boy by a Lincoln priest, so that the boy's skin would not be damaged.[389] One Thomas of York, weak throughout his body, came to the shrine at Norwich 'who guided his steps and supported his feet and frame on two sticks such as are commonly called crutches'.[390] A congenitally impaired man named Humbert 'cast aside the crutches of a paralytic, which he had formerly used when he needed to go somewhere' after his cure at Conques.[391] A woman cured at Norwich suffered from painful limbs and could not make a step without using a stick,[392] while the woman Matilda, discussed above for her efforts in getting to the shrine on foot, normally used a stick for mobility: 'when she wished to go from one place to another she had to support her feeble limbs with a stick and either succeed in getting a little way, or, sometimes, was not able to do even this'.[393] A woman already partially cured before seeking the aid of St Godric used a stick in one hand,[394] while another woman in the same text could not move without a crutch for support.[395] A youth impaired after an accident was unable to walk without the support of two sticks, one under each armpit,[396] as was a man who had been so twisted for nine years that he also needed two crutches,[397] while another youth needed just a single crutch.[398] A woman who had been contorted and twisted in her spine for 22 years arrived at St Godric's shrine on two crutches, dragging herself forwards 'as if on four feet'.[399] Many cases are mentioned in the miracles of St Elisabeth. Some examples include a 12-year-old boy whose bent and foreshortened leg could not touch the ground so that he needed to move around with the aid of a stick,[400] or the boy who could barely sit using an unspecified support, but could walk with the aid of one crutch after a partial cure,[401] or again a man of about thirty who started on his pilgrimage propped up on two crutches.[402] One man who had been lame for almost three years nevertheless managed to reach the tomb of St Elisabeth on his crutches, which he threw away after his cure.[403]

Other objects of everyday life could also be used as supports or mobility aids by impaired people. Again, the following examples are from the miracles of St Elisabeth. After a partial cure, a young man began to upright himself by holding onto a fence and onto other supports and started walking in this fashion.[404] A 5-year-old boy who was lame in all his limbs below the liver was initially only able to crawl with his hands, but after a vow by his mother he began to upright himself holding onto chairs.[405] In the same collection of miracles, an interesting point is made about the adaptation of mobility aids for the specific needs of the impaired individual: a man of about 50 was so crippled in one leg that he could only drag himself about with the aid of two 'specially manufactured' crutches, without which he could not move at all, or else he crawled about in his house.[406] The implication seems to be that this man used his mobility aids for going out, but for one reason or another found it preferable to move around his home environment by crawling.

Besides crutches and sticks, the other most frequently mentioned mobility aids, especially for those people with severe spinal and other orthopaedic impairments, were the so-called hand-trestles.[407] A depiction of this mobility-aid can be seen on the shrine of St Elisabeth itself, where the crippled man receiving alms from St Elisabeth is using hand-trestles.[408] A poor woman who had been bent double came to Norwich with trestles which she held in her hands,[409] and also at Norwich was the case of a boy who begged for his living, 'kneeling on his knees and getting about by trestles which he held in his hands'.[410] A boy who was brought to the Norwich shrine in a litter by his father, 'when forced to move himself, he crept along on his knees, leaning on hand-trestles'.[411] A congenitally impaired man in the St Godric miracles, who had one foot twisted backwards, and whose shins were pliable like marrow without bones, crawled on two 'stools' (*scamnis duobus repens*) and was thus 'carried by his hands from place to place' (*manibus de loco ad locum ferebatur*).[412]

One of the most interesting devices used for a mobility aid seems to have been utilised by one of the saints himself. St Godric, in his old age, suffered from a condition that prevented him from moving in or out of his Oratory unaided. He was supported by a 'triple stick' (*sustentante baculo tripes*),[413] which appears to be a more sophisticated contraption than an ordinary set of crutches. Depictions in illuminated manuscripts sometimes show a device that would fit the 'triple stick' description, but in this case used by infants, as a baby walker.[414] These are three- or four-legged frames, on wheels, which remind one of a modern-day Zimmer frame. Such a three-wheeled walker can be found depicted in a marginal illumination.[415] Interestingly, one manuscript illustration shows just such a type of baby walker, but adapted for height and width, being used by an old woman. This image stems from the fourteenth-century *Hours* of François de Guise.[416] Furthermore, a satirical image on a tapestry, dating from around 1390, depicts a young man, struck down by lovesickness and thereby rendered 'like an infant', also using such a Zimmer frame-type walker.[417] It therefore seems entirely plausible that St Godric's 'triple stick' is a reference to one such adapted baby walker used by an elderly person, in the fashion a modern Zimmer frame would be.

Mobility aid for the orthopaedically impaired could also be provided, as in the case of the visually impaired discussed later, in the form of being led by other people and supported directly by other persons. This was necessary for a woman with pains in her knees who was led to Norwich, where she was cured: 'Thus it came to pass that she who came with her feeble body by the hands of others, when the heavenly medicine did its work, went back safe and sound needing no man's support.'[418] Another woman cured at Norwich 'came supported on one side by her husband Siwate, and on the other by some one else'; the Latin text (*sustentata brachiis*) seems to indicate that she was propped up under her arms by her two helpers.[419] Children, presumably because of their smaller physical size relative to adults, were sometimes carried by their parents or caregivers, as in two examples cited by Finucane: a crippled girl was carried about by her mother on her back or in her arms,[420] in the case of a family destitute enough to beg, and in a wealthier situation, the paralysed daughter of a French seigneur was carried about by her father's squire.[421]

Sometimes the orthopaedically impaired person had no mobility aid to rely on at all, instead having to move around as best as their physical ability would allow them to do. This was the case for a 10-year-old boy who was contracted and hump-backed, so that 'when he wanted to walk, he had to place his hands on his knees or on the ground, and use one or the other for a support'.[422] Another boy, six years old, was also very contracted and could not walk upright, but only if he supported himself with his hands on his knees and bent his head down as far as his knees.[423] In the miracles of St Elisabeth we encounter a hunch-backed man who had become crippled in such a fashion that he could not move, unless he pulled himself forwards on his hands, dragging his legs behind him which were bent backwards and totally lame; after his cure he still needed to prop himself up a little on a stick.[424] Also in the St Elisabeth text is the story of a boy who became unable to walk anymore, due to becoming 'crooked', unless he crawled on his knees and supported himself with his hands.[425] One of the most dramatic descriptions of how a severely impaired person, likened to a 'monster' by the writer, managed to remain mobile is encountered in the same text. A 12-year-old boy, with a hunched back, contorted neck, twisted feet and lame hands had to crawl along on his hands; he was furthermore unable to hold anything, so that everything he was given he carried in his mouth.[426] One may imagine this boy's condition, especially his inability to grasp hold of any objects, to have been similar to that of an impaired beggar depicted in the margins of an illuminated manuscript, who is shown carrying a begging bowl in his mouth – except that this beggar was able to crawl along on hand-trestles.[427] After a gradual cure the boy's legs and knees loosened, and he began crawling 'which he had been unable to do in any way previously',[428] until after another stage in his healing, he was able to support himself on a staff. A severely contracted girl in the St Godric text had to place her knees on the ground for feet if she had to go anywhere at any time.[429] Also in the St Godric text is the case of a man 'who for eleven years had been incapacitated by a weakness of one foot, so that he went about one-legged (*monipes*), not walking but rather through crawling drawing himself forwards (*non gradiens sed potius rependo se protrahens*); he supported all the bulk of the body with the help of the other foot (*alterius pedis totam corporis molem supportabat auxilio*)'.[430] After his cure this man was described as not even needing 'the support of any crutch (*sine omni baculi adminiculo*)',[431] somewhat ironically, since he apparently had no access to a crutch during the period of his impairment.

The texts studied occasionally mention how the visually impaired coped with questions of mobility. Virtually all the mentions of mobility of the visually impaired relate to their arrival at the shrine in question, but since those are the only textual references, and one must infer from these few examples how mobile the visually impaired were in their home surroundings, they have been included here as aspects of personal mobility rather than in the section on transport modes. In the St Foy narratives, a small boy who had been blinded was led by other people to the altar, where he recovered his sight,[432] and a warrior recovered his sight when he was led away from the church after mass,[433] while a widow recovered hers when 'a boy led her by the hand to the holy virgin's abbey church'.[434] Gerbert, who featured in several of St Foy's miracles, had to be led by a stranger to the church for his cure,[435] while a middle-aged man who had become blind overnight was first led home by a guide summoned for him, and subsequently was guided by his small son to the shrine.[436] In the St Elisabeth protocols, a blind woman stated that she had to be led by the hands wherever she went,[437] and a 15-year-old girl had to be led from place to place.[438] Another blind woman said she had no one who would lead her to St Elisabeth's tomb, but she was lucky in that by chance she found three women who did lead her there.[439] An 8-year-old boy with multiple impairments – he was blind, lame and hunchbacked – was led to the tomb by his father.[440] Also led by the father was a blind woman in the St Godric stories,[441] while a man with congenital blindness was just described as being led by others.[442] In the St James text, a man who was punished with blindness had no one other than his wife to lead him around the various shrines.[443]

The Rocamadour narrative mentions three blind people, two of whom were led by their neighbours, while the third was led by his father.[444] At Norwich, we hear of one Ravenilda who was blind and came to the tomb led by another.[445] Another of the St William cases is more detailed: a woman called Gilliva, having been blinded through an accident, came to Norwich guided by her young nephew, who gave her some string and went before her.[446] A most interesting case where the impaired have to rely on and help each other is cited in the St Gall *vitae*, where a lame man (*contractus*) crawling along on his hands led a blind man to the paupers' hostel (*hospitium pauperum*) where both of them stayed until they were cured.[447]

The main method, then, of mobility for the visually impaired consisted of being led by another person. The visually impaired were therefore heavily reliant on mobility aid provided by other people, unlike the orthopaedically impaired, who could use various contraptions on their own accord, without complete dependence on other people. A case where a person who was not physically mobility-impaired was nevertheless aided is cited in the St Ithamar narrative: there a boy who was both mute and deaf was led to the shrine.[448]

In summary, personal mobility, much like the modes of transport used to reach the site of shrines, differed according to the specific needs of an impaired person as well as according to their economic means. If someone was still capable of walking a little, they may have just needed one support, while others needed two crutches, or had to use hand-trestles. The severely impaired people who are described as having to move around by crawling probably had to use this form of mobility not because of negative attitudes to them, or because of economic hardship, but more likely due to the technical limitations of the period in which they lived. It seems that, as in the modes of transport, already existing and therefore familiar objects were modified to act as mobility aids. However, specially designed, 'tailor made' mobility aids will not have been available to all the supplicants, and people made do with whatever objects could be used for the purpose (ordinary sticks instead of the Zimmer frame-like 'triple stick' of St Godric, for example). To a large extent, therefore, and especially so in the case of the visually impaired, personal mobility was dependent on the aid provided by other people – family, friends and neighbours, or even complete strangers.

Because questions of mobility may have made it very difficult for an impaired pilgrim to reach a particular shrine, I will also discuss 'distance' cures, that is cures through votives or by proxy. Votive offerings were sometimes sufficient to heal an impaired supplicant, though at other times the supplicant had to present both a votive offering and make the journey to the shrine in person for a cure to be effective. Votive offerings appear to have a long history: Gregory of Tours already described the pagan sixth-century shrine which the young St Gallus of Clermont found near Cologne; in it there were wooden models of parts of the human body placed there by the 'barbarian' supplicants 'whenever some part of their body was in pain'.[449] In England, Ælfric described the scene at St Swithun's shrine at Winchester, where in the church were votive offerings. The church itself was 'hung all round with crutches (*mid criccum*), and with the stools of cripples who had been healed there from one end to the other on either side of the wall, and not even so could they put half of them up'.[450] Hugh le Barber, who had been barber to the future saint Thomas Cantilupe, related at Cantilupe's canonisation investigation of 1307 how, when he was going blind due to old age, he sent two wax images of his eyes to Hereford to the tomb of his former employer, finally going on pilgrimage to the shrine. With each donation his sight improved, until he was able to play chess again and read the dots on dice.[451] In another case, one John Combe was struck in 1414 with a large stick during a sports game, so that his head was broken open and his shoulder smashed, and in addition he was rendered deaf and blind. He had been bedridden for three months when he received a vision instructing him to have a model made in wax of his head and shoulders, which was to be taken to the tomb of bishop Osmund at Salisbury; John Combe was to pray there as well and offer up the votive image. He did as told and was cured.[452]

In the sources studied in detail one also finds instances of votive offerings left by the supplicants. At Finchale, a woman offered her crutch to St Godric after she had been cured successfully,[453] as did another woman who placed her crutch on the altar after being healed,[454] and a youth placed his crutch at the same shrine in testimony of his healing.[455] At Norwich, too, a mobility impaired man left his crutches there in token of his cure.[456] At Marburg, a man cured after a third visit to St Elisabeth left his sticks behind at the tomb.[457] Votive offerings could also bring about the desired cure. Again at Marburg there are two cases of blind women who obtained a cure after they had made votive offerings in a shape similar to their eyes;[458] one of these women, on regaining her sight, was able to recognise the wax images – the votive offerings left by other pilgrims – hanging above the tomb.[459] Two fifteenth-century images from the shrine of St Wolfgang at Pipping in Bavaria[460] may serve as illustrations. They give a good impression of what kinds of objects (crutches, wax models of body parts) pilgrims presented at a shrine.

Cures could also be effected by proxy. One such proxy was the pilgrim badge. Pilgrim badges were pressed against the relics, shrine or image they were meant to commemorate, which was done by the shrine keeper or the pilgrims themselves. Through this action of making direct physical contact the pilgrim souvenir could absorb some of the shrine's virtues and thaumaturgic powers. This belief in the transference of powers[461] from shrines or relics onto pilgrim signs first emerged in the twelfth century, following reports that people had been healed by souvenirs from the major pilgrimage sites at Compostela, Rocamadour and Canterbury. In the fifteenth century, the Dominican Felix Faber was asked by his friends to take their beads and rings with him on his pilgrimage to the Holy Land, so that he could press their trinkets against every relic and shrine he encountered en route, thereby transferring their healing power.[462] Pilgrim souvenirs therefore allowed curative attempts at spiritual medicine by proxy. 'Since a badge's protective benefits were not restricted to the pilgrim who purchased it, many souvenirs were brought back for sick or disabled relatives and friends who were unable to undertake the journey....'[463]

Proxies could also be other people who undertook the pilgrimage on behalf of the actual supplicant. In the cases of impairment studied here in detail, this situation seems to have arisen because of the severity of the supplicant's physical condition: they were too impaired to undertake the journey themselves, or more often than not they were small children, unable to travel in the first place as well as being impaired. Examples include the case of a congenitally blind boy, who was cured when his parents travelled to Rocamadour,[464] and the severely, multiple impaired boy who was cured gradually after first his father, and then on a second occasion his mother, had made visits to the shrine of St Elisabeth.[465] A woman who was unable to leave the house because of her mobility impairment was cured at home at the same time as her husband, who had made the pilgrimage to Norwich, was present at the shrine of St William.[466] The dangers which sometimes long or difficult journeys posed to the impaired supplicant were recognised by contemporaries, as the following story exemplifies: the parents of a girl who was not only lame in her legs and one arm, but who had also lost control over the movement of her head, were given special dispensation by their local priest to undertake the journey to St Elisabeth's tomb with their multiply impaired daughter. The priest stated at the miracle protocol hearing that the parents had been reluctant to take the girl to the shrine because of the severity of her condition, fearing that she might die on the journey. Had that happened they, the parents, would have had to do penance as if they were the cause of her death, but the priest had reassured them that he would not impose any such penance in the event of her not surviving the journey.[467]

Occasionally, it took more than one visit to the same shrine for a cure to be effective, or the cure took place at home or on the return journey from the shrine; this seems to have been the case particularly with supplicants to St Elisabeth, whose cures sometimes materialised gradually and in various stages.[468] More frequently, the sources mention that a particular supplicant had made completely unsuccessful visits to other shrines, or had only been partially healed at the rival sites. This probably reflects a bias in the sources, in that each collection of miracle narratives has to expound the virtue and efficacy of its saint, one way of which is by demonstrating greater thaumaturgic powers. Matilda, a woman with curvature of her spine, had visited other unspecified shrines until she was finally cured at Norwich,[469] as had a girl from Suffolk whose visits to other shrines failed until she was cured by the relic at Reading,[470] while a young woman was cured in one leg by St Nicholas, but had to wait another six years before receiving a complete cure through St Elisabeth.[471] St Foy cured a man who had travelled around most of Western Europe for four years, doing the tour of the shrines,[472] and at St Gall a boy was cured who had previously been to Rome unsuccessfully.[473] Our Lady of Rocamadour cured a woman who could not be healed by St Anthony,[474] and another woman who was unable to find help even at the church of the Holy Sepulchre in Jerusalem.[475]

Considering that a not insignificant number of pilgrims might have been paying multiple visits to shrines, it is interesting to note that shrines functioned to a degree as quasi-hospitals. An important element in the practical care of the sick often seems to have been provided by the custodians of a shrine. Competition between individual shrines for pilgrims as 'customers' may well have provided an inducement for such care to be given by the custodians, since it was another factor, besides the healing powers of the saintly relics, in attracting clientele. For example, at Reading (where the relics of the hand of St James were) and at Oxford (St Frideswide's shrine) sufferers often remained in the church for some days awaiting their cure, or then stayed on in the church after the immediate cure to convalesce further.[476] Stressing the comparisons between miracle-working shrines and the modern hospital even further, Finucane, imagining the 'bleeding accident victims rushed to shrines', surmises that one may 'see the shrine as a hospital, even as a casualty ward'.[477]

Lastly, as outlined in the introductory remarks to this sub-chapter, it is useful to present a brief discussion regarding the question of the veracity of medieval miracle narratives. Any retrospective modern medical analysis of medieval miracle healings is a futile enterprise from square one. For a start, the terminology used by the writers of medieval miracle accounts is so different from modern medical terminology, it is extremely difficult, if not impossible, to ascribe precise modern medical diagnoses to the conditions presented by supplicants visiting shrines. Diagnosis is difficult even in apparently well-described instances such as possible cases of ergotism. Ergotism, also called St Anthony's Fire,[478] manifested itself in two forms, a convulsive one, and a gangrenous one where flesh putrefied or 'shrivelled', 'dried out' or became 'arid', to follow the terminology employed by medieval texts. In these symptoms ergotism shared its effects with leprosy, with which, however, ergotism appears not to have been confused during the medieval period, or the symptoms conflated.[479] Descriptions of what appear to be three cases of ergot poisoning can be found in a manuscript dated to between 1220 and 1230 of the *Miracles* of St Silvanus of Levroux, where the convulsive form is cured by the saint. The sufferers had contractions in their legs and arms, and in one case so severe that the person's heels touched the buttocks, whilst also experiencing withering and shrinking of hands.[480] The contraction of legs to the buttocks was already observed by canon Henri de Saalma, sacristan of the parish church of Ninove (Belgium) between 1184 and 1191, when people afflicted with St Anthony's fire turned to the relics of St Corneille for help.[481] Later cases were documented in an outbreak of ergotism near Lille in 1749 where a physician described similar symptoms, and during the last recorded episode of ergotism in 1951 where convulsive reactions were observed in two elderly sufferers.[482] Although there seems to be a consistent pattern of symptoms and descriptions across the centuries, nevertheless one cannot assume invariably that in instances of convulsions or contractions described by the medieval texts one is in fact dealing with a disease identified by modern medicine as 'ergotism' – there may well have been a multitude of dissimilar causes for superficially similar phenomena. Then there is the problem of how far the medieval writers were confabulating, even in such apparently 'truthful' texts as the canonisation protocols. I have, in the main, treated the descriptions of people's *impairments* as reflecting 'real', lived experience, while being aware that the narratives of their *cures* may be part of the 'use of miracle-stories as metaphor'.[483]

In essence, therefore, the question 'did miracle healings of impaired people really occur?' is therefore unanswerable. However, one should not just ignore awkward questions, but at least attempt to present a possibility, albeit a speculative one. To do this, I propose to discard the taxonomical approach so often taken by medical historians of trying to match up modern disease diagnoses with medieval descriptions, and instead to investigate the psychosomatic (or even 'sociosomatic'[484]) angle, as a few medieval scholars have sporadically done, notably Henry Mayr-Harting. In his analysis of the healing miracles taking place at the shrine of St Frideswide at Oxford, Mayr-Harting believes that some of the conditions pilgrims were presenting with could be psychosomatic in origin. He concentrates on investigating not just the medical symptoms, but also the actual *process* of the cure, and reaches the intriguing conclusion that the curative process itself, often in spectacular surroundings and in front of crowds of people, was determining the outcome of the healing.

Essentially, the curative process was formed by an interplay between the sufferer, the saint and the attendant crowd. Large numbers of people[485] were present at St Frideswide's shrine, and cures took place in front of these crowds, sometimes during the monastic services. The presence of large crowds, of the impaired as well, is also attested by other sources. For example, after word of healing activity had got around, Ælfric described the scene at St Swithun's shrine at Winchester thus: 'The burial-ground lay filled with crippled folk, so that people could hardly get into the minster; and they were all so miraculously healed within a few days, that one could not find there five unsound men out of that great crowd.'[486] For Oxford, Mayr-Harting cites the example of a hump-backed widow who was cured during such an event, whereby 'all present distinctly heard her back creaking into shape again'.[487] The reaction of these spectators, in their belief and support of miraculous cures, is the deciding factor for Mayr-Harting.

I argue that it is possible to take this idea one step further, and to frame it more theoretically: one can regard what Mayr-Harting describes as the *public* aspect of healing, and contrast this with the *private* healing as carried out by physicians, surgeons, and other medical professionals. Miracle healings at shrines almost invariably took place in a public space (although on a few occasions people were cured during a night vigil when hardly anyone else was attendant) with significant numbers of other people watching and interacting with both the clergy and the supplicants. In contrast, medical treatment was generally carried out at a patient's home, with maybe just a few family members and friends in attendance, and therefore took place on much more private territory. The miraculous cures enacted at shrines were literally 'spectacular' in both senses, in that they were public events spectated upon by the assembled crowds of pilgrims and suppli-cants, and in that they were sensational occurrences, carried out with elaborate rituals which served to enhance their status as 'spectacle' for all the participants.[488] As Peter Brown has pointed out, it is not why people sought cures, but what kind of cures they sought that is important, since 'the history of what constitutes a cure in a given society is a history of that society's values'.[489] Mayr-Harting takes up these insights, and emphasises the ritual aspect of therapy as performed at shrines, especially in that the ritual serves to give the supplicant a status of acceptance for the crowd.[490]

If one wanted to locate more mainstream medical arguments for the possibility of 'miraculous' cures actually having a physical impact, one could, for example, turn to the work of John Wortley, who has examined three case studies of healing in medieval miracle accounts for their medical effectiveness. In general, Wortley acknowledges a placebo effect in the efficacy of relics. Two of his case studies relate to healing by fear. One case concerns the cure of a paralytic man, who was incubating at the shrine of Sts Cosmas and Damian, when in the middle of the night he crawled over to where a speech-impaired woman was also sleeping and started touching her; this prompted the speechless woman to find her voice again, and cry out in fear, while through the noise, the paralysed man also became so frightened, he ran off. Wortley's second case relates to the reluctant healing of impaired pilgrims through fear, in an *exemplum* told by Jacques de Vitry, which I have already discussed earlier. His third case analyses the cure of a paralysed nun through what she believed to be holy water, which in fact turned out to be the water a robber's feet had been washed in.[491] Furthermore, some medical researchers are finding strong 'scientific' evidence for connections between psychological problems and physical illness. Peter Halligan and colleagues published an article looking at the brain activity of modern people who were paralysed due to psychological trauma, and not due to physical injury.[492] The fact that such cases of manifest physical impairment caused by psychological origins are recognised by modern medicine makes one wonder if it was not equally possible for at least *some* of the medieval miracle healings to have been effective due to the psychological causes of impairment, which would then have been curable given the right circumstances, such as public spectacles and public acceptance of a sufferer.

Ronald Finucane has also tried to explain the possibility of actual, 'real' cures taking place at shrines, or experienced elsewhere by supplicants who later reported them to the shrine keepers. He has distinguished between diseases which are self-limiting, or chronic but subject to remission, or psychogenic.[493] Self-limiting diseases he regarded as the minor ailments, such as toothache, indigestion or headache, which would clear up on their own eventually. Impairments, according to this classification (though Finucane does not distinguish impairment from disease), would fall into the categories of chronic disease. So it is suggested that rheumatoid arthritis, which is one chronic disease known to have periods of remission, may have accounted for the many cures of crippled people in the miracle narratives.[494] The third category, psychogenic, covers what Finucane termed the psychosomatic and conversion reactions ('hysteria'), which *can* produce motor and sensory impairments, and which can disappear rapidly or spontaneously.[495] Finucane mentioned that in 'some cases of hysterical paralysis it has been observed that tissues accommodate so that the limb actually becomes immobile or twisted'.[496] He speculated that given the right psychological conditions ('autosuggestion'), coupled with strong belief and the special environment at the shrines, a reversal of impairments caused by psychosomatic diseases might be possible. Such a categorisation runs the risk of dismissing manifestations of medieval impairments as purely psychological and less 'real' than 'proper' somatic diseases, impairments then becoming an imagined condition, the cure of which is more acceptable to modern medical notions, but which is patronising to the medieval sufferers – medieval impaired people cannot all be regarded as hysterics. Furthermore, Finucane posits a strong gender bias among impairing conditions, which reiterates the prejudicial notion that hysterically generated impairments are specific female maladies. He had noted that in his samples of miracle cures, blindness and motor impairments appeared to affect more lower-class women than lower-class men.[497] In itself there is no reason to criticise his findings, but Finucane's explanation for such a gender disparity reinforces modern stereotypes of the 'hysterical female'. He argues that it 'is not unlikely that some cured pilgrims had been suffering from conversion hysteria, and if modern findings about this illness are applicable to the Middle Ages – but only if so – then women would have suffered hysterical debilities more frequently than men'.[498] In more recent scholarship, so-called 'modern findings' which position women as the hysterical, irrational and impressionable gender have come under attack from a variety of disciplines, notably feminist literary criticism, and such scholarship has emphasised the social construction of apparently biological 'facts' (much as has been the case for disability studies).[499] Far more convincing are Finucane's arguments for the gendered differences in causation of impairments which seek the answers in the different lived experiences of medieval men and women, such as women's health risks associated with parturition, or the effect of cultural values which restrict women's nutritional intake in favour of men and children in times of food shortages.[500]

Additionally, there are some cases in the sources studied in detail, where the healing process is a gradual one – no instantaneous 'miracle cure' at the altar – with occasional descriptions of the different stages a supplicant went through in regaining their physical mobility. A new-born boy who had apparently become blind within days of his birth gradually began to make things out when his parents travelled to Rocamadour, and started reaching out for objects held up to him, although he could not yet 'fix his gaze in the same way that someone could who had been able to see from birth'.[501] Most of the gradual cures occur in the narrative of St Elisabeth. On one occasion, the notaries of the protocol saw a boy, who had been mobility impaired, walking with a tottering gait in the manner of a boy learning to walk.[502] On another occasion, a boy who had been speech impaired began to talk after his mother had made a vow to St Elisabeth, however not yet speaking fluently, 'but so, that one was able to understand him after the fashion of children who are learning to speak'.[503] A severely mobility impaired boy, while still at Marburg, began to stretch out one leg and separate his twisted legs first, before on returning home stretching out the other leg; then it took another two days before he was able to get up fully.[504] In the case of another mobility impaired boy it was stated that he was healed gradually, first righting himself up with the aid of sticks, then walking supported by a single crutch.[505] A similar gradual cure occurred in the case of a young man who had lost all powers over the lower half of his body. After a vision in a dream of St Elisabeth, he began to hold himself upright by using a fence and other supports, and started walking in that fashion, so that at the time of the protocol recording 'he walked very well';[506] such a 'cure' reminds one of physiotherapeutic practise more than of spontaneous miracle healing. A very interesting cure is also encountered in the St Elisabeth text, which appears to revolve around a psychological approach, by offering an incentive to the impaired individual. In this case a small boy, 3 years and 6 months old, had been unable to walk. At the tomb, where his mother took him, the lay brother guarding the tomb produced an egg which he held some way away from the boy. The boy then got up and, holding onto the tomb, walked around to the edge of the sarcophagus. The lay brother then moved the egg round a bit farther, so that the boy had to follow him again, 'because of the egg'.[507]

These gradual cures are appealing to the modern medical notion of therapy, precisely because they do not happen spontaneously, and can therefore be regarded as 'medical' rather than 'miraculous'. Speech therapy and physical therapy, in modern medicine, both require time and repeated treatments to be effective. The modern mind is perhaps more readily prepared to accept such gradual 'miracles' as real, than the sudden, abrupt transformation at the high altar or shrine of an immobilised impaired person into an able-bodied, mobile one.

5.4   **Summary**

Although medieval sainthood, miracles and religious healing have been repeatedly studied by historians, the focus of such studies has never been on physical impairment as a distinct subject, but always under the rubric of diseases or ill-health in general. My analysis of a selection of miracle narratives has therefore advanced our knowledge of physical impairment in the period under consideration, by utilising theories of disability studies, which allow us to treat 'impairment' as a separate conceptual category from 'illness'. To place medieval accounts of the miraculous cure of physical impairments within their proper cultural and religious context, the healing function of saints in general was addressed, emphasising the importance that was placed on the healing of impairing conditions in particular (such as orthopaedic and mobility impairments, and sensory impairments). Next, the question of whether such therapeutic miracles were merely a reflection of literary stereotypes was discussed. The healing miracles of Christ and the apostles in the gospels were, to a degree, models for cures performed by medieval saints. With reference to physical impairment in particular, this situation was found to be the case because miracles involved a sense of the supernatural, transcending the normal workings of nature, and physical impairment, as we saw in Chapter 4, was regarded as incurable by normal medical means, leaving recourse to the miraculous as one possible action to take for impaired people. Medieval saints, as imitators of Christ, therefore also transcended nature by working miracles, curing the incurable, that is, impairment, while ordinary medical professionals (physicians and surgeons) could only treat the more mundane afflictions.

Moving on from these general points, the relationship between medicine and miracle was investigated further. It was pointed out that the miracle narratives tended to reflect not, as some modern scholars have assumed, the full range of diseases, illnesses and impairments that medieval people might have suffered from, but only those conditions which were found to be difficult to treat or cure at all by normal medical means. This statement was substantiated by evidence from the sources, in that it became clear that many supplicants at therapeutic shrines had tried normal medical treatment unsuccessfully prior to turning to cures of a miraculous sort. Seeking the aid of saints and their curative powers, therefore, was not invariably the first treatment method medieval people applied to their diseases, illnesses or impairments. Earthly medicine and divine medicine interplayed and complemented each other, it seems.

Not all miracle accounts were about straightforward healing, though. In some instances, the curative miracle also involved a moral message or spiritual meaning. This was found to be the case in some miracles concerning transgression and punishment, whereby the protagonist of a miracle story might be initially punished for specific deviant behaviour, only to be cured once this behaviour was recognised and renounced upon. However, a number of miracles made no mention of transgression or punishment, but conversely emphasised that the cause of a person's impairment was purely accidental, both in the modern sense of the word (as the result of an accidental injury) and in the medieval philosophical sense (as an accident of 'nature'). Notions of sin as the cause of physical impairment were therefore not invariably expressed in the *miracula*.

The most valuable aspect of the miracle narratives I studied was the fact that they carried with them incidental information about the lived experience of medieval impaired people. Some of this information was more of a theoretical nature, such as the themes of defectiveness, liminality or burdensomeness of impaired people, while other aspects covered a more practical angle, providing us with evidence concerning questions about the livelihood of impaired people, or what mobility aids may have been available to them. The philosophical concept of an impaired person as 'defective' emerged in the narratives in some cases of severe physical impairment, although the overwhelming majority of *miracula* made no such statements.

Of great importance was the concept of liminality with regard to impairment (a topic also covered in Chapter 2), whereby the impaired person is seen to occupy an ambiguous, in-between space between conceptual categories, and between real social positions; it was therefore very interesting to find that some of the miracle narratives also regarded the (severely) impaired as liminal figures, positioned half-way between life and death. Equally interesting and important was the discovery that many of the impaired protagonists in the narratives were described as being unable to perform certain functions, mainly related to unaided movement and the inability to earn a living through work – it is in the *miracula*, alone out of all the sources I have studied in relation to the rest of my research, that one finds medieval concepts that come closest to our modern notion of the impaired as 'disabled'. Asking questions whether, historically, one can speak of 'disability' or whether one is just dealing with 'impairment', was, after all, one of the crucial contributions of modern disability theories.

Connected with notions of the impaired as defective, liminal and 'disabled' was the description of impaired persons as a burden to others, and as an object of mockery, which was found in some miracle narratives, albeit very rarely. Somewhat more often, the impaired were described as impoverished, having to beg for a living, or reliant on private and public acts of charity, although this tended to affect only those pilgrims who were suffering from what we term severe impairments, or those who had lost connections to their family and social environment.

With regard to practical measures, it was found that the miracle stories offered up a wealth of information concerning mobility of the impaired, covering both questions as to the extent of personal mobility and what means to aid such mobility were available to them, as well as methods of travel and transportation of the more severely impaired. Because not all pilgrims could make the journey to a therapeutic shrine themselves, miracle cures through votive offerings and by proxy were also discussed. It was noted that some pilgrims had to make repeat journeys to shrines before they managed to obtain a cure, while others travelled to a range of different sites before being healed.

Finally, a speculative discussion of the veracity of medieval miracle narratives was conducted. Some historians have tended to dismiss all miracle healings as fabrication, while others took the equally narrow view that such miracles only cured psychosomatic disorders. A more fruitful approach has been to look at the interaction between sufferer, saint and shrine, which placed greater emphasis on social and cultural factors than on medical ones alone. In the end, the question as to whether medieval therapeutic miracles 'actually' happened still stands, and the answer depends very much on the viewpoint of the modern writer.

6   Conclusion

The premise of this book lay in making a conceptual distinction between physical impairment as a 'real', physiological condition, and between physical 'disability' as a socially constructed or cultural condition. Such a distinction removed the a priori assumption that all physically impaired people in all societies, whether different historically or different geographically, are always regarded as disabled. Based on this theoretical concept, I researched what theoretical approaches and attitudes to physical impairment existed in the western high Middle Ages.

In summary, the results of my research in the preceding chapters demonstrate that 'disability' is a theme which has been neglected by historians in general, particularly as far as the medieval period is concerned. Disability has frequently been considered to be an unchanging part of the 'human condition'. Some types of medieval historical sources themselves (such as chronicles and works of historiography) omitted to mention the impaired, since they were not deemed to constitute a suitable subject for narratives about deeds done by the great and powerful. Modern disability studies, developed out of sociological theory, were also found to be inadequate, for different reasons. Although this time such theories were very suited to explaining and theorising disability in a modern context, the sheer lack of any sense of period or awareness of historical issues concerning anything prior to the nineteenth century meant that these theories became, in effect, redundant as far as the medieval period was concerned. Theories derived from disability studies are very *useful* as conceptual tools, allowing us to make the important distinction between impairment and disability, but are almost *useless* as far as research into non-Western, pre-industrial, or non-Classical cultures is concerned. Here theories developed by anthropologists and ethnologists have been far more fruitful, mainly due to the fact that these scholars have had to work with a variety of different cultural assumptions, not just their own familiar ones. One might even say, borrowing a concept from ethnology, that medical and medievalist historians, as well as modern disability theorists, have taken an etic approach to impairment in the Middle Ages, while anthropologists and ethnologists, taking an emic approach, have managed to develop a more suitable theoretical apparatus for studying cultural variance.

Turning our attention to medieval philosophical and theological notions of impairment, it was found that ideas revolving around impairment demonstrated a strong ambiguity as far as connections between physical impairment and spiritual sin were concerned. In the biblical tradition, the New Testament had already shifted the emphasis from impairment as punishment to impairment as the focus for Christ's healing activities. In the Middle Ages as such, both notions, of impairment (and, in a way, *all* illness) as the result of sin, and impairment as something that required physical healing, existed in an ambivalent tension. An important medieval concept concerned the deviation of the impaired body from the culturally constructed norm, in the sense that an impaired body was also perceived of as a disordered and challenging body. In the afterlife, medieval notions seemed to negate the impaired body: bodies were never thought of as being resurrected with the physical defects or imperfections they may have had in life. This demonstrated crucial differences in ideas about identity and personhood between medieval and modern notions of physical impairment.

In medieval 'scientific' discourse, that is in writings derived from medical sources and texts on natural philosophy, impairment was treated either as a condition that required an aetiological explanation, or as a potential condition that required prevention. The reason for this is that medicine, medieval as well as modern, could actually offer very little to the impaired in the way of therapeutic measures. Aetiologies tried to ascribe the causes of impairment to humoral imbalances, to astrological reasons, to deviant sexual practices, and to the maternal imagination. Congenital impairment, attributed to deviant sexual behaviour of the parents as well as to humoral reasons, did not invariably reflect the 'sins of the parents' onto the child – again, medieval attitudes were ambivalent on this matter. With regard to preventative measures, medieval medical methods centred mainly on surgical techniques intended to prevent wounds, injuries and fractures from leading to permanent, incurable impairments. Besides textbook medicine, medieval people also had recourse to what we would now term 'complementary', 'alternative' or 'magical' medicine.

Miraculous cures achieved at the shrines of saints offered far greater possibilities for impaired people than medical therapies. Cures of impairing conditions were seen to constitute one of the main miraculous activities of saints, according to my own and other researchers' studies. Saintly healing was, to a degree, modelled on the healing miracles of Christ in the gospels, in which texts one already found the cure of those people with (incurable) impairments, rather than the cure of mundane afflictions, which earthly medicine could tackle just as well. However, medieval impaired pilgrims often tried such earthly medicine first before seeking miraculous cures. Sometimes a miracle cure followed on from repentance after sustaining an impairment in punishment for a particular transgression, but equally a number of miracle stories made it quite clear that a person's impairment was the result of accident only. Again, the perceived relationship between sin and physical impairment emerges as a tenuous and ambivalent one in the high Middle Ages. Miracle narratives were also found to be the only distinct corpus of sources that provided incidental information with regard to the lived experience of impaired people. They provide a wealth of social, economic and cultural information about impaired people, most importantly concerning notions of the impaired as liminal figures, and of the impaired as 'disabled' in the modern sense, as being presented with physical obstacles to making their own living and reliant on others (reliance on others also emerges on a more practical level, in connection with questions about the personal mobility of the impaired).

Historians, as Charles T. Wood has remarked,[1] are primarily concerned with observable processes of change over time, while subjects that do not require historical explanation, in other words unchanging subjects, do not arouse the historian's interest. I have found very little change – with one notable exception: the decline of healing miracles – in relation to physical impairment over the period, *c.*1100–*c.*1400, which has been the focus of this book. There has been little evidence of intracultural variance, as anthropology has expressed it, if one takes the view of western medieval Europe as a cultural entity. Throughout the period, attitudes to and notions of physical impairment remained relatively static. Within such attitudes, there may have been ambiguities and even contradictory notions (e.g. the question of sin and impairment), but one cannot identify a single period or event that firmly positioned impairment in one conceptual category or another. In a sense, one cannot even find too much intercultural variance, between medieval and modern Western notions of impairment, with regard to perceived links between sin and physical, particularly congenital, impairment. Public figures in our modern society, as was seen in Chapter 1.2, are still capable of speaking of sin and congenital impairment in the same breath, and modern medical aetiologies have in fact reinforced notions that sins of the parents manifest themselves in their children, except that now such 'sins' are not defined as sexual transgressions, but as 'irresponsible behaviour', especially by the mother during pregnancy (smoking and consuming alcohol, for example).[2] We are, to echo Umberto Eco, culturally 'still living the Middle Ages'.[3]

Similarly, there was found to be a lack of any great distinctions between the way different types of sources treated notions of the impaired. Intellectuals, such as Albertus Magnus, whom we might now regard as more of a theologian than a scientist, were equally at home writing about 'science' (i.e. natural history or medicine) as about theology. Conversely, figures such as Henri de Mondeville, whom we think of first and foremost as a surgeon, that is, a scientist, were also versed in concepts derived from philosophy and theology. In other words, no significant difference in attitudes was displayed by the medical and the religious discourses. Making distinctions between the two disciplines betrays a modern, if not to say etic, approach to medieval culture. An emic approach, in contrast, allows us to overcome such modern assumptions regarding the separation of 'science' from 'religion', and lets us recognise that medieval notions of these categories were far more fluid.

As to the one notable change, which forms an exception within otherwise relatively static conceptual systems, the decline of healing miracles, this may have also impacted on attitudes to the physically impaired. Whereas in religious terms the early Middle Ages looked to the saints for the connection between God and humankind (through the process of intercession), from around the year 1000 onwards a different order emerged. The emphasis became ever more strongly placed on the sacerdotal mediation between God and the normal believer. Writing in the thirteenth century William Durandus, in his *Rationale*, was important for further spreading the idea of greater sacerdotal powers.[4] More priestly intermediation and less important (and perhaps less accessible) saints could possibly explain the decline in healing miracles. Religiosity, furthermore, becomes more spiritualised in the course of the later Middle Ages, hence miracles become less 'practical' in the sense of curing people's physical ailments, but become more rarefied and spiritual (visions, ecstatic experiences). The cults developing around the Eucharist, Christ's body and Christ's wounds in the later Middle Ages also contributed to this spiritualisation of religiosity, paradoxically thereby making later medieval religiosity more corporeal. Bodies of all sorts mattered more in the later Middle Ages than in the earlier period. The body of Christ as in the feast of Corpus Christi became important and popular, female mystics experienced religious ecstasy through their bodies (especially through mutilations of their bodies), and the decaying body came to feature prominently on funerary monuments.[5] Later medieval saints and mystics (and the flagellants) were voluntarily marked physically in imitation of Christ's body. In contrast, real, living physically impaired people had received their impairment, wounds or mutilation involuntarily. As later medieval religion became more corporeal in this spiritualised sense, and especially as the suffering, mutilated, deformed or decaying body was interpreted through deeply religious sentiments, so conversely actual impaired people, who had not voluntarily mutilated themselves, but who had become impaired by chance, lost social and cultural status. The voluntarily disabled (displaying religious mutilations or other bodily sufferings) needed to distance themselves from the common, unfortunate debilitated body. Healing miracles gave way to visions instead.

Recent theories of agency and of the rise in importance of the individual over the collective group may also go some way to explain the change, if not to say break, in attitudes toward miracles and the actions of saints. While throughout the medieval period the human body was perceived as interacting with the environment in the widest sense, the manner of this interaction changed from what Harald Kleinschmidt has called a heterodynamic mode to an autodynamic one. In the earlier Middle Ages there were 'heterodynamic impacts flowing onto a person from the physical environment and/or from other persons'.[6] Ordinary people were therefore acted upon (by forces outside of their own bodies), whilst those with status (secular or religious elites) acted on and for others. In this sense the relic of the saint acted on the supplicant seeking a cure. Kleinschmidt expands these ideas by stating that everyone was regarded as capable of seeking protection and tapping into sources of energy from the physical environment, especially from supernatural or divine agencies. This way it was possible for the individual to overcome obstacles posed by the physical environment, by other persons or groups. However, from the eleventh century onward 'the emerging hilltop castles and urban communities of towns and cities created small segments whose inhabitants were expected to act autodynamically as individuals, and they were regarded as capable of relying more on their own bodily energies than on the assistance or protection of others'.[7] Saintly intercession for (physical) assistance could therefore be deemed part of the old, superseded heterodynamism. Interestingly the change from heterodynamic to autodynamic agency occurs in the eleventh century, which makes it contemporaneous with the rise of sacerdotal authority and corporeal religiosity mentioned above – all reducing the intercessory importance of saintly relics for physical cures.

Finally, the question of whether we are dealing with 'impaired' or with 'disabled' people during the medieval period requires a tentative answer. According to the majority of the sources I have studied, we can only speak of impairment, but not of disability, during the Middle Ages. The one notable exception was provided by a few of the miracle narratives, where views were expressed concerning an impaired person's inability to sustain themselves economically, their reliance on aid by other people, and (rarely) the idea that some impaired people were a burden. As far as 'intellectual' texts of the Middle Ages are concerned, one must conclude that although in reality there were probably as many physically impaired people, proportionately, as there were in other societies, including our own modern world, there were very few medieval disabled people.

Appendix
Medieval miracle narratives

The titling of a miracle within a particular collection follows the scheme originally used by the printed edition of that collection. Page references relate to citations from the modern editions used. For further details on each saint, the manuscript sources and the modern editions used, please refer to the relevant introduction to each miracle narrative.

V   Miracles *in vitae* from St Gall

Some *vitae* of saints in manuscripts from St Gall, produced between the ninth and eleventh centuries, provide interesting details concerning the healing activity of men and women of God. The *vitae* have been translated in part and discussed by J. Duft, *Notker der Arzt. Klostermedizin und Mönchsarzt im frühmittelalterlichen St. Gallen*, St. Gall: Fehr'sche Buchhandlung, 1972, and it is this German edition the extracts here have been based on. The extracts are comprised from the following texts:

- a life of St Gallus, an Irish monk who came to the region of Lake Constance in around 610 and died *c*.650, known as the *Vita sancti Galli* (here abbreviated as V G(W)) composed by Wetti, a monk of Reichenau, between 816 and 824, and with another version by Walahfrid Strabo (833/4) (here abbreviated as V G(S)); furthermore a fragmentary form exists of this *vita*, known as the *Vetustissima* (abbreviated V V) of around 771 (see Duft, pp. 17–18);
- a *vita* of St Otmar (d. 759), composed in St Gall by the deacon Gozbert, and revised by Walahfrid Strabo 834–8, known as the *Vita sancti Otmari* (abbreviated V O); also a *Relatio de Sancto Otmaro* (abbreviated V RO), written by Iso of St Gall 864–7 (see Duft, pp. 18–19);
- and a *Vita sanctae Wiboradae* (abbreviated V W), of the anchoress and *inclusa* Wiborada, who died in 926 during the invasions of the Magyars, partly written in the tenth century, with additions of the eleventh century (see Duft, p. 19).

Vetustissima

V V 5

A crippled man (*paraliticus*) called Maurus in Arbon was so contracted together that he could no longer walk by his own means; he was healed by the clothing of the recently deceased saint.

Vita sancti Galli, *version by Wetti*

V G(W) 33

Deaf people (*surdi*) were healed by the wax of miracle-working candles.

Vita sancti Galli, *version by Walahfrid Strabo*

V G(S) II.13

Healing of a man who had become blind and deaf through a long period of sickness, and who was brought to the tomb in a cart.

V G(S) II.26

A man who became crippled after being struck by lightning (*violentia fulminis ictus*) was healed at the tomb.

V G(S) II.27

A deaf-mute man (*surdus et mutus*) was healed there after blood poured from his mouth and ears.

V G(S) II.29

A nun with twisted arms (*brachia contorta*) was healed.

V G(S) II.31

A man crippled in all his limbs (*debilis membris omnibus contractus*) was healed, under great pains, in the crypt of St Gall.

V G(S) II.37

A girl blind from birth (*caeca*) was carried to the monastery by her mother, and received her sight there.

V G(S) II.39

The withered and twisted hands of a girl (*manus aridae et curvatae*) were revitalised.

V G(S) II.41

A mute man received his voice.

V G(S) II.42

A boy lamed in all his limbs (*membris omnibus contractum*) was healed.

V G(S) II.43

A girl suffering from lameness (*paralisi*) received the strength to stand.

Vita sancti Otmari

V O 10

A deaf-mute (*surdus et mutus*) man with two wax tablets, which he always carried about with him, to rattle with in aid of begging sustenance for himself, placed these on the tomb of Otmar, fell into a deep sleep and awoke healed.

V O 13

A lame man (*contractus*) crawling along on his hands led a blind man to the paupers' hostel (*hospitium pauperum*) at St Gall, where both of them stayed the night, and both were healed at the tomb.

V O 15

A cleric whose fingers were so contorted [perhaps by some form of arthritis?], that the nails dug into the palm of his hand up to the bone, was healed with great pains at the tomb.

Relatio de Sancto Otmaro

V RO 11

A beggar who was sinistrally lamed was directed to St Gall in a dream, otherwise his foot would have to be amputated (*pedem eius sese abscissurum esse*).

V RO 12

A mute man fell down on the ground in front of the tomb, whereupon blood gushed from his mouth, and through the shock ('durch den Schrecken') he found his tongue.

V RO 13

A boy from Orléans who was lame at the joints in almost all his limbs, and who was crippled (*omnibus paene membrorum juncturis contractum atque conglobatum*), travelled with his father on a small push-cart ('Schiebkarren') first to Rome, and subsequently to St Gall, where he was healed in 864 with great pains.

V RO 15

On the occasion of the translation of St Otmar in 867 a mute man received his faculty of speech, due to his spirit being moved ('aus seelischer Bewegung').

V RO 18

A person with a shortened and crippled shin (*tibia*) was healed with a cracking sound, as if wood was breaking.

Vita sanctae Wiboradae

V W 8

In her youth Wiborada cared for and nursed the sick and the impaired (*aegrotos ac debiles*).

V W 43

A merchant from Zurich, who had a grave illness of the eyes (*oculorum dolore graviter laborabat*), was healed by the blood of the saint.

F   Miracles of St Foy at Conques

St Foy was an early Christian child martyr; her relics had been kept at Conques since 866, when the monks of the Benedictine abbey acquired them in an act of *furta sacra*. During the eleventh century, Conques experienced its heyday of popularity and pilgrimage, with a gradual decline setting in during the twelfth century. The first two books of the collection of St Foy's miracles, the *Liber miraculorum Sancte Fidis*, were written in the early eleventh century by Bernard of Angers, while the remaining books are by anonymous authors writing in the middle of the eleventh century. Bernard of Angers, unusually for a collection of *miracula*, arranged the miracles not by chronological sequence, but in an order by subject matter, and the later anonymous authors more or less stuck to his scheme. The emphasis in the *miracula* is not just on the 'normal' activities of a saint (healing incurable illnesses, freeing prisoners, delivering people from shipwreck), but on 'unheard of and new miracles' of St Foy, such as bringing back to life dead animals or reinstating the eyes of a man who had had his eyeballs ripped out over a year earlier. Bernard of Angers states at one point that his intent was not to list every miracle that occurred, but that he 'concentrated on the miracles that were worked to take revenge on evil-doers or on those that are in some way new and unusual' (F I.9, p. 69).

The English translation used here, *The Book of Sainte Foy*, translated with an introduction and notes by Pamela Sheingorn, Philadelphia, PA: University of Pennsylvania Press, 1995, is based on the printed edition (Auguste Bouillet (ed.), *Liber miraculorum sancte Fidis*. Collection de textes pour servir à l'étude et à l'enseignement de l'histoire, fasc. 21, Paris, 1897) of a late-eleventh century manuscript now at Sélestat in Alsace, Bibliothèque Humaniste MS lat. 22, together with further miracles from other manuscripts. Other miracles of St Foy, here given as F L.3 and F L.5, were probably composed in the first half of the twelfth century (from an English manuscript of the second half of the twelfth century, London, B. L., MS Arundel lat. 91).

F 1.1

Guibert, servant of Gerald, had his eyes torn out by the roots by Gerald; at Conques a year later, his eyes were restored to him during a vigil at the shrine. Guibert stayed at Conques, where the abbot put him in charge of selling wax to pilgrims. However, Guibert took up with an 'unchaste woman' (p. 50) and was punished for this by being blinded in one eye, which was cured once Guibert repented; he lapsed a second time, and again was blinded in one eye by St Foy, only to be cured yet again once he repented. Apparently this 'tit-for-tat' went on for some time, until Guibert 'lost the service of the other eye' (p. 50), which made him reconsider, so that he sought to become a monk. He 'was fortunate enough to regain his eyesight. But even after so many chastising scourges Guibert was still unable to restrain his lust. It is reported that he sank into the same mire, although no bodily punishment followed' (p. 50). At the conclusion of this miracle, the author, Bernard of Angers, compares it favourably with the miracle told in the Gospel about the man born blind [John 9:1–7], even going so far as to state that this miracle was 'much more marvellous by far' (p. 51). Sheingorn remarks that in a similar miracle conducted by Saint Benedict, the paralytic peasant who was cured was also struck with his original affliction each time he sinned by fornicating (p. 290 note 18).

F 1.2

A similar miracle, in which a man named Gerbert had his eyes gouged out by a local lord, and then had his sight restored at Conques. He became a devout man living in the monastery. Bernard of Angers attached a moral to the end of this miracle, possibly in comparison with the behaviour of Guibert in the previous one. He said: 'Though their restoration was contrary to nature, his eyes shine now just as they did before, not like glass but like flesh. But to prevent the happenstance that he might be corrupted by arrogance or by the seductive counsel of those near him – and might wish to return to the secular life, through divine will the sight of his left eye began to disappear almost completely afterwards' (p. 55).

F 1.7

Bernard of Angers commented on the previous miracles and attested their veracity. In discussing the cure of the two blinded men, he said: 'If I wished, I would be able to keep on writing a great many miracles about them. For when they begin to sneak off to worldly affairs, divine power immediately hinders them. Either by blinding an eye or by disabling a limb, God forces them to stay where they are. Moreover, Guibert, just as I said above, was unable to control his lust, and every time he was sullied with a prostitute he experienced the retribution of divine vengeance' (pp. 67–8).

F 1.9

A widow's blind daughter was healed during a night watch at the shrine.

F 1.15

A 'poor girl who had been crippled in all her joints and had been carried to Sainte Foy's monastery' (p. 80) was cured completely. She stayed near the monastery for some time afterwards to work for her food and lodging, employed as a weaver by a woman. When the girl refused to stand up and leave her work during a procession for the saint, she 'began to be made pathetically deformed throughout her whole body. She became so misshapen that it was just as if she had never been healed but had remained bent and crooked, wholly deprived of the function of her muscles. Her body was completely drawn together and she didn't have the strength to let go of the tools of her loom – the very shuttle was held fast in her clenched hand.... [she] could speak only hoarsely because her condition greatly restricted her voice (though she had been able to speak normally before)' (pp. 80–1). She was carried behind the procession, and kept vigil for several nights, so that she was 'transformed a second time from a cripple to a person who could stand upright' (p. 81).

F 1.28

The relic of St Foy had been taken to a synod convened by the bishop of Rodez, as had other reliquaries of saints, which were all arranged in tents and pavilions on a meadow near Rodez. 'A boy, blind and lame, deaf and mute from birth, had been carried there by his parents and placed close beneath the image ... After he had been left there for about an hour, he merited divine medicine. When he had received the grace of a complete cure, the boy stood up speaking, hearing, seeing and even walking around happily, for he was no longer lame' (p. 98).

F 1.29

'At the same synod a man who was blind and lame spent the night in vigil before the image of Saint Marius the Confessor in order to be cured' (p. 99). The man was told in a vision to approach St Foy, which he immediately did. '[W]hen the man rushed into the entrance of the pavilion, at once his blood vessels regained strength and his muscles were invigorated. What had been bent became straight. Also the veil over his pupils split apart, and after a sudden and violent discharge of blood came very clear light. And then he was completely healthy, for the right hand of the heavenly doctor had treated his body' (p. 99).

F 2.1

The same Gerbert who had had his eyes restored, but later became blind in his left eye (F 1.2), experienced another miracle revolving around the restoration of his sight. In a brawl started by another man he had his healthy, right eye poked out, so that he was now totally blinded, and had to be led by a stranger to the church of St Foy. This time it took three months of prayers and vigils before Gerbert's eye was restored.

F 2.4

St Foy's relics were taken in procession into Auvergne. While there, many miracles happened, including the cure of a deaf-mute named Stephen, 'on whom nature herself had inflicted his defects while he was still in his mother's womb' (p. 121). During the procession Stephen 'began to push his fingers into the passage-ways of his ears with great force and to rub them quite vigorously. Soon spouts of blood from these openings, along with a bloody stream that rose up from his throat, broke through the obstacles that were blocking his voice and his hearing', and he spoke. 'But he had never heard the sound of a human voice. Therefore it is apparent that his ability to bring forth words he had never heard is beyond human understanding and had a divine cause' (p. 122). Stephen became frightened by the unfamiliar noises of chanting, bells and so on, and nearly became mad, trying to escape from the people that held him. 'In his frenzy nothing comforted or consoled him until the din ceased. It would have been better for him to have remained a deaf-mute but with a rational mind than to be cheated of the gift of human intelligence and turn into a madman in circumstances like these. But the miracle was perfect, for he recovered his senses and was sound both in mind and body' (p. 122).

A 'little old woman' whose entire body had been afflicted by rheumatism for six years was also cured at this procession, even though she had lived at Conques all her life and had seen other people from elsewhere receive cures at the shrine. Her miracle is very detailed and contains a lot of information about literary stereotypes and prejudices, it is therefore worth citing in full.

For the beginning of this miracle story please see p. 164

> While they were denouncing her in this way, the old woman sprang up with a sudden leap and without any feeling of pain. She had been cured with miraculous swiftness. Walking completely upright with firm steps, she praised God. I saw her myself afterward in the village of Conques, where she lived as a servant in the house of a respectable widow named Richarde. Cheerful and healthy, she had ample strength to do her work. This miracle caused great joy for all, and even for those who were mocking her. But these must have been ignorant and stupid schoolboys if they didn't know that Christ deigned to cure an old woman who had a curvature of the spine for eighteen years, [Luke 13:11–13] and an old man who lay paralysed in the portico of a pool for thirty-eight years, [John 5:2–9] both of whom had given up hope of a cure long before. As to these miracles, it seems very appropriate and in accordance with my reasoning that the Lord had delayed the healing of this woman for such a long time, either on account of her own sin, or so that His works might be shown in her. But now the Compassionate One looked on her and He wanted at least to confound those who were deriding her, so He helped her on her bed of sorrow [Psalms 40:4 (41:3)] (pp. 122–3).

Another of the miracles concerned a girl with multiple impairments. 'Then there was a girl, a native of Auvergne, whom nature had thrust out of her mother's womb into the light, blind, deaf and mute. Also her fingers were not separated from her palms, so that her hands were perpetually closed into fists. Some time before, at Conques, Sainte Foy had granted her a triple miracle, for she transformed eyes, ears and mouth into working organs. But she left the birth defect of her fists' (p. 123). The girl had heard about the procession, and in the morning after the procession, 'while all the others were watching, of their own accord her fists opened little by little and the fingers quivered, one by one. The hands that had been inflexible and not suited for work were unbound and reshaped by the highest Craftsman' (p. 124).

F 2.7

A man called Raymond was injured terribly by a sword wound, so that 'his nose was cut in two about halfway down, his jaw was severed on one side and on the other almost cut off to the middle, and the root of his tongue was separated from his throat. Below his eyelashes such a huge hole gaped that the sight of his divided face with the bones hanging down was terrifying. His friends and vassals carried him home and watched over him, half-alive, for almost three months. Because Raymond had sustained an incurable wound, his life was more of a loathsome burden than a pleasure to his friends. Since his mouth was no longer able to take food, they dripped thick liquids over the gaping hole that I mentioned' (p. 130). After a long time in this state Raymond decided to have himself carried to

Conques, communicating by signs and nodding his head. During the night he was completely healed after a vision of St Foy.

F 2.13

The brother of the author Bernard of Anger had 'contorted' limbs, with a 'brutal wrenching of his limbs' (p. 139), and he too is healed by St Foy. The 'contortion' here seems to be an acute illness, not a chronic one, and appears to have nothing in common with the many cases described as 'contorted' or 'contracted' in other miracle collections.

F 3.3

A young man was stabbed in the eye while pursuing some robbers. 'He was stabbed through the center of his eye with such force that the exit point of the lance was discovered behind his ear. . . . Eventually the wound festered and his whole head swelled up. Since the discharge from the wound was blocked up inside, he was afflicted with intolerable pain and near to death's destruction' (p. 147). After vowing a gold ring the young man was cured: 'For the sealed-in pus erupted from the wound with a great stench and flowed in long gushes of putre-faction until all the swelling of his head diminished and it returned to its natural size. It was declared that divine compassion brought it about. Shortly thereafter he recovered so completely that no deformity could be seen on his face except a modest scar' (ibid.). It is interesting to note that there is no mention of whether the man recovered his sight or not, bearing in mind that the first miracle in the collection deals with the spectacular restitution of a man's entire eye. This mira-cle here seems more concerned with the swelling of the head than with the inevitable loss of sight in the one eye that must have ensued after such a wounding.

F 3.6

A middle-aged man had to spend the night in the open in Normandy, keeping watch over some horses. He was exhausted and so 'gave in to sleep'. When he awoke the next day he could no longer see the horses, because he had become blind overnight. 'A guide was summoned for him and he made his way home by groping. There he remained for many days. Although he knew that he deserved his blindness, it occurred to him that he ought to travel to the various churches of the saints' (p. 151). He even travelled to Rome, but to no avail; then he had a dream in which he was told to go to St Foy, which he ignored, and remained blind for two years. Eventually he did go to St Foy, guided by his small son. At the shrine he recovered his sight: 'Struck by severe pain in his temples and other parts of his head, he leaned on the shoulder of a peasant standing next to him. Even with the peasant supporting him, he was scarcely able to stand on his feet. After this pain so much gore was seen to gush forth from each of his closed eyes that his clothing and beard were completely befouled with clotted blood. Then, realizing that a miracle had given him the gift of restored sight, he lifted up one eyelid and, as his sight increased little by little, he was able to recognize shapes and things opposite him and to point at them with his finger' (pp. 151–2). It is not made clear why the man 'deserved' his blindness; maybe his blindness is punishment for some transgression, perhaps for falling asleep instead of watching over the horses? A similar miracle, where the impairment/illness occurs after spending the night asleep out in the open is recorded in the miracles of the Hand of St James (at J XX).

F 3.10

The lord of a castle, one Robert, tried to attack one of the monks of St Foy's monastery, and in punishment he was struck blind, and also had his entire body stricken and his mouth wrenched back toward one ear, so that he had to be carried home on a litter 'in this repulsive condition' (p. 159). After repentance for his attempted acts, the man was fully cured.

F 3.14

Another lord, Reinfroi, and 50 of his men were struck blind when they tried to seize some land belonging to St Foy's manor. Again, after suitable acts of repentance, his eyesight was restored. (And presumably that of his fifty followers, although the text omits to mention this.)

F 3.17

Another lord, Siger, and all his children either died miserably or were impaired in punishment for Siger's 'great hostility' to St Foy. Siger died of a 'wretched illness', three of his sons died soon afterwards, and a fourth son was 'deformed by a paralyzing disease that forced him to follow his brothers to an ignominious death', one daughter was also paralysed and died destitute, and another daughter along with her children 'contracted a disease that caused swelling and sores', suffering great pain [*elephantino morbo ulcerosa pena dampnatur crudelissima*] (pp. 166–7, and p. 299 note 35).

F 3.22

The daughter of a peasant, about seven years old, was paralysed 'from her waist to her feet'. The peasant carried his daughter on a horse-drawn pallet to St Foy's shrine, where she was cured during mass. With the crowd of pilgrims attendant, the 'little girl suffered a little more intensely with pain in her limbs, and afterward all the pain had disappeared and she regained complete health. For at the same moment the joints in her back became connected, her muscles stretched out straight, and the soles of her feet were strengthened; in this way her two legs were restored immediately from their paralysis' (p. 173).

F 3.23

A young man 'who from birth had made no human sound' (p. 174) was brought to the shrine by a warrior. After a night vigil, the boy was cured at sunrise. A year later, the same warrior brought another mute man to Conques to be cured. And on a third occasion, the warrior overtook a mute man named Gozmar on the road to Conques. 'Gozmar turned toward him and began to ask alms from him by moving his lips' (p. 174). Gozmar was taken to the shrine, where he was cured.

F 4.3

A boy of almost five years old had the pupils of his eyes pierced with sharp, pointed sticks, and was left for dead, in an act of vendetta by the relatives of a man whom the boy's fugitive father had killed. The boy was rescued by the men of the village and taken to the church door, where he was instructed 'that with the others who were sick or injured he should beg alms from the people coming to pray. For several months he sought contributions there' (p. 184). One day he was led by people to the altar, and gradually recovered his sight. 'He reached out to touch the forms of things opposite him as if by the dim light of a dark moon, then he began to cry out with boyish glee that he could see a little. The way he was shouting brought to memory the man about whom it was attested that after his sight was restored by the Savior he saw men who looked to him like walking trees. [Matthew 8:24] That little boy was like him, as I say, for with scarcely any delay the light continued to increase and he saw everything so clearly that he both recognized by sight and named whatever was shown to him' (p. 184). The boy lived from monastic support for the rest of his life.

F 4.10

A warrior named Rigaud was wounded in such a way that his right arm was pierced by a sword and the sword buried itself deep in his side. 'After this severe wound his arm was so paralyzed and numb that he felt no pain when a red-hot iron was placed in his hand, though this experiment was tried rather often' (p. 198). Rigaud became depressed and wanted to die 'rather than to drag out a disgusting and useless life with his body in such a shameful state' (p. 198). At a visit to St Foy's shrine Rigaud regained the use of his paralysed arm.

F 4.12

A paralysed girl was to be brought to the shrine, but she was abandoned by those who were meant to take her on the other side of the river from Conques. She had to beg alms off passers-by, and at night she was menaced by wild animals. She had 'no strength to hold them off either with her hand or with a staff. Since no one took pity on her and carried her to the monastery, she remained for many days in this wretched state. Finally it was God's will that the senior monks of the monastery be moved to mercy. They ordered that she be carried to the monastery on a pallet. For a long time she could be seen lying there at its main entrance, at the most 'beautiful gate of the temple,' in the same way that the lame man later healed by Peter [Acts 3.2] once sought alms from those entering the Temple to pray there' (p. 200). Finally, towards evening of Palm Sunday, the paralysed girl was 'lifted up from the ground and walked to the holy virgin's tomb' (ibid.).

F 4.13

A man named Humbert was brought by his parents to be cured. 'His mother's livid nature had sent him forth from her womb in a condition in which his lower body, from the kidneys down, lay lifeless' (p. 201). He spent many years at the shrine, supported by alms, until during a vigil after the feast of the Assumption 'intense pain shot through his useless limbs and he began to wail and cry out.... Suddenly there was a cracking sound and his twisted limbs were stretched out straight. Through his invocation of the holy virgin the disabled body he had dragged around since he left his mother's womb was now healed. And so he cast aside the crutches of a paralytic, which he had formerly used when he needed to go somewhere' (p. 201).

F 4.14

A warrior named William suffered a head wound, and as 'a result his eyesight faded and then he became completely blind, but after he appealed to Sainte Foy he found eye salves effective and regained his sight.' Some days later William intervened in a brawl and was stabbed in the eye, resulting in great pains in his head, and again, blindness. After receiving some holy water from St Foy's shrine to be poured over his head, the pain went away 'but his sight was still very dim' (p. 202). William then went to Conques in person, and after mass on the day of St Foy's feast, he was led from the church. 'It seemed to him that he could make out human shapes as one does in the wavery light of dawn, but he couldn't really tell who they were' (ibid.). He returned to the altar, and there his sight was fully restored.

F 4.15

A woman mourned so much over the death of her spouse that she wore out 'her eyes with her tears until they clouded over in blindness' (p. 203). She wandered to many shrines, but remained blind for nine years. After a dream she went to Conques. There, during her stay in the guest house, 'a pain like an unbearable migraine headache [*dolor intolerabilis migraneo*] began to pound her head, and like a Bistonian woman who had drunk deeply of wine she rolled her head back and forth on her bed without stopping. Finally a boy led her by the hand to the holy virgin's abbey church and there she soaked the dust with streams of tears. But, wondrous to see! and contrary to nature, her tears turned to blood, which flowed down in waves and lay in red clots on the ground. After this gush of blood stopped, a tiny spark of light gradually began to light her eyes and she distinguished the shapes of things inside the church. Before sunset she could see everything clearly' (ibid. and p. 302 note 50).

F 4.17 'About a Warrior Who Had a Shriveled Hand Caused by a Wound'

A young warrior 'suffered a serious wound in his side from a lance. He was treated by the unskilled hands of physicians who erred in bandaging the wound too quickly. In so doing, they trapped putrefying, congealed bloody matter inside his body and it began to infect his internal organs. And since the confined fluid inside him had no outlet it raged on the inside and his body swelled up on the outside' (p. 206). After a dream, in which St Foy caused the wound to emit bloody matter, the man woke up to find this had actually happened, and he was cured. The writer seems to have got a little confused at this stage, as the chapter heading speaks of a withered hand, but the miracle itself makes no mention of anything other than a festering wound.

F 4.24

Hugh the master mason, who was working on the church, had his lower legs crushed by a cart carrying stones from the quarry. The bone of his leg was 'curved back like a sickle. Lamenting wildly at this, [the fellow workers] invoked the medical assistance of Sainte Foy. Then the injured master mason himself grasped his bowed leg with both hands and straightened it as easily as if it were made of warm wax' (p. 219). After his instantaneous cure, Hugh then completed his job of taking the load of rocks down to the church.

F L.3

The relics of St Foy were carried in procession to her church at Tanavelle and this attracted the local populace. 'Each person who was sick or physically impaired was carried to the procession as it passed, and several of them were restored to their former good health at once' (p. 248). On the third day of the procession St Foy showed herself to be the 'equal of Paul and even of Peter' (ibid.), by making a lame old man walk again, as the apostles had in Acts 3:1–11. A 'boisterous group of young people from Brioude' was en route to the procession and they came upon an

> old man who was very decrepit and extremely aged. From his youth he had been unable to use his arms and legs. In addition he suffered from a condition that had developed at the same time, namely that his limbs were stiff and unbending; he could neither move them to walk nor sit with any comfort. Since he suffered from such a physical impairment and had to struggle with it every day, he lacked any means of support and patiently joined the ranks of poor beggars. When he heard that his companions [the young people] were hurrying to the holy virgin's procession, he turned to his faith in her and

wanted to put to the test what he had heard about her long before. But since he couldn't walk, he eagerly asked them to take him to her and to expose him to the favor of her miracles, which could end the misfortunes governing his life. Through God's will his companions believed that he could be cured. They were deeply moved by his plight, so they prepared a beast of burden to transport him, placed him on it, and conducted him to the town of Talizat. They quickly heard from people who were coming back from there that the stewards of the holy image who had brought it to the region had already decided to return to Conques. They hesitated, not knowing what to do. Because they were uncertain about trusting faith, they made a bad decision. They made up their minds to set the lame old man down where he was, so that they might more easily hurry to the saint, who for them was not Faith but a martyr, or at least a virgin. And so he was left alone without shelter, but not without help. . . .

When the man realized all at once that he had been left without any assistance, I believe that he began to be very sad, not unreasonably, and he became thoroughly upset and distressed by sorrow. Who could describe today the tears that he shed as he began to pray to Sainte Foy? . . .

As he ceaselessly called on Sainte Foy, immediately through God's will the old man stood up straight, his feet firmly on the ground. He wasn't tottering around, as usually happens in such cases, since what he asked from Foy he received firmly through his faith. The new, old man came to us swiftly and nimbly on his own feet – for we were about two miles away from him – so that he could tell us what had happened. . . . And so that he could add physical proof to his assertion that he had been cured, he still had some signs of his former malady. But in addition proper witnesses were found, namely, the people who had taken him to Talizat. It was easy to see that he walked with quivering steps and it was not surprising, since he was not accustomed to running and the length of the journey had exhausted him. He helped to carry the holy virgin's reliquary with his aged hands, which he was using as if they were new although it was clear beyond a doubt that they were spotted with age (pp. 248–50).

The writer of this miracle makes some puns on religious faith and Foy's name 'Faith'. The story is also reminiscent of other miracles in which the protagonist is abandoned by the people taking them to the site of the saint's healing relics, for example F 4.12 in this collection, or L.5, before receiving a cure.

F L.5

William, a young military man, became ill during a campaign after eating poisonous foods in desperation for lack of proper food. He also drank water from a stagnant pool due to his intense thirst. He had sweat 'pour from his thoroughly enfeebled body, his stomach swelled up, the color of his face changed, and little by little his limbs began to contract terribly. Not even the physicians could decide whether his condition ought to be called dropsy or paralysis. As time passed and William was under the constant care of doctors, the part of his body from the kidneys upward regained its normal functions. The rest was completely lifeless' (p. 254). One day William, accompanied by two servants, decided to do the tour of saints' shrines in the hope of finding a cure. 'Or, if he was not to be cured, he wanted to hasten his death through the hardships of travel. For it is said that members of the nobility deliberately prefer to exile themselves and leave home rather than to be viewed with disdain by their kin' (pp. 254–5). William wandered all around the Frankish, Germanic, Celtic, Belgic and Ligurian regions. On his way back from the shrine of St James his servants abandoned him. Eventually he came to Conques and was cured at the shrine: 'All at once his skin split open, the structure of his muscles firmed up, blood ran down everywhere; the sick man immediately regained his health and stood on his feet. I learned this from none but William himself, who told me that he had spent four years in his paralyzed condition' (p. 256).

I   Miracles of St Ithamar at Rochester

Ithamar is one of the least known English saints, yet even he had a collection of miracle stories centred on his twelfth-century shrine at Rochester. The historic person of Ithamar was bishop of Rochester from 644 to his death *c*.655.

The full treatise on his miracles exists in one manuscript, Cambridge, Corpus Christi College, Ms. 161 (a collection of saints' lives written in the late twelfth or early thirteenth century), although in the fourteenth century John of Tynemouth included an abbreviated version in his collection of English saints' lives, the *Sanctilogium*. The modern edition of the text is by Denis Bethell, 'The Miracles of St Ithamar', *Analecta Bollandiana*, 89, 1971, pp. 421–37.

I II   Two blind people cured

An aged monk had an eye disorder [*oculis debilitatus*] (an alternative reading gives: struck by blindness [*cecitate percussus*]). He tried the medical treatment, but this failed to give him back his sight [*Cui medicus quibusdam medicinalibus instrumentis cum oculorum secreta rimaretur et crebris punctionibus ageret ut telam subtilissimam pupillis offusam quovis modo eicere posset, non solum nichil ei profuit, verum tantillo quod supererat luminis extincto, damno cecitatis vim nimii doloris adiciens, duplici senem affecit infortunio.*] The monk implored for the help of St Ithamar, and after experiencing a nocturnal vision, he went to the shrine of the saint and his sight was restored. Another blind man was also cured at the shrine (p. 430).

I III

A woman suffering from a weakening illness [*materfamilias, et erat languor fortissimus*] (p. 430) went to the shrine after having a vision, offering a candle to the saint. There she was cured, arising from her sickbed [*de lecto languoris surgit*] (p. 431).

I IV

The husband of the woman just cured (I III) also fell victim to a weakening illness [*decidens in languorem*] (p. 431), and he too was cured.

I V

An aged priest suffered from a blinding infirmity [*infirmitate cecutienti*] (p.431) and was cured in a vision of St Ithamar, in which the saint touched the eyes of the priest with his hands like a physician [*manuque protensa quasi medici functus officio, oculos . . . tetigit*] (p. 431).

I VI

A bishop was healed by the saint of an eye disorder [*oculorum dolore*] (p. 431), which his doctors could neither remove nor assuage [*Aderant medici, arte et labore plurimo agentes, ut dolorem ei aut tollerent aut lenirent*] (p. 431).

I XIII

A boy who was mute and deaf [*mutus et surdus effectus est*] (p. 435) was cured after he had been led to the shrine of St Ithamar [*ad illum deductus est* (alternative reading: *ad tumbam sancti Yhtamari deductus est)*] (p. 435).

I XVI

A woman, poor in material things but rich in faith, was young but badly deformed by nature [*mulier quedam, pauper quidem rebus, sed fide dives, etatis ut videbatur iuvenilis, sed nature vitio deformis*]. She was hit by a double calamity [*gemina est assecuta calamitas*], in that she could barely hear and not at all speak [*Audire parum poterat, loqui nichil*]. With difficulty could she understand anything, and she could only make herself understood by nodding [*Vix intelligebat aliquem, nulli ipsa nisi nutibus intellecta*] (p. 436). She went to the shrine, where in front of the spectators a mixture of spit and blood flowed from her mouth. The people pleaded for her, and after many days and the celebration of many masses, when the Lord's Prayer was recited, her ears were suddenly opened and the binding of her tongue was loosened, and she spoke [*Nam subito aperte sunt aures eius et solutum est vinculum lingue illius, et loquebatur*] (p. 437). The writer of the miracle account then embarked on an interesting discussion of the veracity of this miracle. It was pointed out that some people may doubt the miracle was 'for real', because it may be regarded as impossible for a woman, who had never spoken an intelligible word before, to suddenly speak perfectly. The potential doubters were referred to an analogy with the miracle of Balaam's ass (Numbers 22:28), which spoke suddenly in human voice: If for someone the cure was seen to be doubtful or incredible, in that suddenly without instruction or the use of experience the woman received the faculty of speech, let the doubter attend to him (i.e. God) who has formed human words in the ass of the prophet [*Si cui sane dubium vel incredibile videtur, ut tam subito sine doctrine vel usus experientia loquendi facultatem acceperit, attendat quis asine arioli illius verba humana formaverit*]. Furthermore, the doubter is to be let know that for God nothing is difficult, and nothing against nature is impossible to do for the author of nature [*et sciet quia Deo nichil est difficile, nichil contra naturam nature auctori factu impossibile*]. While the monks talked among themselves about this miracle, a secular priest arrived and then related the story of how a boy with an eye disorder was also healed by St Ithamar, when his mother donated a candle to the saint, after which the boy could at first see a little [*visu paulum recuperato*], and then could discern everything clearly [*nunc omnia clare discernit*]. After eight days, the woman cured of her speech and hearing impediment came to the shrine bearing a candle to make thanks for regaining her health. Among the people surrounding her were those who had discussed the miracle on an earlier day with the priest, constantly affirming that they had heard not even one word from her either in jest or serious [*Stabant autem et illi quibuscum diu conversata fuerat, constanter affirmantes ne unum quidem verbum se ab illa vel ioco vel serio audisse*]. They had apparently on many occasion out of curiosity tried to get the woman to say something, both by forcing her and by deceit [*cum multotiens aut vi aut dolis curiose agerent*], to establish whether the woman was really mute or not [*quatinus an vere muta esset explorare potuissent*] (p. 437). Again, the writer of the miracle account goes to great lengths to point out that the woman really was completely mute up until the miracle. Finally, she told the surrounding people that she came to the shrine after having a vision while asleep in her bed.

W   Miracles of St William of Norwich

St William was a boy from Norwich who was believed to have been ritually sacrificed by the town's Jewish population in 1144. Shortly after his death, people began to report miracles worked by or through William. Thomas of Monmouth, the author of the *miracula*, was a monk at the Benedictine monastery in Norwich; he first appeared in the monastery around 1150, but related the story of St William from the saint's childhood onward; the last event he recorded dates from *c.*1172. The miracles recorded in his text therefore span the period from 1144 to around 1172, and Thomas appears to have composed his text in 1172–3. The miracle account has been edited and translated by A. Jessop and M. R. James, *The Life and Miracles of St William of Norwich by Thomas of Monmouth*, Cambridge: Cambridge University Press, 1896, based on a manuscript in Cambridge, University Library MS Add. 3037, folios 1 to 77 recto, dated to somewhat before 1200.

W II.viii   Argument for veracity of miracles based on cure of disabled

Thomas of Monmouth argued against the sceptics, who regarded the miracles of St William as fictitious, that the miracles would not have lasted for so long nor been so frequent if they were not true. 'But we have seen full many people labouring under various inconveniences, blind, dumb, deaf, lame, hump-backed, bent, going on all fours,[1] people with swellings, with the dropsy, with ulcers and wens,[2] mad people and many others of both sexes diseased with every sort of complaint, cured by the merits of the holy martyr William' [*Nempe uidimus quam plurimos uariis per multum tempus laborantes incommodis, cecos, mutos, surdos, claudos, incuruos, contractos, scabellarios, turgidos, ydropsicos, ulcerosos, gutturnosos, furibundos, aliosque multos utriusque sexus diuersis languoribus morbidos sancti martiris Willelmi meritis curatos*] (p. 86).

W III.vii   Cure of arthritic woman

Claricia, wife of Gaufridus de Marc, had been suffering for some years from kidney pain and pains in her knees, which could not be cured by physicians even though she spent a lot of money on them [*Hec per aliquot dolore renum ac genuum laborauerat annos, nec per aliquos, licet in illis multum expenderit, curari potuit medicos.*] (p. 132). She was led to the shrine by others, and bent her knees as far as she was able to touch the stone of the tomb, and was healed. 'Thus it came to pass that she who came with her feeble body by the hands of others, when the heavenly medicine did its work, went back safe and sound needing no man's support' [*Sicque factum est, ut que manibus alienis corpore inbecillis aduenerat, celesti operante medicina, nullius egens adminiculo incolumis rediret et sospes.*] (p. 132).

W III.xiv   Cure of arthritic woman

Alditha, wife of Toke the chandler, suffered from an illness where her limbs were racked with pain, and she could not take a step without using a stick nor do any sort of work using her hands [*nec sine baculo gressum figeret, nec omnino aliquid operis manibus efficere posset*] (p. 147). She was cured after dedicating a candle to the saint.

W III.xvi   Cure of boy born dumb

Colobern and Ansfrida of Norwich had a boy about seven years old who was dumb from birth [*a natiuitate mutum*] (p. 149). The parents were advised in a dream to take the boy to the shrine, which they did. There they prayed and dedicated a candle, and once the boy had kissed the tomb, he turned round to his parents and 'suddenly broke forth in his mother tongue asking that they might go back home' (p. 149).

W III.xxii   Woman cured of gout

A certain Ida had been afflicted by gout so badly that it had spread from her knees to her arm and right shoulder, so that she could only get to the tomb of the saint with difficulty and with the help of others; after her cure she was able to go away alone.

W III.xxiv   Woman cured of weakness in limbs

A certain Goldeburga was so ill so that when she came to the shrine her limbs could hardly support her; after a few days she obtained a perfect recovery.

W III.xxvii   Cure of boy from immobility

Roger and his wife Godiva brought their 10-year-old boy to the shrine. The boy was unable to make a single step, and for a long time had been incapable of moving or turning himself [*Hi filium decennem toto corpore inbecillem attulerunt, quia gressu proprio illuc uenirenequaquam poterat, quoniam a multis idebus se mouere seu conuertere impotens erat*] (p. 158). The boy's condition was likened to that of one almost dead [*fere emortuum*] (ibid.). He was laid on the tomb, and after prayers and a short while he was much better, insomuch that he could now turn about unaided.

W IV.ii   Cure of blind man

Gurwan the tanner, in the days of famine and pestilence, had in his house a blind man along with other poor persons [*famis et mortalitatis diebus cum aliis in domo sua pauperibus cecum quendam ipse habuerat*] (pp. 167–8). The blind man was told in a dream that after having three masses sung he would recover his sight, which happened.

W IV.v   Woman cured of gout

One Botilda, wife of Toche the baker at Norwich, had for a long time had such severe pains in her feet that she could not put her foot to the ground. She was unable to leave the house, so her husband went to the saint's tomb instead; her cure took place at home at the same time her husband was at the shrine.

W IV.ix   Medical versus miraculous cure

William the sacrist (who was the subject of a miracle at III.xiii, not cited here), was ill again. In a vision to another monk, St William said that William the sacrist must 'first vow to me that he will never henceforth take any medicine except this of mine' [*mihi uouere uolo se nullam ulterius alteram preter huiusmodi meam suscepturum medicinam*] (p. 175). William drank holy water in which the teeth of the saint had been washed, and recovered for a while, only to get worse again. The doctors 'kept advising him to take measures for his safety, and try some medicine' [*crebro illi a medicis suggerebatur ut sibi scilicet consuleret, ac medicine remedium attemptaret*] (p. 176). The sacrist was bound by his vow, but his pains got worse, and 'he yielded to the advice of the doctors and sought refuge in the deceits of medicine' [*medicis persuadentibus tandem heu consensit, et fallacis medicine asylo se contulit*] (ibid.). Needless to say, William the sacrist was punished for his vow-breaking and died four days after taking the doctors' medicine.

*W IV.xi   Crippled woman cured, and cure
of blind woman*

Among many people healed 'a woman of Norwich called Ada who had been ill
for a whole year [*iam annuo egrotauerat languore*], came supported [*sustentata brachiis*]
on one side by her husband Siwate, and on the other by some one else' (p. 181).
'Also, Ravenilda wife of William of Hastedune, who had gradually lost her sight
through the long weakening of her eyes, came to the tomb of Saint William, led
by another, and rejoiced at the full recovery of her sight' (pp. 181–2).

W V.xiv   Cure of a bent woman who walked with trestles
[de contracta muliere scabellaria sanata]

A poor woman from Bury St Edmunds, who had been bent double for many
years, came to the shrine [*muliercula...per multos contracta...annos*] (p. 205). She
walked to Norwich with trestles which she held in her hands [*hec manualibus gradiens
scabellis, prout potuit*] (p. 205). She came as near to the tomb of the saint as she could
because of the press of people and prayed. 'Scarce had she ended her prayer
when she was seized with a sudden and acute pain, her sinews were stretched with
a loud cracking, and herself stretched to her full length' [*Vix orationem terminauerat,
cum subito correpta dolore acerbe angustiatur, neruisque crepitu magno distensis et ipsa distenditur.*]
(ibid.). She suffered for a while from severe pain, and after it ceased, she rested,
and then after an hour arose 'whole and sound' (ibid.) in front of witnesses.

W V.xv   Cure of contracted woman

A woman from Flordon became affected by parturition such that with her sinews
all contracted her whole body was in a weakened state, so that for many days she
was unable to feed herself with her hands nor walk on her feet [*et ea dolore partus
atque angustia contractis membrorum neruis tantam corporis incurrit imbecillitatem, ut multis
postea diebus neque se ipsam manibus pascere neque pedibus posset ambulare*] (p. 206). After
remaining in this condition for a long time, she was set on a horse with the help
of her husband and others, and brought to the shrine, near which she was set
down. After three hours there she was cured. 'And so, she who had come sad
and in need of others' help, went away in joy trusting to her own feet' [*Et factum
est, que tristis et aliene opis aduenerat indigua, leta cum suis regreditur gressibus propriis
confisa*] (p. 206).

W V.xvi   Cure of contracted and mute girl

A girl of seven, who was contracted and dumb [*contractam ac mutam*] (p. 207), was
brought to the shrine by her mother. She was placed by the tomb, and when
someone happened to bring an egg to the site, she said 'Look, mother I've got an
egg!' (ibid.). Witnesses confirmed that they knew the woman and her daughter,
and had often seen the contracted and mute girl.

W V.xvii   Cure of girl blind, deaf and dumb from birth

A poor woman was told in a vision to bring her daughter, who had been born blind and mute [*ab ortu cecam et mutam*] (p. 208), to the saint's shrine. At the tomb, the film which had covered the girl's eyes 'like the skin of an egg' parted [*albugine que uirginis oculos tanquam oui membrana obduxerat dissoluta*] (p. 208) amidst bleeding from the eyes. Bystanders lit a candle and waved it to and fro in front of the girl's face, and she 'followed it with her eyes in whatever direction it was moved' (p. 209). Then followed another 'test' of the girl's new-found abilities:

'We then put away the candle, and produced an apple. She took it and admired it, and when her mother said in English: "Eat the apple, daughter, eat it!" she repeated the words, under the impression that she had answered her mother, as not yet knowing how to say anything but what she had heard some one else say. So that I conjecture that she had not only been blind and dumb, but deaf as well' [*Auferentes denique candelam, exhibuimus et pomum. Qoud apprehensum cum admiraretur, Anglica lingua mater ait: Comede, filia, comede pomum. Ad hec dum eundem puellula sermonem retexeret, se matri respondisse credidit. Necdum aliud loqui nouerat, nisi quod ab alio audiebat. Vnde conicimus non illam tantum cecam et mutam, immo fuisse et surdam.*] (ibid.).

Thomas of Monmouth uses this miracle to point out that it was so great, that from that day on 'a pious devotion to St William took root in the hearts even of unbelievers' [*deuotio incredulorum radicauit in cordibus*] (ibid.).

W V.xxii   Cure of woman impaired by swollen knees

Goda, the wife of Copman of Norwich, came to the tomb to seek relief of her affliction; she had been troubled by kidney pains, and the pain had descended to her knees and made them swell, so that her knees were 'the size and shape of pots' (p. 216), and she could no longer walk. In addition, her left eye swelled up to the size of an egg. She had herself carried to the shrine, where she was cured.

W V.xxiii   Woman cured of deafness

Alditha, wife of Thoche the chandler,[3] had been growing deaf over the years 'to such an extent that you could only make yourself heard by putting your lips close to her ear' [*obsurduerant aures adeoque inualuerat incommodum, ut nisi tuum illius auribus os applicares ab ipsa nequaquam audiri posses*] (p. 218). Thomas of Monmouth points out the social implications of her deafness perceived by the woman:

'She was consequently afraid to go out, and only talked to her own family, fearing lest the reproach of her deafness should be detected by others, and bring derision upon her' [*Vnde et in publicum prodire uerebatur, et non nisi domesticorum utebatur alloquiis. Timebat enim ualde ne surdiciei sue obprobrium aliene quandoque noticie prodiret in risum*] (ibid.).

She went to the shrine, where she prayed and stopped both her ears with the cloth that covered the tomb, and at once she could hear again.

W VI.viii   Cure of blind woman

Gilliva, daughter of Burcard a carpenter, lost her vision through an accident and had been blind for three years. In addition, she had problems with her eyelids, so that for that entire time her eye lashes were always closed as if glued together. Her young nephew gave her some string and went before, guiding her to Norwich. At the shrine she began to pray but was interrupted by an attack of pain in her eyes and head. Eventually, after blood came from her eyes, the pain subsided and she could open her eyelids and see again after three years.

W VI.xi   Cure of wonderfully contracted woman

A woman called Matilda had been afflicted since her youth by a sorrowful debility [*debilitas dolenda*] (p. 242). Thomas of Monmouth gives a detailed description of her condition in anticipation of the great miracle that is necessary to heal her:

'Ever since then, in fact, she had been so weak of body, that owing to the curvature of her spine she was quite doubled up, her legs twisted together, and her knees pressed one against the other. The consequence was, that when she wished to go from one place to another she had to support her feeble limbs with a stick and either succeed in getting a little way, or, sometimes, was not able to do even this. Peter, the priest of Langham, a vill of the Bishop's, had long housed her by way of charity, and supplied her with food and clothing. If she ever desired to visit some shrine for the recovery of her health, he used to have her taken there laid like a sack across a horse' [*Facta est siquidem ab ea etate adeo corpore imbecillis, ut curuata dorsi spina, et ipsa fieret curua, et cancellatis cruribus innexa uicissim colliderentur genua. Vnde contigit, quod si quandoque de loco se ad locum transferre uoluisset, imbecillia baculo membra sustentans, uel gressus modicum proficeret uel nonnumquam nec in modico preualeret. Hanc Petrus presbiter de Langeham uilla episcopali per multum tempus elemosine gratia in domo sua tenuit, pauit, et uestiuit. Quam si quandoque recuperande sanitatis gratia sacra uisitare loca concupisset, illus equo ad instar sacci pleni in transuersum deportare faciebat.*] (p. 242).

These other shrines proved ineffective, and she decided to go to Norwich, setting out with her stick. 'Each step was hardly a finger's length, and there was considerable delay between them, so that one watching her progress would judge her to be slower than any tortoise' (p. 243). When she finally got to the cathedral, she felt the soles of her feet 'pricked as if by thorns' (ibid.), and then in front of the shrine she was racked by pain, so that she writhed and rolled on the ground, after which she managed to get up, and still feeble, made her way along the screen of the shrine by clinging to the shafts, until she reached the tomb itself. She had Peter the priest called to dispel the doubts of sceptics, and asserted that she had indeed been the subject of a miracle.

W VI.xii   Cure of hump-backed and contracted boy

The son of Godric of Wortham was ten years old and afflicted by a weakness [*imbecillitas*] (p. 244) which daily increased upon him. 'The disease infected all his limbs: the sinews were dried up and contracted: his spine was bent, and a hump grew on his back. From being upright the boy became crooked; his stomach was pressed against his knees and, when he wanted to walk, he had to place his hands on his knees or on the ground, and use one or the other for a support. The doctors who were consulted did him no good' [*Percurrente per artus molestia, arefacti nerui contrahuntur, et incuruata dorsi spina dorso gibbus innascitur. Fit itaque puerulus de recto contractus, et adherente genibus uentre cum ambulare proponeret, applicatis ad genua uel terre palmis, ipsa uel ipsam pro podio haberet. Medici frustra laborantes adhibentur*] (pp. 244–5). The boy was brought to Norwich in a hand barrow [*manuali uehitur uehiculo*] (p. 245), and was placed by the tomb of the saint. At that instant the sinews stretched themselves, the boy was racked with pain, and in a short time he rose up and walked back with his father in an upright fashion. But after some days the weakness returned, and the boy had to be taken to Norwich again, where he was cured completely this time.

W VII.i   Man cured of loss of speech and sight

Reimbert, seneschal to the abbot of Battle, had fallen into a serious illness 'which increasing deprived him alike of speech and sight' (p. 263). He remembered the tomb of St William he had once seen at Norwich and 'setting him before his mind's eye, he invited his help with the tongue of his heart' [*ante mentis oculos ponens cordis lingua qua potuit eius sibi opem inuocauit*] (p. 264). He was instantly cured. The invocation had to be made with the heart's tongue, since a 'proper' invocation through the spoken word was now impossible for Reimbert.

W VII.ii   Youth cured of palsy

A youth called Schet, son of one Eilmer, living in Yarmouth, had long been afflicted with palsy. The same day he was brought to the shrine 'the string of his tongue was loosed, speech restored to him, and health to his strengthless limbs' (p. 265).

W VII.viii   Many impaired persons cured

'I have also very often seen persons come there who were lame, blind, deaf, or dumb, and many others sick of divers diseases, and have known most of them to be cured' (p. 269).

W VII.ix   Cure of boy blind, deaf and dumb from birth

In 1156 a woman of Repps brought her son to the shrine who was blind from birth, also deaf, dumb and weak in all his body, and 'deprived of the use of his limbs' (p. 270); on the same day he was cured.

W VII.x   Cure of a contracted boy

A boy who from infancy had been contracted became upright. The boy had lived many years in Norwich and begged at many houses there, 'kneeling on his knees and getting about by trestles which he held in his hands: for the power of walking was denied him, inasmuch as his sinews were dried up, his knees contracted, and his calves wasted away' [*genibus innixus et manualibus gradiens scabellis.... Arefactis siquidem neruis, contracto poplite, ac desiccatis tibiis, usus illi negabatur gradiendi.*] (p. 270).

W VII.xi   Cure of a second crippled person

One Thomas of York came to the shrine, who was 'very weak throughout his body, who guided his steps and supported his feet and frame on two sticks such as are commonly called crutches' [*debilis quidem uiribus et toto imbecillis corpore, duobus quos uulgo potentias uocant baculis gressus utcumque dirigens, et imbecilles artus sustentans.*] (p. 271). He obtained the healing at Norwich, 'in token of which he there left his crutches' [*ibique in signum sua podia dimisit*] (ibid.).

W VII.xii   Cure of a contracted woman

A poor contracted woman, always seen by others to be doubled up [*neque quisquam illam nisi contractam se uidisse testabatur*] (p. 271), was also cured at the shrine.

W VII.xiv   Cure of a crippled girl

An 8-year-old girl from Norwich called Agnes had suffered from birth severely 'from gout' [*podagre ciragreque*] (p. 273) in her hands and feet. She was 'unable to raise herself or even to turn from one side to the other without assistance. To make matters worse, the sinews in her neck were contracted and her left cheek adhered so firmly to her left shoulder that you saw the one imbedded in the other, and the neck could not be bent in any direction whatever without bending the shoulder. All these afflictions therefore she suffered: walk she could not with her gouty feet, nor touch anything with her contracted hands, while the adherence of her head to the shoulder deprived her of the wonted power of seeing, standing, turning, nay, eating: for when she had to take food, it was cut up on the ground or on a trencher, and she lay down and fed like a beast, able only to eat what her tongue or teeth caught hold of. In this absolutely helpless state she was turned, raised and moved about by others' help' [*Non se propriis ualebat uiribus eleuare, neque absque adiuuantis adminiculo a latere in latus quandoque conuertere. Neruis quoque in ceruicem contractis, ad augmentum incommodi, humero sinistro sinistra mala tam inseparabiliter adherebat, ut alteri alterum incastrari cerneres atque in nullas omnino partes inflexo humero ceruix flecti preualebat. Multiplex igitur incommodum, pedibus podagricis incessus, manibus contractis attactus, capitique humero coherenti consuetudinarius uidendi, erigendi, conuertendi et comedendi negabatur usus. Quotiens enim manducandi perurgebat necessitas, cibo super terram uel asserem comminuto, humi procumbens, et ad instar pecudis oppetens, id solum poterat manducare quod lingua uel dentibus contingebat attingere. Toto igitur impos et imbecillis corpore alienis uertebatur, erigebatur, et circumferebatur manibus.*] (p. 274). The girl was brought to the shrine, carried in her mother's arms, and was immediately healed.

W VII.xv   Cure of a contracted girl

Hathewis, daughter of Edwin the priest of Taverham, was contracted and weak in the limbs; she was cured at the shrine.

W VII.xvi   Cure of another contracted girl, and three boys

One Huelina of Rochesburch, whose heels from birth adhered to her back by a 'vice of nature' [*cui ex nature uitio pedum tali natibus adheserant*] (p. 275), was brought by her father to the shrine 'in a wheeled vehicle of the kind called a litter (civière)' [*in uehiculo rotatili aduehitur, quod ciueriam appellant*][4] (ibid.). On the same day a boy called Baldwin was brought by his father, 'also in a litter with wheels' [*itidem in ciueria aduehitur rotatili*] (ibid.); 'the sinews of his feet and legs from the knees downwards were wasted and deprived him of the power of walking. However, when forced to move himself, he crept along on his knees, leaning on hand-trestles' [*cui arefactis a genibus infra pedum et tibiarum neruis, usus negabatur gradiendi. Quandoque tamen sed cum necessitas ingruebat, genibus innixus scabellis ibat manualibus.*] (ibid.). Both the girl and boy were healed fully at the shrine.

Not many days after, a boy named Herbert who was blind and mute from infancy [*a primeuo cecus et mutus tempore*] (pp. 275–6) was brought to the shrine by his parents, and was cured. Also a certain Ralph, son of Richard of Hadeston, who was weak in all his limbs [*membris omnibus imbecillis*] (p. 276) was brought to Norwich by his friends and was cured.

M   Miracles of the Virgin Mary at Rocamadour

Citations are from Marcus Bull, *The Miracles of Our Lady of Rocamadour: Analysis and Translation*, Woodbridge NY: Boydell Press, 1999, using reference to book and chapter in which the miracle occurs (e.g. I.5) and the page number in that edition. Only those miracles which, in their context of impairment, have something unusual or otherwise interesting to say are described or cited more fully. The collection of miracles at Rocamadour in Quercy, southern France, was made in 1172–3. The English translation is based on a manuscript at Bibliothèque nationale, Paris, MS lat. 16565.

The *miracula* are divided into three books. In total, the *miracula* relate 126 miracles: 53 in book I, 49 in book II and 24 in book III. Of all the 126 miracles, there are 37 miracles, or 29 per cent of the total number, relating to healing and cures of impairments and other illnesses: blindness has eight cures (at I.3, I.16, I.21, I.23, II.9, II.18, II.19, II.36), hearing and speech impediments have nine cures (at I.6, I.26, I.33, I.35, I.39, I.45, II.5, II.15, II.48) and paralysis and contraction have eleven cures (at I.4, I.22, I.38, II.5, II.9, II.15, II.24, II.32, II.46, III.11, III.21). A further number of miracles relate to the cure of ailments other than impairments, namely: epilepsy with two cures (at II.24, II.13), possession and/or madness with seven cures (at I.5, I.28, I.35, I.41, II.10, II.16, II.40), and fevers with two cures, inflammations, growths, or ulcers with 11 cures, diverse injuries with 16 cures, and various or unspecified diseases with 14 cures. If one takes into account these cures as well, together with the impairments, then all healing miracles amount to 80 of 126 miracles, or 64 per cent.

The remaining miracles relate to protections (48 per cent), punishments (21 per cent), and offerings (35 per cent). The percentages add up to a sum greater than 100 per cent, since many miracles are counted more than once, as they feature in more than one category, for example miracle I.5 appears as a cure for possession, a punishment, and as an offering miracle.

M I.3   Cure of blindness but punishment for breaking vow

A woman who lived in Vienne had been blind for a long time in both eyes. She vowed she would go to the Virgin's church [at Rocamadour] if her blindness was cured. This happened, but the woman put off performing her vow. In punishment, a sharp bone from some meat she was eating blocked her throat. The *miracula* state that the virgin 'inflicted a harsher wound upon her' (p. 103). Only when other people prayed for her did the Virgin relent and the bone was knocked out of the woman's throat. The woman of course then went to Rocamadour.

M I.4   Paralysis as punishment

Some robbers assaulting a man on pilgrimage had their hands 'paralysed and shrivelled' (p. 104) when they tried to steal his money. The robbers were frightened, prayed to the Virgin and repented their deeds, and even their intended victim the pilgrim prays, and the robbers were healed.

M I.6   Muteness as punishment

A man was on pilgrimage from the Toulousain, entrusted with money offerings for the Virgin by other pilgrims, but he kept some of the money for himself. 'To prevent him from perishing for such a crime when examined at the Last Judgement, he was deprived of the use of his tongue in the here and now' (p. 105). Only pleas from his companions could help the man. After he revealed where he had hidden the money, he was changed back from being mute again.

M I.15   Shrivelled arm cured

'Count Robert of Meulan fell off his horse and landed on his right arm, which became dislocated at the shoulder joint. it was put right thanks to the skills of doctors. After some time had passed, he happened to fall on the same arm, which was dislocated more seriously than before at the same joint. Doctors applied poultices which did absolutely no good, and they lost hope that the arm would get better; it hung down behind Robert's back as if it were shrivelled up, and nothing the doctors could do would make it lift up' (pp. 112–13) Robert prayed to the Virgin and made vows, and suddenly he 'began to move the arm and to wave it around' (p. 113).

M I.16   Blind boy cured

In the province of Reims, Robert, known as 'the Lean', had a son who when he 'was two days old – if that – he became permanently blind' (p. 113). His parents vowed to go to Rocamadour. After eight days of travelling there, the little boy 'who had never seen anything, gradually began to make things out. Moreover, he started to reach out his hands when something was held up to him. But because he still had fairly small pupils, he could not fix his gaze in the same way that someone could who had been able to see from birth.'

M I.17   Speech-impediment prevented

'During a battle a knight who was in his sixties was hit in the mouth by the hilt of a sword and had four of his front teeth knocked out. To prevent himself from becoming an incoherent-sounding object of universal derision, he eagerly prayed to the glorious Mother of God for the teeth to be restored' (p. 113). His teeth were restored, white as ivory.

M I.20   Woman cured of dropsy

A woman named Hathvidis, who had been ill with dropsy for seven years, could not be cured by doctors' treatments. She had been so swollen up that 'two people could scarcely put their arms around her on account of her great size' (p. 115). She was cured after praying.

M I.21   Three blind people cured

Three blind people lived in same village in the diocese of Clermont. Two were taken to Rocamadour by their neighbours, one was cured in the church, the other on the way home, after a mixture of complaining that his friend was cured and he not, and also by not despairing and continuing to ask for the Virgin's help. 'And so it happened that this man, who hitherto had needed to be led by a guide, now became his own guide, . . . he became able to walk ahead of the group and lead the others' (p. 115). The third blind person from the village was cured after his father took him on pilgrimage. The father confessed he had sinned in putting off the journey, and the blind son was cured after three days.

M I.22   Woman first punished by being
crippled then cured

In Burgundy a woman did work on the feast day of St Anthony, and her hand suddenly seized up. Asking for a cure at the altar of her local church dedicated to

St Anthony did not bring success, so she went to Rocamadour. There she was cured. 'And her arm, which had become withered, made a noise similar to the sound of a fence being broken' (p. 116) while the cure took place in the church.

M I.23   Child blind since birth cured

Childless parents, the woman being already quite advanced in years, were granted their wish for a child at Rocamadour, but the resulting boy was born blind. His mother lamented this, but weaned the child and brought him up. Then the parents travelled to Rocamadour again, this time to ask for a cure for their boy, which happened.

M I.24   Knight harassing pilgrim punished with ergotism

A knight harassing a pilgrim was punished by a burning, called 'infernal fire' [= ergotism] in his foot. The burning was so fierce that the knight had not just his foot consumed by it, but the lower leg right up to his knee. 'The knight was afraid that his whole body would burn away, so he had his leg amputated at the knee. Straight away the fire crossed over into the other foot and began to consume him with great intensity, until finally he lost both feet and was left maimed' (p. 118).

M I.26   Mute woman cured

'A noble woman, Paschors of Romans, had for a very long time lost not only the faculty of speech but also the ability to make any sound at all' (p. 118). At Rocamadour, she placed herself by a corner of the altar, where the guardian of the church tried to push her away, because he thought she was being a nuisance. He even went so far as to hit her on the head with his rod in an attempt to drive her away from the altar. She persevered, being 'greedy for health', and while the Magnificat was being sung she was cured and joined in the singing.

M I.33   Girl deaf and dumb since birth cured

Huga was deaf and dumb since birth, but now of marriageable age. She then went to the shrine with her father, mother and sisters. After praying, she could hear the church bells, and 'on recognizing Gerbert, the guardian of the church with whom she had been staying, she called out to him using his name.... the girl was speaking clearly and distinctly...' (p. 122).

M I.35   Man is both dumb and mad

For insulting the Virgin, a squire was 'deprived of all his bodily strength and became both dumb and mad' (p. 123). He was restrained with difficulty. Physicians came and tried to heal him, 'and laboured long and hard without success. When they had exhausted all their means of healing they pronounced the squire incurable' (ibid.). At the shrine he was healed and the Virgin released 'the bond which held his tongue' (p. 124).

M I.38   *Cripple cured by a vision*

Gerbert of Creysse 'was so crippled that his knees dug into his chest and his ankles stuck to his buttocks' (p. 126). He had himself carried to Rocamadour in a basket, there he begged for food from other pilgrims. While asleep, he was 'overcome by the great pain in his body'. He had a vision, in which the Virgin and the martyr George pulled him upright, and he was cured.

M I.39   *Deaf and dumb woman healed*

'For a long time Polilia, who was deaf and dumb and came from Périgueux, lived in the village of Rocamadour with a poor woman called Juliana. When she wanted to get food, whatever she could come by, she used to stand outside the doors of the villagers' dwellings, tapping on the doorposts or the doors themselves and not stopping until the inhabitants were moved by her wretchedness to take pity on her' (p. 126). When she heard of the healing of Gerbert the cripple (M I.38), she immediately sighed in the direction of the shrine, but 'it was with weeping and moaning that she expressed herself because she could not speak' (ibid.). She too was healed.

M I.45   *Knights lose powers of speech*

Two knights of Henry II on campaign in Ireland 'lose the power of speech because of the inclement air, the change of diet and the fact that they had to drink water from rivers' (p. 130). They wanted to go to Rocamadour, but because 'they were unable to speak, the two men were obliged to make an inner vow' (ibid.). The Virgin 'restored their ability to speak and made the mute talk once more' (ibid.).

M II prol   Prologue to the second part

'... let us call to mind the man from Burgundy who was grey-haired, illustrious and sound of judgement; the man from the region of Troyes; the woman from Pavia; the woman from Gascony; someone from Nevers; someone from Montélimar. All these regained their sight; not all of them did so right here in our church, but they all claimed that it was through the suffrages of our church, and they had many witnesses with them. Let us call to mind the woman from Beaucaire who recovered her senses; the woman from Burgundy who regained the ability to speak; someone from the Rouergue who had long been crippled and had long lain near the church but was then made upright... However, the notary was unwell on the days when these things became known, and so did not write down in the correct manner and with proper headings those miracles...' (p. 137).

M II.5   *Mute and paralysed woman cured*

'A woman from Saint-Guilhelm-le-Désert near Lodève was a mute whose mouth was twisted back towards her ear and whose arm was shrivelled up' (p. 143). She was taken to the shrine and cured there.

M II.9   *Thieves punished by blindness*

Three pilgrims were attacked by thieves; the Virgin 'seized hold of the servants of iniquity...and took away their sight, which is a human being's most cherished asset. She also paralysed their hands and rendered them immobile like statues, out of pity leaving them only with the use of their tongues so that they could ask for mercy and express heartfelt penitence' (p. 146). The thieves pleaded with the pilgrims, and the Virgin 'restored the thieves' senses and returned their bodies to their former health' (p. 147).

M II.15   *Badly mutilated woman abandoned then cured*

A woman, Stephana, was badly attacked and mauled by wolves. She was found by the people from her village the next day, but 'she had been so ravaged that it was scarcely possible to recognize in her a human form.... She was terrifying to behold, even for those who were her close relatives. Yet who is there I can call 'relative' considering that they swiftly and mercilessly rejected her? Her tongue could not move to form words. And when food was placed in her mouth it came out of holes in her throat and chest, leaving her with just a distant, thin taste. Because her nerves were contracted and her limbs damaged, her knees became stuck to her chest. And the wounds, from which considerable amounts of flesh had been removed, could not be covered over with her remaining skin. Although it says in the Bible that *no one ever hates his own flesh, but nourishes it and cherishes it, as Christ does the church* [Ephesians 5:29], people decided that this deformed member had to be removed from the body as something useless and putrid' (pp. 151–2). The villagers then dumped Stephana in a cart and took her at night to a remote village, where they abandoned her. 'When the people there looked at her they thought that she was some kind of monstrosity' (p. 152). These other villagers, too, abandoned her, and in the end she was fished out of a river by a knight. The knight had her placed in a barn, 'removed from contact with people because the stench and frightfulness of her wounds were an assault on the sight and smell of those attending to her' (ibid.). The knight looked after her, and she recovered 'thanks to the attention of doctors and the fortifying effects of food' (ibid.). But she was not cured completely. 'The sick woman felt that none of the doctors' medicines or poultices would make her well. By means of hand signals, head movements and whatever weak sounds she was able to make she begged to be carried to Rocamadour. The journey there took a very long time because she was poor and on her back; but finally she was carried to the church...As we said earlier, she was at that time bent over and could not lift her head to breathe' (p. 153). Stephana persisted with her prayers and she was cured.

M II.18   *Blind man cured*

The peasant William Boarius 'lived quietly from the fruits of his labours . . . he did not have it in mind to harm anyone, and he did not take from his neighbours what was theirs. Nonetheless the hand of the Lord fell heavily upon him: he was deprived of his sight, and for six years or more he remained blind. . . . The skill and hard work of physicians did not work on him, failing to restore to him any degree of sight. They were astonished how it could be that only his sight was affected when the rest of his body was perfectly healthy' (p. 154). William's wife had heard of Rocamadour and vowed to offer a candle as tall as William if he was to be cured; she also threatened to burn the very same candle if he was not cured. William was cured immediately.

M II.19   *Pregnant woman blinded in labour*

A woman from Burgundy was pregnant, and went into labour in the hospital of St John the Baptist in Jerusalem. During the birth she lost the use of her eyes. Her husband took her to the church of the Holy Sepulchre, but their prayers were not answered there. Only when the husband and wife vowed to make a pilgrimage to Rocamadour was the woman cured straight away. 'They praised and glorified the star of the sea who lights up the blindness in our minds with the radiance of her humility and repairs our bodies in all their many different infirmities' (p. 156).

M II.24   *Knight punished with epilepsy and paralysis*

A young knight from Gascony was a gambler, irreverent, and blasphemous, so that God 'brought his heavy hand down upon him by giving him the falling sickness' (p. 156). 'Up until that moment this man seemed to be soaring through the clouds and considered himself second to no mortal being. But now he lies frothing at the mouth in agony. He gnashes his teeth, he contorts his mouth, and his eyes stare terrifyingly. He clenches his fists, and there is no use in his limbs as if they were dead' (pp. 156–7). The man was unable to find a doctor who could cure him, so he decided to go to Rocamadour. There he prayed and was cured, after vowing not to commit the sorts of crimes any more for which people held him responsible. After returning home, his father-in-law accused him of acting more like a monk than a knight, and the man eventually was convinced by the arguments and broke his vow. 'His illness then returned. In full view of the many people who were there he began to foam at the mouth and collapsed onto the ground, falling more heavily than he had done before. His right arm and right hand – the one he used to throw dice – became withered, as did the middle part of his body, which became paralysed. . . . The man screamed that he would be fortunate if he departed this life, in that he had become *scorned by men and despised by the people* [Psalms 21:7]. He said that he would have been better off if he had never drawn breath: better that than be afflicted by a destructive illness and daily die a hateful death' (p. 161). His relatives did not give up on him, and he returned to Rocamadour a penitent, where he mortified himself, stripping naked, rolling around on the ground and kissing the feet of the other pilgrims. He was then completely cured.

M II.26   *Withered arm in punishment*

'Renald Belloz, a guardian of the church, threw a stone at a sparrow which was trying to fly into the most holy basilica of Rocamadour. He lost the strength in his arm, and it remained withered for the rest of his life' (p. 163).

M II.32   *Young man's paralysis cured*

A youth from Montpellier was 'gravely stricken by paralysis and, on the advice of his physicians, was carried to the baths. Whereas only part of his body had been withered up till then, when he was brought back from the baths his whole body was now desiccated and crippled. He was immobile, like a statue, and he could not feel anything. His eyes were permanently closed, his mouth was twisted back, and he could not do anything with his hands: he appeared to be dead yet did not die' (p. 166). He was just about breathing and 'was not properly alive'. His relatives made a life-size wax effigy of him to send to Rocamadour, which worked, because '[a]s soon as this was done, the youth came back to life' (ibid.).

M II.36   *Blind woman cured*

A woman from the Auvergne had lost her sight for about seven years. At Rocamadour, she was more concerned 'about the sort of sight which can be recovered and lost than about the vision of the Lord which, when the burden of the flesh is laid aside, will endure without diminution' (p. 169). She spent days near the altar, and even had to be 'restrained by the brethren of the church because her spirit had become more fervent and her complaining was sometimes too shrill, and also because they found her voice irritating and excessively loud' (ibid.). She persisted, and at Lauds when the lights were first extinguished in the church (to mark the blindness of the Jews), so that it was as dark in there as it was for her, the woman's eyes were rekindled at the same time as these lights were rekindled.

M II.41   *Incurable leg-ailment cured by miracle*

Godfrey the son of Count Hartmann in Germany had an illness in his legs for a year. He was so debilitated that he was confined to his room. 'When one limb hurts, the others do so too because the parts of the body are joined in such a way that one part cannot be damaged without injury to all the others. ... Medical science was ineffective and quite useless because no remedy existed to make this sick youth better. His family had lost hope for his recovery, particularly because a long-lasting illness is said to be incurable' (p. 172). After promising to travel to Rocamadour, Godfrey got better.

M II.46   A cripple cured

'Raymond, from Couserans, had been a cripple since childhood and had lost his strength throughout his body. He was weak and thin, and he had such slender joints that his stiffened limbs and wrinkled skin made him only just resemble a real person' (p. 175). His parents frequently prayed for him, and when they had some candles made of the same length and thickness as their son's legs, he was healed.

M II.48

In the same house as Raymond (M II.46) and another very sick person (M II.47) there was yet another impaired person: 'In this same house there was also a deaf woman. As she witnessed the sorts of cures which were happening, and being herself in need of divine aid, she prayed and regained her hearing' (p. 176).

M III.3   Dropsical man, neither dead nor alive

Gerald of Saint-Michel was swollen all over his body and diagnosed as having dropsy. For two-and-a-half months he ate nothing apart from some cherry juice and water. 'Day in, day out people expected him to die, for the attentions of physicians did nothing to cure him. His condition utterly defeated the experts' knowledge. Contrary to nature, or rather exceeding the bounds of what is natural, his bodily substance came to resemble soil, and he lay like a lopped tree. He was dead yet unable to die' (p. 183). After Gerald vowed an annual money payment and his relatives prayed, he was cured.

M III.10   Making a silent vow

A merchant who was robbed and badly wounded turned to the Virgin: 'even though he was unable to open his mouth because of the circumstances in which he found himself, in his heart he turned to and called upon the Lady of Rocamadour' (p. 187). God not just restored the man back to health, but revived him from the dead 'not by means of the trifles of physicians, but thanks to his Mother, Our Lady' (p. 188).

M III.11   Blasphemous knight is crippled

Senorez, a knight from the Périgord, had gone on pilgrimage to Jerusalem and other shrines. When he came to Rocamadour, he criticised the votive offerings in wax, asserting the models had been fraudulently placed there by the monks and not by visiting cured pilgrims, saying that at the other shrines he had been to he had not seen this sort of thing. For that 'Senorez was struck down in all his limbs and became paralysed' (p. 189). After being punished with this affliction for more than two months ('a long time'. as the text puts it) he repented, but apparently he did not deserve a cure just yet. After more repentance and praying he was cured: 'While he was making [his] devout confession, the knight's sinews grew stronger and his joints eased so that he was able to stand up and return to perfect health' (p. 190).

M III.13   Cure of epileptic

'A citizen of Milan called Brancus was laid low for four years by the falling sickness. He prayed to the Blessed Virgin; and his prayers were answered. He then came to the church of his liberator, with his father, and recounted the miracle' (p. 190).

M III.21   Paralytic woman cured

'Guillelma of la Boisera, from Grenoble, was crippled by paralysis in the middle part of her body. She was ill for a long time, and nothing that anyone could think of, nor the treatments of doctors, could do anything to cure her. She was in the flower of her youth, but her great illness had made her thin and shrivelled before her time' (pp. 195–6). She had heard about Rocamadour, and after praying for a cure and vowing to go to the shrine, she was cured immediately.

J   Miracles of the Hand of St James at Reading

The miracles occurred in the later twelfth century, but were recorded in a thirteenth-century manuscript, now at Gloucester, Dean and Chapter, MS 1, ff. 171v–175v. The edition and translation was made by Brian Kemp, 'The Miracles of the Hand of St James', *Berkshire Archaeological Journal*, 65, 1970, pp. 1–19. For the Latin text, Prof. Kemp kindly allowed me to see his transcript of the manuscript text.

The author of the miracle accounts seems to have had a basic knowledge of medicine, that is humoral theory, and some anatomy (as in the detailed description of people's twisted limbs). Reading abbey did possess some medical texts that would have been available to the writer of the miracle accounts, although Reading had fewer such texts than one would expect from evidence in other abbeys. In a book list made between *c.*1180 and 1190 (in other words, around the time the miracles were being recorded), the following title is mentioned: 'Liber de physica, Passionarius scilicet, qui fuit abbatis Anscherii in uno uolumine'.[5] Also at Leominster Priory, which was a daughter house of Reading, in a similar book list one finds the entry 'Medicinalis unus anglicis litteris scriptus'.[6] It is therefore possible that the recorder of the miracles may have had a rudimentary knowledge of medical terminology, if not of medical practice.

J III

John the clerk was struck dumb and remained so for some length of time. He was cured on the feast day of St James, when 'he came to Reading to entreat the creator of nature in respect of his own defect of nature' [*Qui predicta predicti apostoli solempnitate pro nature defectu nature supplicaturus auctori, Radingiam venit.*] (p. 7).

J VII

A ghost frightened Alice of Essex so much that when she returned home, her hair stood on end, and she 'lost her reason' [*confunditur sensus*]. She threw some fire into her face, and became 'seriously disturbed, as though she had gone mad' [*et tanquam in insaniam versa, agitari enormiter cepit, omnemque gestum et motum insanienti simillimum pretendit*]. During her sleep, her left arm withered and became attached to her abdomen. The combined effects of the relic of the hand of St James and holy water poured over her arm cured her. The curative process involved pain, and it took two to three hours for her withered arm to come away from her abdomen, with torn skin hanging from her arm, and her arm swollen and aching badly. She recovered after considerable time in the church, with 'no trace of her disability remaining any longer on her' [*nullo pristine infirmitatis inditio nullo debilitatis vestigio in ea ulterius remanente*] (p. 10).

J X

The withered hand of a monk of Reading was restored; he 'could neither raise his hand nor keep hold of anything he might grasp' (p. 10).

J XII

Concerning a girl from Suffolk: 'nature had so condemned this girl from birth [*Hanc autem adolescentulam a nativitate sua ita natura dampnaverat*], that from her knees down she appeared to have no firm bones in her shins and could not bend or straighten her knees. For her shins were full of flesh and skin and could be folded over like gristle and pulled round with her arm' (p. 11). She had tried cures at other shrines but they had failed, and it was only the relic at Reading that helped her. Her shins immediately hardened and became as strong as if they had bones in them, and she was able to walk in a short while.

J XIII

Concerning William, a boy from Reading: 'from his birth nature had so punished him by the awful laws of her indignation, that, with both legs shrunken, he was regarded as a spastic [*que ab ineunte etate diris indignationis sue legibus natura ita multaverat, ut contracto utroque poplite, spasmum pati putaretur*]. Moreover, his legs were so thin that they appeared no thicker than a human thumb' (p. 11). His lameness was cured, his withered and shrunken sinews slackened and became moist, and his bones 'began to grow and harden' (ibid.). 'Hitherto he had been unaccustomed to standing upright and incapable of walking and so he was afraid to trust himself, because he lacked confidence in his ability and strength. After a little while he mastered the basic principles of walking and climbed up the steps to the altar, a difficult operation for the feet of a disabled person' (p. 11).

J XVIII

Gilbert, a keeper of hounds, was overly fond of hunting and was punished by blindness for hunting on St James' day. His blindness was incurable by ointments or remedies. '...he began to become a burden to those among whom he had previously been very popular [*cepit fieri onerosus quibus prius fuerat gratiosus*]. In his adversity he found few friends, in his poverty very few, and in his blindness scarcely any physicians [*Raros enim amicos repperit adversitas, paucissimos paupertas, fere nullos medicantium cecitas*], as in the saying, 'when you are successful you will number many friends; in bad times you will be alone'. Bound by poverty and grief he sat in darkness...' (p. 13). Barely his wife remained loyal to him; she guided him around various shrines, unsuccessfully, until eventually he was cured by St James.

J XX

Ysembla, a young girl, slept out in the open one summer and thereby 'disabled her body and lost her agility. In fact, her left side from the sole of her foot to her shoulder had withered and lost all living movement. Her hand was shrunken and paralysed and hung motionless from her side close to her back. Her foot was bent round and, incapable of acting as a foot, was so twisted that (her main foot bones took the place of her heel, her toes were in the place of the bones, and the nails of her shoe were where her toes should have been)[7] [*Pes circumflexus pedis officium diffitens ita pervertebatur ut calcis crates cratis articuli articulorum locum clavellata usurparent*]. And the girl, being thus made useless to herself and pitiable to others, was harassed by her stepmother with many insults and taunted with abuse of various kinds' [*Haque puella sibi facta mutilata, aliisque miserabile a noverca sua plurimis lascessita iniuriis, variis affecta obprobriis*] (pp. 14–15). She was compelled by her 'evil' step-mother to try and find a cure at the shrines of saints. In a vision she was told to go to Reading, at which she protested: 'But...I have not seen Reading, nor do I know your [St James'] monastery. And how can I go there when I am crippled and weak, ignorant of the way and penniless? No, I shall not go nor will I tire myself out any more to no purpose' (p. 15). She ignored her vision, and returned home still uncured, where her 'evil' stepmother harangued her: ' "Aha, you went away a cripple and, look, you have come back a cripple. Go away from me" ', she said, "and crawl where you will, for you shall certainly not stay under my roof" (p. 15). The girl was taken in by an aunt, who immediately realised the impor-tance of the vision, and sent the girl off to Reading with only one coin which the aunt had, so that the girl could purchase a candle with the money. In the church at Reading she 'threw herself on the pavement and, letting out the most piercing cries, screamed in all directions. She shook her head about, banged her head and dashed her body against the stone with so little consideration for herself that one might have thought that she wished to destroy herself...' (p. 15). After three hours the cure started, her limbs coming back to life so that she moved from a sprawling to a proper posture; later there was lots of coughing and vomiting which cleared 'the fluid which had harmed her' (p. 15). The girl then returned home completely cured.

J XXIII

A woman from the Oxford region was confined to her bed for two years, 'bent up and shrunken' [*curva et contracta*] (p. 17). She was set in a two-wheeled carriage by her brother and sent to Reading. On the way there she was cured and arrived in Reading on foot (walking, presumably, and therefore no longer needing the carriage).

G Miracles of St Godric of Finchale

St Godric died in 1170, and Reginald of Durham had still been able to visit the aged Godric (he lived to be around 100 years old) during his lifetime to collect materials for the *vita* written by him. After Godric's death, Finchale priory where he had been a hermit became the site of a shrine for some while. The printed edition of the *vita* used here, *Libellus de Vita et Miraculis S. Godrici, Heremitæ de Finchale, auctore Reginaldo Monacho Dunelmensi*, ed. J. Stevenson, Surtees Society, 20, 1845, is based on a manuscript in the Bodleian Library, MS Laud. E. 47, otherwise marked 413.

There are 225 miracles in total in the collection of Godric's *miracula*. Of these, 71 miracles (32 per cent) relate to the cure of mobility-impairing conditions, 44 (20 per cent) relate to the cure of blindness or other eye disorders, 20 (9 per cent) relate to deafness in one or both ears, 11 (5 per cent) relate to speech impediments or muteness, 16 (7 per cent) to insanity and 6 (3 per cent) to epilepsy. So a total of 168 out of 225 miracles, or 75 per cent, relate to impairments, insanity or epilepsy. The remaining 57 miracles (25 per cent) deal with various activities ranging from cures of other illnesses, such as fevers, tumours or 'weakness', to cures of animals, or visionary miracles.

From the Vita

G lxxxv   quanta denique corporis debilitate detritus sit

Magnæ denique aetatis senio succrescente, cœpit paulatim vir Dei vires corporales amittere; at tamen aliquantulum erga spiritualis desiderii exercitia sollicitius pervigilanti animo Domino vacare. Adeo quidem seniles ejus artus ætatis prolixæ multitudo detriverat, quod ipse solus etiam pedes, vel sustentante baculo tripes, de mansiuncula Oratorii sui egredi vel ingredi non valebat. Elevabatur proinde, reclinabatur et efferebatur, manibus alienis, qui jam sibi subvenire non poterat, viribus corporeis deficientibus propriis. Unde aliquando tanta confectus est ægritudine, quod ei dies sui transitus nobis videretur imminere (pp. 186–7). Godric was believed to be at death's door by some of the brothers, but he recovered little by little.

G cxxii

Godric cured the swollen feet and shins of a man by telling him to rise and walk in the name of Christ [*In Nomine Jesu Christi Nazareni, surge et ambula*] (p. 245); this is reminiscent of Christ's healings in the Gospels, where Christ had told paralytic and lame people to 'rise and walk' (e.g. Matthew 9:7, Mark 2:12 and John 5:9).

G clviii

Godric cured one of the brothers of a tumorous swelling in the left foot, which had affected the monk so badly that he could barely get up out of his bed [*vix de lectulo potuisset exsurgere*] (p. 300).

From the Miracula de Sancto Godrico

G 1	epilepsy in a little girl
G 2	boy with contracted arms and blind since age of four
G 3	mad young man
G 4	gout for ten years in a woman
G 5	loss of use of arms for two years
G 6	vertigo?
G 7	quotidian fever
G 8	epilepsy and lunacy in a woman
G 9	fever
G 10	woman blind for five years
G 11	woman paralysed in all her limbs
G 12	man with gout
G 13	paralysed woman, could not move to do any work
G 14	weakness cured
G 15	priest's daughter, deprived of hearing for half a year in one ear and totally deaf in other ear
G 16	woman bent over and contracted for seven years, with hands on her knees, half cured by St Thomas, so that she used a stick in one hand but the other hand was still stuck to her knee, also went to St Andrew in Scotland, but was only cured at Finchale, where she offered her crutch and a candle on the altar
G 17	girl paralysed from birth
G 18	headache
G 19	pain in thigh of woman, could not move without a crutch for support, after her cure placed crutch on altar at Finchale
G 20	woman swollen in all her body
G 21	tumour in chest
G 22	blind woman
G 23	another blind woman
G 24	ruptured abscess

G 25   woman deaf for thirteen years

G 26   woman with impairment in her feet, so that she could not move anywhere save with the help of others

G 27   paralytic man

G 28   man who had lost all movement of his shins and was incapable of walking, with contorted and contracted feet

G 29   woman with film in front of her eyes

G 30   swelling in shins

G 31   woman who was deaf for four years, only heard when people shouted in her ear

G 32   chest pains

G 33   woman freed from demon

G 34   girl cured of long-standing blindness

G 35   blind woman

G 36   woman could do no work for three years because of paralysis

G 37   girl, 2 years old, with contracted right hand and foot, so that she could not move for half a year

G 38   weakness cured

G 39   woman deaf in one ear for sixteen years

G 40   female demoniac

G 41   boy with painful tumour in knee

G 42   man blind for two years

G 43   woman with one hand and arm withered and stiff since birth, could not move it, also had tumour

G 44   weakness, due to pain in shins

G 45   woman who was infirm in all her limbs, and deaf in one ear

G 46   youth injured on a building site, so that his spine was broken in three places; was bedridden for many months; ended up contracted and humpbacked, unable to walk without the support of two sticks under each armpit [*duobus baculis sub alterutri lateris axe suffultus*]

G 47   woman paralysed for three years

G 48   infirm woman

G 49   insane woman

G 50   woman with hands contracted from birth, so that she could not move any object

G 51   insane woman

G 52   woman swollen all over her body

G 53   white doves in a vision

G 54   woman paralysed from birth

G 55   man blind for half a year

G 56   woman blind for a year

G 57   man with gout for two years, unable to walk

G 58   headache

G 59   woman who had lost ability to speak

G 60   shepherd with contracted hand

G 61   ruptured abscess
G 62   woman paralysed in all her body so that she was unable to move
G 63   woman with withered arm for three years
G 64   woman blind for two years
G 65   youth with weakness of the knee for two years, so that he could not move without a crutch; the crutch was placed at the shrine in testimony of his healing
G 66   woman unable to move her arms, legs and entire body for five years; unable to move herself without the aid of others
G 67   girl born deaf and mute
G 68   man bedridden with weakness; brought to the shrine in a cart
G 69   monk with tumour
G 70   boy born mute
G 71   woman deaf for four years in both ears
G 72   woman infirm for seven years
G 73   woman lost movement and use of one arm for half a year
G 74   woman blind for fourteen years
G 75   another blind woman
G 76   woman deaf from birth
G 77   woman deaf for six years
G 78   another woman, deaf in both ears for five years
G 79   blind woman
G 80   woman mute for four years
G 81   woman blind for two years
G 82   woman with heartburn
G 83   woman became deaf so that she could not hear anything
G 84   woman deaf for a long time
G 85   paralysed woman
G 86   woman mute from birth; also had contracted arms and hands
G 87   paralysed woman
G 88   deaf woman
G 89   woman with headache and chest pains
G 90   demoniac youth
G 91   woman unable to use her hands, and unable to walk
G 92   priest of the shrine freed from withered arm, barely able to move it
G 93   woman who had lost use of one hand
G 94   woman mute and deaf for five years and four months
G 95   insane girl
G 96   woman with contracted hand and foot
G 97   man deaf in one ear
G 98   man blind for four years
G 99   blind woman
G 100 woman with film in front of her eyes
G 101 woman blind for twenty-three years
G 102 woman with contracted hand

G 103   youth with incurable tumour in feet and legs, whom no medicine could help or cure [*pedum et tibiarum tumorem incurabilem... quem nulla medicinalis industria mitigare vel curare*]

G 104   woman mute for ten years

G 105   woman blind for six years

G 106   woman deaf for one year

G 107   person bedridden for three years due to weakness; cured of diverse infirmity [*de infirmitate diversa*]

G 108   woman blind in one eye for forty years

G 109   another woman blind in one eye for one year

G 110   woman with contracted hand for four-and-a-half years

G 111   boy with weakness, described as half dead

G 112   insane and demoniac woman

vl13   woman blind in one eye for five years

G 114   another blind woman, led by her father

G 115   woman with weakness and tumour in her knee, incurable by medicine

G 116   woman who for twenty-two years had been contorted and twisted in her spine, also had a hunched back, needed two crutches to support her, dragged herself forwards as if on four feet [*sis sese protrahens quadrupes*]

G 117   man so twisted for nine years that he needed two crutches to move about

G 118   woman blind for a long time

G 119   woman with film obscuring her eyes

G 120   boy who was weakened so that he could not move without other people's aid

G 121   another boy unable to walk, brought on horseback

G 122   feverish woman

G 123   woman blind for sixteen years

G 124   woman with hands contracted since the age of 16

G 125   woman with weakness

G 126   infirm man healed by a vision

G 127   infant boy healed who would not suckle

G 128   boy healed of illness

G 129   boy with pustules in his eyes

G 130   woman with large abscess like a humpback

G 131   woman with one contracted hand, incurable

G 132   woman with cancerous fistula

G 133   woman blind for a long time

G 134   insane man

G 135   paralytic man, brought by his mother on horseback

G 136   person with obstruction of chest

G 137   woman blind in one eye

G 138   insane woman

G 139   woman unable to walk, brought in a cart with driver

G 140   little boy born blind

G 141   blind man

G 142   woman had a stroke, fell down in the street as if she was mad, was helped back indoors by others, could speak again after a while, but was contracted in one hand, her fingers bent in towards the palm of her hand, also was infirm in all her body; was taken to shrine by her servants; was healed after incubation at the shrine

G 143   resurrection of a boy

G 144   lamb contracted from birth

G 145   contracted man healed, all his limbs were immobilised and inflexible

G 146   blind woman

G 147   feverish woman

G 148   elderly blind man

G 149   woman deaf from birth

G 150   bedridden, weakened man

G 151   demoniac woman

G 152   girl with cancer in her mouth

G 153   epileptic man

G 154   insane man

G 155   boy blind for two years

G 156   baby boy who nearly died during difficult birth

G 157   man who had lost (the use of) one leg for seven years and whose right knee was contracted

G 158   man with contracted knees, deprived of (the use of) all his members

G 159   woman blind for nine years

G 160   man fell hard, broke the bone of one leg, his knee, and his shin, so that no doctor could cure him; at the shrine, the worn-away bones re-integrated themselves

G 161   woman with swollen chest

G 162   woman with swollen belly as if pregnant

G 163   woman blind in one eye since birth

G 164   person with swelling or tumour in chest

G 165   boy had one foot so contracted that it did not touch the ground; the other foot was lame (clubfooted), so that only the ankle touched the ground

G 166   woman unable to walk for many years

G 167   man lost all use of one arm for three years, could not move or flex it

G 168   girl with body swollen, by a tumour, so that she was half-dead

G 169   young knight who had been wounded in Normandy

G 170   demoniac and mad girl

G 171   man cured of leprosy

G 172   woman cured of leprosy

G 173   boy who had been brought up in the hospital of St Peter (an orphan or foundling, perhaps) was contracted in all the members of his body; one of his hands and one arm were contracted, and so twisted to be like woven thread [*in modum intexti funiculi intorta*]; his legs also were contracted

G 174   a monk with an illness spreading from his shins to his kidneys

G 175   woman blind in one eye for many years

G 176 small boy swollen as far as his skin would stretch

G 177 another small boy with a swelling and tumour

G 178 man who lost his shoes on way to shrine, found them again

G 179 youth was for many years hindered by a great illness, had lost the use of hands and arms due to drying up of these limbs, was sickly and pale, and suffered from convulsions

G 180 maddened cattle

G 181 blind man

G 182 woman with hands and arms contracted since birth, and also legs with similarly contorted feet, was brought by others to the shrine

G 183 woman with worms, fistulas and many holes in her thigh

G 184 woman mute and deaf since birth

G 185 woman with pains in head so severe that she was compared to a demoniac by those who saw her

G 186 woman suffering daily from fits

G 187 man with incurable ulcer in his thigh, unable to work, unable to move without aid from other people, taken to shrine by his friends

G 188 woman with entire body swollen

G 189 woman with headaches since birth, finally lost sight in one eye

G 190 youth had lost use of his limbs, spent many years bedridden, half-deaf, blind and weak, has sight restored in one eye at shrine, and regained use of his limbs a little

G 191 woman half-dead from a tumour

G 192 priest blind for a year and a half

G 193 simple-minded and half-witted man [*homo simplicissimus et idiota*] who held office of shepherd at Finchale had vision of saint

G 194 cleric with strange illness whereby it felt as if he had living things crawling around inside his navel

G 195 carpenter cured of illness making him bedridden

G 196 epileptic girl

G 197 youth with tumour in his lower legs

G 198 boy with bad cough, nearly dies

G 199 woman with badly swollen body

G 200 woman with cardiac pains (heartburn)

G 201 cleric who had a fever for two years

G 202 knight with pleurisy, and unable to digest food

G 203 cleric who had vision of the saint which cured him of pains in the legs rendering him unable to walk

G 204 leprous girl

G 205 woman lost ability to walk, nor was able to move or could do any work properly, was taken to shrine on horseback by her husband

G 206 insane man

G 207 man with contracted limbs

G 208 cure of half-dead sheep

G 209 miracle of a rainbow

G 210   youth with congenital deformity, whereby his hands were contracted so that it appeared they were connected to his upper arms, and as if they were covered with one skin [*alteram manuum suarum ab ipso ortus sui primordio semper contractam habuit, adeo intorte ad superiora brachii connexam et astrictam ac si unius pellis operimento counitæ compaginata fuisset*]; he had also become mute and deaf; miracle occurred in 1175

G 211   a prophecy of the saint

G 212   miracle of the saint's book drenched by rain

G 213   knight with illness (swelling) affecting his head and neck

G 214   girl with contracted leg, the heel of the right foot stuck to her buttocks, and all of her right shin was attached to the back of her thigh, her left foot was contorted and she was in pain if she tried to walk; it was necessary for her to place her knees on the ground for feet if she had to go anywhere at any-time [*genibus pro pedibus super terram oportuit ipsam repere, si aliquando alicubi debuisset ire*]; she was healed perfectly after two days at the shrine

G 215   woman who drank poison which caused her body to swell

G 216   seven year old boy who had been mute from birth

G 217   boy who was mute and lame, appeared to be more burdensome for his parents and all his friends [*onerosior sibi et cunctis amicis suis apparuit*]

G 218   man who for eleven years had been incapacitated by a weakness of one foot, so that he went about one-legged [*monipes*], not walking but rather through crawling drawing himself forwards [*non gradiens sed potius rependo se protrahens*]; he supported all the bulk of the body with the help of the other foot [*alterius pedis totam corporis molem supportabat auxilio*]; after being healed he could walk without the support of any crutch [*sine omni baculi adminiculo*]

G 219   miracle of youth who had barley growing out of one ear, which had rooted itself in his ear, causing him headaches and deafness

G 220   youth suddenly struck blind in one eye for working in the fields on a Sunday

G 221   man who had been born contracted, he had one foot going backwards [*alterum pedum retrogradum habuit*] (foot twisted backwards), the other was curved back and was bandaged to the back of the leg [*alium vero recurvum at ad crurum fines posterius obligatum*], his shins could twist and bend to any place like marrow without bones [*tibiæ vero ejus tortæ et flexuosæ quolibet, velut medulla sine osse*]; he crawled on two stools (hand trestles) [*scamnis duobus repens*] and he was carried by his hands from place to place [*manibus de loco ad locum ferebatur*]; in addition he had the thumb of his right hand in the middle of his palm as if it was affixed by the roots [*Præterea et pollicem manus dexteræ in medio palmi quasi radicitus infixum habuit*], whose sharp nail nearly penetrated the back of the palm on the outside [*cujus unguis acuta posteritas propemodum palmi exteriora penetravit*]; his hand was totally useless for any other task, and he had begged for his living for many years

G 222   *Alius quidam miser, qui forte hoc non peccati sui meritispertulit, ab utero matris cæcus natus fuit. Nam sicut ex rerum exitu postmodum patuit, fortassis nec ipse neque parentes ejus peccaverant, ut pæna peccati vindice, cæcus nasci debuisset. Unde eo manifestius Dei opera in istius curatione debebant mundo propalari, quo hujus flagelli exitum, peccati meritis id non exigentibus, secretiori Dei judicio dignus fuerat experiri. Hic, aliis ducentibus, ad viri Dei sepulchrum est perductus, et sequenti nocte postquam venerat, ab omni cæcitate est liberatus. Et quia ad lucernam Dei confugit, lumen oculorum ab ipsa percipere meruit, sanusque et videns, Sancto Godrico medicante, rediit, qui nunquam antea lumen cæli videre prævaluit; sicque sanctus Dei Godricus cæcus nato medicus probatissimus est effectus, qui vivens in corpore nunquam aliqua medicinalis artis peritia fuerat imbutus.* 'A certain other unfortunate person, who by chance had brought this about and not by merit of his sinning, had been born blind from his mother's womb. For just as it became clear a little while later from the outcome of these things, perhaps neither he himself nor his parents had sinned, when punishment for the sinning was claimed, he was obliged to be born blind'.

The text continues by stating that this was connected with making evident the works of God, being in his care, to be made manifest to the world.

'He, led by others, was brought to the tomb of the man of God, and in the following night after he had arrived, he was freed of all blindness. And since he sought refuge with the lamp of God, from the same one he earned to receive the light of his eyes, and healthy and seeing through the medicine of St Godric, he returned, he who never before had been able to see the light of heaven; and so Godric the holy man of God has proved himself to be the most effective physician for a man born blind, [Godric] who never while he was living in his body had delved into any knowledge of the medicinal art.'

G 223   man born mute
G 224   man with distended body due to tumour
G 225   wife who had been blind for 15 years, during which time she gave birth to three sons, whom she never saw until she was cured at the shrine

E   Miracles of St Elisabeth at Marburg

During her lifetime St Elisabeth of Hungary (1207–31) was concerned with providing charity for the poor, the sick and other needy persons, so much so that iconographically, after her status of sanctity had been confirmed, she was often depicted in the company of people displaying the symptoms of what we would now term physical impairment: visually and orthopaedically impaired people are especially frequent.[8] It is therefore not surprising that a large number of the miracle cures attributed to St Elisabeth should revolve around orthopaedically impairing conditions, the *contracti, claudi, contorti* and *gibbosi* mentioned in the Latin texts.

St Elisabeth was canonised in 1235, and as part of her canonisation proceedings the miracles worked through her relics were used as evidence for her sanctity. Collections and examinations of miracle reports were made in 1232–4, resulting in the *Libellus de dictis quator ancillarum S. Elisabeth confectus* and in the *Miracula sancte Elyzabet*, the latter containing 106 miracle accounts. It is the miracles related in these protocols that are dealt with here. In discussing the miracle protocols, I have relied on the edition with analysis and German translation by Jürgen Jansen, *Medizinische Kasuistik in den »Miracula Sancte Elyzabet«. Medizinhistorische Analyse und Übersetzung der Wunderprotokolle am Grab der Elisabeth von Thüringen (1207–31)* (Marburger Schriften zur Medizingeschichte Band 15), Frankfurt a. M., Bern and New York: Verlag Peter Lang, 1985. The miracle protocols were collected in two sections, which Jansen termed MI (Miracula I, for the first reports by the commission for sanctification in 1232/3, with 106 miracles) and MII (Miracula II, for the 1234 commission reports containing a further 24 miracles). For the sake of brevity not all the miracles dealing with impairments will be fully described, but only those of special interest, either because of the amount of detail on the condition they describe, or because of the information they provide on contemporary attitudes to the impaired. However, I have listed all the miracles here, by title or brief description, because of the statistical inferences it allows one to make regarding the occurrence of specific disorders, which follow later.

1. Orthopaedic problems

Fifty-four miracle reports deal with 'sickness' of the limbs, and thereby constitute the single largest category of miracles. Sometimes the impairments are described vividly, for example, six of the pilgrims were so disabled they could just about crawl, four people needed a crutch to support themselves, two could not walk upright any more, and some pilgrims had to be transported to the shrine by others. Most pilgrims were 'ill in all of their body', only in 7 cases is there mention of damaged lower limbs (leg impairments), and in 2 cases impaired upper limbs, also 3 cases of unilateral paralysis. The protocols are relatively precise in their descriptions of impairments, and often refer to the physical consequences of such conditions. For example, in 5 cases it is mentioned that the legs were 'drawn back to the bottom' and seemed to have grown together with the posterior, and in three pilgrims the leg on one side was so foreshortened that it would not touch the ground anymore. Seven cases mention the pain the person concerned felt. Six persons were described as hunch-backed, and four people were shaking uncontrollably 'in the whole body' or in their hands and feet (Jansen, pp. 16–23).

Children and young people formed the majority of persons seeking a cure, and of these most fell into the 1- to 5-year-old age bracket. In five accounts Jansen can find evidence for congenital impairments (p. 21).

The healing process after the visit to the shrine could ensue immediately and spontaneously in some patients, while in others it took up to half a year for a full cure to have effect. The miracle commission witnessed a young man, who nominally had been healed, still walking with the wobbly gait of a child which is just beginning to learn to walk (p. 21) – an observation on the gradual healing and rehabilitation of those nervous or orthopaedic disorders that do actually improve over time.

In 27 cases the protocols mention a single orthopaedic impairment: 15 lame persons (*claudus*), six contracted, deformed or twisted people (*contractus*), often synonymous with 'crippled', two paralysis cases (*paraliticus*), one crooked, bent or twisted person (*curvus*), and one with a swelling (*inflatus*).

In 20 cases the protocols mention multiple impairments: four lame and hunch-backed (*claudus et gibbosus*), three hunch-backed and humped or swollen (*gibbosus et strumosus*), two lame and mute (*claudus et mutus*), two lame and ulcerous (*claudus et infistulatus*), and two hunch-backed and contracted (*gibbosus et contractus*) people. There was also one person each who was lame and humped or swollen (*claudus et strumosus*), lame and swollen (*claudus et inflatus*), lame, blind, deaf and mute (*claudus, cecus, surdus et mutus*), hunch-backed and crooked or bent (*gibbosus et incurvatus*), hunch-backed and deformed (*gibbosus et distortus*), hunch-backed, crippled and swollen (*gibbosus, contractus et strumosus*), and bent and mute (*curvus et mutus*).

In six cases the protocols mention a non-specific impairment: two people unable to walk (*impotens ad gradiendum*), one person having the head resting on the shoulder and a shaking arm (*habens caput ad scapulam reclinatum et brachium tremulum*), one infirm or weakened below the belt (= the lower limbs) (*infirmus ad cingulo deorsum*), one having weakened or debilitated limbs, hunch-backed and swollen (*debilia membra habens, gibbosus et strumosus*), and one was healed in hands and legs (shins) (*sanata in manibus et cruribus*).

2. *Eye disorders*

Eye disorders are dealt with by 21 of the protocols, 15 of which concern blindness in both eyes and 6 concern persons who were blind in only 1 eye. Many different symptoms are described, including 3 cases of children who were blind from birth. In the case of blindness acquired later in life, there are descriptions of the gradual loss of sight of the pilgrims concerned, for example how they could no longer see the light of day, the sky, the moon, or the fire, or how they needed to be guided by others (p. 48). Quite often there are dramatic healing descriptions, involving blood or another bodily fluid gushing from the affected eye(s) (Jansen, pp. 47–9).

3. *Speech impairments*

Five accounts deal with the phenomenon of speechlessness. Among the miracles relating to orthopaedic disorders (see category 1), there are also four cases where the person was mute in addition to having an orthopaedic impairment, and one of the epileptic pilgrims was mute as well. Speechlessness is therefore never men-tioned on its own, but always in conjunction with the other impairments. The descriptions of the cases of speechlessness are fairly basic, in that they purely men-tion the fact that a person was mute without providing further medical details, as was done for eye disorders (though one case refers to a three-and-a-half-year-old girl who was congenitally mute, whereas another miracle mentions a person who could already speak fluently for some time before they became mute). The healing of speechlessness is also described sparsely, namely as part and parcel of the cure of the other impairment: people are healed of their orthopaedic impairment and simultaneously, or later in their homes, they receive the ability to speak (Jansen, pp. 56–7).

4. Impairment through accidents

See miracles MI 25, MI 75, MI 89, MI 92, MI 70, and MII 20 and MII 24. These miracles relate to the kind of injuries sustained in the home or at work, that is, what we might term occupational injuries. Of these, two cases relate to fractures, and one case to a hernia, another case deals with a man who accidentally hit his knee with an axe, and in one instance a woman had injured her knee after getting knocked down by a pig (Jansen, pp. 69–72).

5. Epilepsy

Epilepsy is mentioned in 14 miracles of the protocols. Symptoms are described as including falling down, hitting out and/or flailing of arms and legs, foaming at the mouth or gnashing of teeth, opened staring eyes, and a general stiffening of the body. Again, as in the orthopaedic cases, most pilgrims were under 20 years old, and of these the majority fell into the 1–5-year-old age bracket. Sometimes mention is also made of the duration of 'fits' and of their frequency (Jansen, pp. 32–5).

6. Mental disorders

Only 5 cases are described, of which 4 concern persons who were *furiosae* and 1 concerns a possessed girl. The 4 *furiosae* exhibited behaviour that the miracle protocols deemed abnormal (Jansen, p. 41).

Miracles in protocol MI

MI 1

Cure of 5-year-old boy who had been born blind.

MI 2

Resuscitation of dead boy.

MI 3

Nine-year-old girl with swellings in lower and upper legs, also with hunch back, so that she had to wander around her village begging for alms bent over so far that her hands rested on her knees. Her stepfather carried her on his back in a basket to St Elisabeth's tomb. In a vision during a dream the girl was told by St Elisabeth to 'rise up and walk' (p. 160: *Stehe auf und gehe umher*), an allusion to the apostle Peter's of healing, who spoke the same words to a crippled man (Acts 3:6).

MI 4

Sixteen-year-old girl lame in arms and legs, had to be moved, laid down and carried by other people.

MI 5

Twelve-year-old boy, who became lame in his right leg, which became bent and foreshortened, and could not touch the ground so that he needed to move around with the aid of a stick, also had a withered left hand.

MI 6

Resuscitation of a drowned 18-year-old student.

MI 7

Resuscitation of a three-and-a-half-year-old boy found dead.

MI 8

Nine-year-old boy who had an abscess when six weeks old causing one of his eyes to become blind due to a film growing over it.

MI 9

Nine-year-old girl with sores.

MI 10

Resuscitation of 4-year-old boy drowned falling into a well (he had gone out to play with other boys unsupervised, as his father was bedridden due to illness, and his mother was in labour, or had just given birth).

MI 11

Five-year-old girl with the flux.

MI 12

A young woman with her legs flexed at the knee, so that she could only lie on her side, was cured in one leg by St Nicholas; she could thereafter move around bent over double. She had to wait another six years for a cure through St Elisabeth: at the tomb she waited eight days, until she was laid over the tomb and felt a pain in her contracted leg which immediately was stretched out and healed, causing her to almost faint in fear. Next day she was again carried to the tomb, for the pain in her bent back, and nearly fainted again during the miracle.

MI 13

Resurrection of the stillborn boy from a pair of twins a woman gave birth to, the girl twin had been born alive and well.

MI 14

A woman suffered from nasal polyps for 12 years, at the same time she joined the heretical sect of the poor of Lyon [= Waldensians], of whom none could cure her, only after she renounced her heresy and had confession was she cured. Her condition was so awful that she appeared deformed and even her own son became reluctant to share a house with her, since she 'insulted people's senses of sight and smell' (p. 171, *Sie verletzte nämlich den Gesichts- und Geruchssinn der Menschen*).

MI 15

A 13-year-old boy had been lame since birth, with weak shins and hardly any posterior, so that he could not walk at all and could barely sit using a support, also his hands and arms trembled so much he could hardly eat and drink by himself, even his eyes shook; all these conditions had affected him since birth. He was taken to the tomb tied to the saddle on a horse, and placed on the tomb. After his cure he had to use a crutch at first, but was healed so much that the trembling in his eyes, arms and hands stopped, and he returned home after his shins had a chance to develop enough for him to be able to stand unsupported. He was able to walk unassisted on level ground, and only needed one crutch to deal with sloping ground.

MI 16

Twenty-year-old insane woman.

MI 17

A woman with [bladder] stone.

MI 18

Insane woman cured after three visits to the tomb.

MI 19

A woman was bedridden with 'weakness' and needed help from others if she had to move out of the bed. She was carried to the tomb in a carriage. After it broke en route, she continued using two crutches, something she would have been incapable of earlier, until she was fully cured at the tomb.

MI 20

A girl had been mute and incapable of walking for five years.

MI 21

A man of 40 years or more of age developed spots (*macula*) over his pupils, so that he could see only very little; he often strayed off the path and wandered through the fields, for which he was laughed at by others going along the path. He finally became completely blind for four weeks before being cured at the tomb.

MI 22

A 4-year-old girl became so weak that her limbs, when touched, made a sound as if they were dry wood. She grew a hump on her back and a swelling on her chest, and could no longer stand on her feet.

MI 23

Epileptic man.

MI 24

A 4-year-old boy became epileptic and simultaneously became mute, though he had spoken fluently before. He was ill for twelve weeks before being cured.

MI 25

A man of about 30 injured his knee with an axe, as the protocol witnesses could still observe on him, so that he had to remain bedridden from October [1231] until Easter the following year [11 April 1232]; in addition he believed he also had the illness called 'antrax' so that the wound was made worse and he feared for his life as well as worrying about his wound healing. After vowing to go to the tomb of St Elisabeth, the pain in his leg immediately began to lessen, so that during Pentecost [30 May 1232] he was able to start his journey propped up on two crutches, even though before he had hardly been able to touch the ground with his injured leg. Returning from the tomb, he was cured fully and threw away his crutches.

MI 26

A girl of about 16 had for three years had such weakened eyesight that during a waning moon she could not see anything, and during a waxing moon she could see but a little. In addition, she could not follow the path she was meant to walk along. After commencing her journey to the tomb, the film covering her eyes broke and so much liquid issued forth that her mother could barely keep the flies away from her face.

MI 27

A 6-year-old girl with mental illness.

MI 28

A young man of nearly 22 lost all powers over the lower half of his body, below the belt, so that he could not move himself unless he pulled his torso along by one hand and dragged the rest of his body after it. He also had a large hump on his back, and severe pain in his lungs. He was placed in a wagon and taken to the tomb, where he spent three weeks until his hunch back was cured. After returning home in a two-wheeled carriage, he complained to St Elisabeth that he would in future not come to her if he was unable to walk of his own accord. After a vision in a dream he then began to upright himself holding onto a fence and onto other supports, and started walking in this fashion, so that at the time of writing the protocol he walked very well (p. 180, *und jetzt geht er sehr gut*).

MI 29

A man became ill in his leg, which developed a large swelling like a statue; one leg became so bent that he could not touch the ground with it, and he had lost all sensation in that leg as if it was a dead limb. After two visits to the tomb he started to improve, and he was completely cured on a third visit, leaving his sticks behind at the tomb. A witness in the protocol testified he had seen the man lying ill for twenty weeks, after which he saw him weakened and supported on crutches, and then saw him healed after the visits to the tomb.

MI 30

A 9-year-old girl had been ill with the flux since she was 18 weeks old, and had also at one point developed an abscess above one eye, which shrank after nine weeks but left behind a piece of skin covering her pupil; this skin also disappeared after a year, but the girl still remained blind for the next four years, until cured at the tomb of her blindness and the flux. Several female witness testified for the protocol that they could tell the girl remained blind even after the spot (*macula*) in her pupil had disappeared, because they performed a test whereby they asked the girl to cover her good eye and try to see with the other one, which she could not.

MI 31

A 13-year-old girl's left hand had been swollen so much for three years that she could barely make any use of it; her arm became swollen as well up to her elbow and ulcerated. After her mother made a vow to St Elisabeth, the girl's arm and hand gradually began to get better.

MI 32

Severely epileptic girl, one-and-a-half-years old.

MI 33

A boy aged three-and-a-half had been unable to walk since childhood (p. 183, *von Kindheit an*) since he was paralysed from the waist down, but was cured at the tomb. After his mother took him there and placed him on the ground, the lay brother guarding the tomb produced an egg which he held somewhat away from the boy; the boy got up and holding onto the tomb walked round to the edge of the sarcophagus. The lay brother then moved round a bit farther, so that the boy had to follow him, because of the egg.

MI 34

A 6-year-old boy became ill two years after his birth. He gradually began to contract (p. 184, *zusammenzog*) so that he could not walk upright, but only if he supported himself with his hands on his knees and bent his head down almost as far as his knees. He also had a hump on his back the size of a new-born's head. After the father made a vow, the boy began to upright himself, and the hump on his back began to reduce itself, so that by the time the protocol notaries saw the boy, it was only half the size of an egg.

MI 35

Epileptic girl.

MI 36

Epileptic boy.

MI 37

A 1-year-old boy cured of swollen and closed eyes.

MI 38

A 40-year-old woman became blind for a year, during which time she could not differentiate the day[light] from the fire, and had skin and fleshy tissue covering her eyes, as others told her. She added at the protocol hearing that she had to be led by the hands wherever she went.

MI 39

Woman cured of pustules.

MI 40

A woman aged over 30 had been paralysed in nearly all limbs of her body for three years. Often lying in bed, she could only stand up with great pain and walked with great difficulty and very slowly, so that in a room of thirty paces she had to pause two or three times, trembling in all her limbs.

MI 41

Epileptic boy.

MI 42

A girl had been unable to walk from birth until the age of four-and-a-half, since her arms and legs were withered and her skin was wrinkled 'like a folded up rag' (p. 190, *nach der Art eines zusammengefalteten Lappens*).

MI 43

Epileptic 10-year-old girl.

MI 44

A 3-year-old boy was lame in such a way that one leg was always placed below the other one, and his knees appeared to be joined to his belly; also, puss discharged from the skin in his belly and from his legs, so that the smell was hardly bearable. He could neither crawl nor walk, nor move himself, and was in this condition from the feast of St Catherine [25 November 1231] until the beginning of Lent [24 February 1232]. When his mother vowed to take a wax candle to the tomb of St Elisabeth, the boy became able to right himself up with the aid of sticks. Both parents then went to the tomb (without the boy), and on their return they found their boy walking supported by a crutch; he was healed gradually.

MI 45

A man was lame in his limbs for a year and sixteen weeks, so that he could only move his feet, legs and arms with great difficulty. Since he found no cure with others, he finally went, with great physical effort, to the tomb of the lady Elisabeth, hoping for grace (p. 192, *Da er aber keine Heilung bei anderen fand, ging er endlich, sich die Gnade erhoffend, mit großer körperlicher Anstrengung zum Grab der Herrin Elisabeth*). There he was immediately and completely healed, and he no longer begged as before but provided for himself through the work of his hands (p. 192, *und er bettelte nicht mehr wie vorher, sondern ernährte sich von der Arbeit seiner Hände*).

MI 46

A 5-year-old girl had been robbed of the faculties of sight, hearing, speech and walking for sixteen weeks. On the day her parents made a vow she started to become better and gradually became completely well again.

MI 47

Resuscitation of a 2-year-old drowned girl, after her 6-year-old sister had dropped her into a river while their mother was absent.

MI 48

A hunch-backed man from Frankfurt had also been crippled for a year in such a fashion that he could not move unless he pulled himself forwards on his hands, dragging his legs behind him which were bent backwards and totally lame. He was a beggar who had nothing, and openly begged for alms of the faithful in church, and was led to the grave of St Elisabeth (p. 194, *da er Bettler war, und nichts hatte, in der Kirche öffentlich von Gläubigern Almosen bettelte, ist er so zum Grab der erwähnten Herrin geführt worden*). Having returned home, he was freed of his hunch back, after which he returned to the tomb, this time getting fully cured, just propping himself up a little on a stick. Three of the protocol witnesses referred to this man as a servant (*Diener*) whom they saw begging within the church for necessities – was he a metaphoric servant of God, or a domestic servant who became unemployable for the duration of his impairment?

MI 49

Resuscitation of a 26-year-old man drowned in naturally hot baths.

MI 50

A 15-year-old girl had been blind the last two-and-a-half years, after waking up one morning suddenly blinded; she had had to be led from place to place.

MI 51

A 16-year-old boy had suffered from great pain in his thigh, knee and shin, so that he became bedridden [on 11 November 1231], unable to walk and had to be carried about by other people until Christmas, when he started walking, weakly and using crutches. After making a vow, he set out for the tomb the Saturday before Pentecost [28 May 1232], and because he suffered constantly he barely managed ten miles in eight days (the distance from his home to the tomb). He stayed in the hospital for four weeks, made daily visits to the tomb, but was not cured. As he was setting out for his return journey he managed a distance of three bow shots from the hospital when he sat down to rest, together with some other equally sick companion. He fell asleep and had a vision that someone was pouring water over him. After he awoke, he asked his companion why he had allowed someone to pour water over him. His companion answered with a smile that he should get up and put the crutches aside, since he hoped the boy had been healed. The boy immediately stood up, discarding one crutch while walking a little using the remaining crutch, and noticed he felt better. Then he returned to the tomb carrying both crutches over his shoulder, said his thanks and returned home cured.

MI 52

A 40-year-old woman suffered from a 'weakness' in her hands, causing them to swell up and tremble constantly, so that when she was eating she could move her hands to her mouth only slowly and with difficulty, and for four years she could do no work whatsoever. After the first two years in this condition, she also fell victim to a weakness in the legs, her knees displaying large swellings, and her shins below the knees were so weak and lame that she could no longer stretch out her legs. She completely lost her ability to walk and had to be carried by others. She added, that were hot coals to fall on her feet she would be unable to move or withdraw her feet of her own accord. She was taken to the tomb in a vehicle, and was carried from the vehicle to the tomb by others, where she was healed and became able to stand and walk again. Her husband, one of the witnesses, said that he himself often carried her with his own hands while she was ill and cared for her.

MI 53

Epileptic 19-year-old youth.

MI 54

The maidservant of a burgher of Limburg took the burgher's son to the tomb, in fulfilment of the parents' vow, to heal their son, who had a hunch back, swollen glands, and who could not lift his head from his shoulder.

MI 55

A 2-year-old boy was so lame in one arm and one leg, that he could not make use of these limbs; he also had a growth on his chest. He was carried to the tomb by his mother, and on the return journey he began to stretch his arm, becoming fully healed by the time he got home.

MI 56

A girl began to fall ill when she was 14, developing three lumpy growths on her thigh and another growth on her upper arm, the veins in her legs and one arm hardened, and her legs and that arm became totally lame. She also lost control over her head, so that she could not keep it upright any more. She could neither walk, nor stand, nor sit. After being brought to the tomb and laid on it, she was able to sit, and returning home, she gradually became better. After being taken to the tomb a fourth time, she was able to control the movements of her head again and regained the use of her limbs, so that she could walk, spin and do other work. The three lumpy growths in her leg also vanished, and the fourth one started to recede, so that by the time of the protocol it was only half the size it had been. One of the witnesses, the priest of her village, added that the parents had been afraid of taking the girl to the tomb because of the severity of her condition, fearing that she might die on the journey. Had that happened, they, the parents, would have had to do penance as if they were the cause of her death, but the priest had reassured them that he would not impose any such penance on them if she should die.

MI 57

A woman aged 20 woke up after a midday nap to find she had a twisted eye and twisted mouth. She could no longer close her eye which trembled constantly, could hold neither spittle nor drink in her mouth, and her teeth appeared to be all disfigured, after a part of her entire face was twisted. Her illness lasted eight weeks, and she was healed completely within seven days at the tomb of St Elisabeth.

MI 58

An 8-year-old boy had been unable to walk for seven years. He began to walk at home after his father had sent a wax image to St Elisabeth. The notaries of the protocol saw the boy walking, with a tottering gait in the manner of a boy learning to walk.

MI 59

An 18-year-old man was woken up by his master to go and do his normal work and found he was bereft of all strength in his limbs below the belt. He was taken by his brother to the portal of the basilica in a carriage drawn by two horses (*Zweigespann*), from where he was carried to the tomb. On the return journey he began to convalesce, and after eight days was completely cured so that he was able to perform his normal tasks.

MI 60

A 15-year-old boy with crooked eyes, one faced upwards, the other downwards, and twisted mouth.

MI 61

A boy who was lame in one leg for two years, so that this leg remained smaller than the other from below the knee onwards, finally staying a span shorter than the other leg because of the infirmity. The knee was also very swollen.

MI 62

A man of about 50 was so crippled in one leg, he could not sit properly. He could only drag himself about with the aid of two specially manufactured crutches, without which he could not move at all, or else he crawled about in his house. He remained in this condition for about a year.

MI 63

Girl of three-and-a-half who had been lame and mute since birth.

MI 64

A 2-year-old boy had swellings, a hunched back, and his legs were so crippled that they appeared grown together with his bottom; he was healed after being brought to the tomb.

MI 65

A three-and-a-half year old boy had been unable to walk all his life. When the witness, his aunt, was asked as to why the boy could not walk, she said she did not know exactly, but she thought it might be due to an illness, 'since he had beautiful limbs but very tiny legs' (p. 205, *denn er hatte schöne Glieder, aber sehr winzige Beine*). The boy threw away his crutches and some while later began to walk freely after a candle had been donated to St Elisabeth.

MI 66

A 7-year-old girl had humps on her chest and on her back for two years, and for three-and-a-half years she had been disfigured by her upper lip which grew over her mouth to the extent of three fingers' breadth; also her face became so swollen that her eyes were no longer visible, and her feet and legs also became swollen, so that for two years she could not walk.

MI 67

Dropsical woman; an 'experienced physician declared her to be dropsical and incurable' (p. 207, *ein erfahrener Arzt erklärte sie für wassersüchtig und unheilbar*).

MI 68

A 4-year-old girl had been unable to walk 'since childhood' (p. 208, *von Kindheit an*). When the notaries asked her parents whether she had any other infirmities, they answered no, but the girl had been weak in all her limbs and would eat earth and coal, and also burnt bread in small amounts. After being healed from her lameness, she also started eating all manner of foods.

MI 69

A man, then aged 20, somehow fell ill and became lame in one leg; he remained in this condition for one year. It took him five weeks to manage the 20 mile journey to the tomb, where he was healed, because he found it so difficult.

MI 70

When a boy was 13, he became ill so that he was weakened in his legs, and his legs began to twist themselves around each other 'like the parts of a rope are interwoven with one another, so that if one pulled them apart, they returned to each other again and went back to their original position' (p. 209, *wie die Teile eines Seiles miteinander verflochten sind, so daß sie, wenn man sie auseinanderzog, zueinander zurückkehrten und in die Ausgangslage zurückgingen*). Parts of the boy's neck were so contorted that the upper part was facing the chest and the lower part was facing the back. He also had a hump on his back and two bones were beginning to show through on his thigh. In this condition the youth spent eleven weeks at the tomb until he was healed on the feast of St Martin [11 November 1232] (which may be significant, since iconographically Martin was often associated with a crippled beggar). He began to move one leg and to separate it from the other one, or rather to stretch out the one leg since he was still lying in a vehicle. After he had returned home, he stretched the other leg in the same fashion. Afterwards he was able to get up after another two days, stretched out and healed so that only a small distortion was visible. Various witnesses testified they had seen the boy disfigured so dreadfully and horribly, and it appears that he remained within the hospital enclosure during his entire stay at the site of the tomb.

MI 71

Girl with pea stuck in her ear for fifteen-and-a-half years.

MI 72

A 9-year-old boy began to become crooked and started walking bent forwards, and a hump the size of a large pot grew on his back, so that finally he was only able to move himself on hands and knees. This condition lasted for half-a-year, until he was carried to the tomb, where he began to feel better once offerings had been made and was healed completely within seven weeks.

MI 73

Dropsical woman.

MI 74

Boy cured of a discharge from his nose which had also deformed his lower eyelid and the entire eye for two years.

MI 75

A man had fallen from a tower and had fractured his spine in three places, and also his sternum had fractured twice and one of his shins. For three weeks he was in such pain and agony that it was necessary to wrap him in linen sheets, since he could not bear to be touched by hands or to be moved. After making a vow he began to be able to walk with the aid of crutches, and within three-and-a-half months he was completely healed.

MI 76

A woman was completely blind for one year, so that she could not see the light of the heavens. She had no one who would lead her to the tomb of St Elisabeth, but by chance she found three women who led her. She made [votive] offerings similar to her eyes (p. 213, *den Augen gleiche Opfer*) and regained her sight in one eye to such an extent that she was able to recognise the wax images hanging above the tomb, and then the gilded images on the curtain. She returned home, but developed a pain in the other eye, which was healed once she had made a second journey to the tomb.

MI 77

Epileptic woman.

MI 78

Towards the end of his fourth year, a boy became so ill that he got a weakness in his limbs and his hands were lame; a hump grew out of his back, and a film of skin covered his eyes so that he could not see the light of day. He remained lame, hunchbacked and blind until he was eight years old, when his father led him to the tomb. At the tomb he opened his eyes, and immediately the flesh on his legs and his posterior began to renew itself, the bonds of his nerves and sinews were loosened, and his hunch back began to shrink. The hunch back had not completely vanished by the time of the protocol.

MI 79

A 9-year-old boy had had fistulas on each foot for four years, his legs were withered and he was so lame that he could not walk without a stick. After a vow by the mother, the boy began to walk gradually without his stick, until his condition improved so much that after he had thrown away his stick he was able to walk steadily and without impairment.

MI 80

Epileptic boy.

MI 81

Epileptic girl.

MI 82

A 12-year-old boy had a hunched back, as if his back had been broken, and his neck was strangely contorted towards the hump, so that when the boy's father on occasion scrutinised him he shrunk back as if from some monster. The boy's feet were so twisted that the ankles were turned towards the soles of his feet; furthermore he had lame hands. Everything that one gave to him he carried in his mouth and he crawled along on his hands, since his shins were also lame and appeared to have grown together with his posterior. His knees joined together with his belly, and he had one eye pulled up very high while the other eye was pushed down very far. Similarly parts of his mouth were twisted inhumanly, and he had fistulas on his feet, his thighs and his shins, so that illness appeared in thirty-four places. For five years he lay bedridden like that. In the next two years he nourished himself sometimes with the one, sometimes with the other hand. Apart from that he remained contorted in all his body parts as before. After the father had gone to the tomb, he returned to find his boy with 'loosened legs and knees, crawling, which he had been unable to do in any way previously' (p. 218, *mit gelösten Beinen und Knien, kriechend, was er vorher auf keine Weise konnte*). Thereafter the boy began to support himself on a staff, pulling his left leg along as before. After the mother had made a journey to the tomb, she found the boy walking without the staff which he had discarded. The boy was completely healed in his feet, his hands, his back, his legs, and his eyes and mouth, only the hunched back remained but much smaller.

MI 83

Girl cured of flux.

MI 84

A 50-year-old woman had been blind in her left eye for three years. She was cured at the tomb, but in turn her other eye became darkened and she returned home. After weeping her right eye was healed.

MI 85

A woman had been unable to see for two years, she could not differentiate between the day, the sun or the fire. She was healed eventually at home after an initially unsuccessful visit to the tomb.

MI 86

A 5-year-old boy had been healthy for one year of his life and sick during the other four years, so that he was lame in all limbs below the liver; wherever he was laid down he remained unless he was able to crawl with his hands. During that time he was also unable to speak. He was healed when his mother vowed to make annual offerings to St Elisabeth, when he immediately began to upright himself, holding onto chairs and finally he began to walk and also to speak, though not yet fluently 'but so that one was able to understand him after the fashion of children who are learning to speak' (p. 221, *sondern so, daß man ihn nach der Art der Kinder, die sprechen lernen, verstand*).

MI 87

An 8-year-old girl became swollen in all of her body and her legs became paralysed as far as her posterior. After the mother had visited the tomb, the swelling continuously receded and the legs became more pliant, so that the girl was walking on crutches even though she was unable to bend herself almost to the knees. One Sunday, after she had been led on her crutches to some other girls, she very soon stood up and returned home without her crutches, about which the other children rejoiced with her.

MI 88

A 9-year-old girl had a spot (*maculam*) in one eye for seven years during which time she could not see anything; she was healed after her father had visited the tomb.

MI 89

A 30-year-old woman had been injured in the knee so badly by a pig that she was bedridden for eleven weeks. After the wound had healed, she still could not walk with the lamed leg, apart from with the aid of crutches, and so she went for eight months. Then, with great difficulty, she visited the tomb of St Elisabeth, and on her return she immediately began to get better gradually, so that after fourteen days she could walk upright and without any impairments. One of the witnesses added that during her impairment he often helped lead her to the table of her master (*Dienstherrn*) by whose alms she was sustained.

MI 90

A 5-year-old girl had lame legs (shins) and lame feet, and from wherever she was placed she was unable to move herself, neither walking nor crawling. She was healed after being taken to the tomb by her parents.

MI 91

A girl, now 5 years old, had been born with very weak eyes, so that she could hardly recognise the path. After one-and-a-half years she became completely blind, so that she could not see the light of day at all any more. Her grandmother and some other relatives made a vow, and within three days the girl regained her sight completely.

MI 92

A man who got a hernia after leaping from a cart during harvest time, became unconscious and also lost the ability to speak.

MI 93

At the age of only 15 weeks a girl began to have a contorted back, so that on both the back and the chest she developed a tumour like a hump; she remained mute until her third year, and a knot grew on each arm. After being taken to the tomb the girl was completely cured.

MI 94

A woman with cancerous growth between her eyes who went to the tomb after she could not be healed 'by any art' (p. 225, *durch keine Kunst*).

MI 95

A 16-year-old boy had had fistulas for seven years, so that much pus issued from his shins, his thighs and his shoulders. When he was 16, he also became weakened in the legs and in his whole body so that he could do no work and could only walk with difficulty, supported on crutches. He was healed after visiting the tomb.

MI 96

A girl blind in one eye due to a white spot.

MI 97

A boy, now four-and-a-half years old, had been healthy for three-and-a-half years of his life. Then he became so sick that he became crooked, as if a hunched back wanted to grow, and his neck became twisted unilaterally; lastly, he had been unable to walk any more the past two months, unless he crawled on his knees and supported himself with his hands. He was cured when his mother smeared him, as if it were a salve, with earth taken from the tomb.

MI 98

The 12-year-old son of a knight fell ill, so that after three days the flesh began to wither away from his legs and hips, and eventually only skin covered the bones below his bottom; he lay bedridden for a year and five months, completely immobilised, and where he had been carried he remained unable to move. The day after the boy's parents had made a vow, the boy was being carried from one *reminata* to another and fell to the ground, with people trying to pick him up. He told them to leave him lying there on account of a dream that St Elisabeth would heal him, and immediately the boy got up and walked about.

MI 99

An 18-year-old woman had been blind in her right eye for six years, and with her left eye she saw so little that she could barely discern the light of day. Then she became totally blind in her left eye also. On the way to the tomb of St Elisabeth with her mother the young woman vowed to serve the saint in perpetuity, and was immediately healed.

MI 100

A woman of nearly 60 had been blind in her left eye for seven years. She apparently became blind when she was lying-in, on the third day after having given birth, due to a malign spirit in the shape of a boy, who crouched in the fire, and after the apparition had vanished, she found herself blinded. She was healed immediately upon setting out for the tomb, having vowed offerings in the shape of her eyes. Her husband corroborated what she said to the notaries, except that he did not see the spirit by the fire, but he heard her screams 'due to the presence and imagination' (p. 229, *wegen der Gegenwart und der Einbildung*) of the spirit.

MI 101

A man of about 40 had fallen ill in such a fashion that the nerves of his left leg began to contract, so that the foot of the same leg appeared to have joined together with his posterior. The flesh of the entire leg had also withered and disappeared, so that this entire bone was only covered by skin. Also, his back was so weakened below the belt that he could not move himself in any way. He lay 'like a [piece of] wood' (p. 229, *wie ein Holz*) from Pentecost [30 May 1232] until the Sunday after Epiphany [16 January 1232]. He was healed after making a vow, upon which he was immediately struck by a great pain in his back and in his withered leg, and after he had stretched out his leg, he got up without hesitation and walked without the aid of support. He added that while he was experiencing the great pain, the nerves in his back and leg began to clink and clatter.

MI 102

Insane man aged 50.

MI 103

Dropsical and inflated woman of around 50.

MI 104

Dropsical woman whose physicians declared her incurable.

MI 105

A 20-year-old woman had had great pain in her eyes for three and a half years, and eventually became totally blind. She spent four-and-a-half years blind, with her eyes closed and her eyelids as if bound. She was healed after a vision on her return journey from the tomb.

MI 106

A boy, now 4 years old, had a hump growing out of his back and a growth on his chest the size of a new-born boy's head. After he had had this deformity for half a year, his legs contracted and became so weakened that his legs withered away and his knees swelled up, and the soles of his feet and his shins appeared to have joined together with his posterior. 'And so he lay 1 year and 3 weeks like a monster' (p. 233, *Und so lag er 1 Jahr und 3 Wochen wie ein Ungeheuer*). His mother vowed she would donate her son to St Elisabeth as her perpetual servant if he was healed. The next morning the boy began to walk straight, and both the hump and the growth had disappeared, thereafter he was healed in all parts of his body.

Miracles in protocol MII

MII 1

Cistercian monk of around 18 years of age who became epileptic.

MII 2

Twelve-year-old boy cured of epilepsy.

MII 3

Cistercian abbot with ulcerous leg.

MII 4

Epileptic student.

MII 5

A man was plagued by pain in one of his legs for twenty years and longer, and somewhat less in his other leg, leaving both legs bloody and red. He started getting better two years before the protocol, after making a vow to St Elisabeth, and he was completely healed within the last half year. His 18-year-old daughter attested that since she 'started developing reason' (p. 237, *anfing Verstand zu haben*), she had seen her father in that condition, and she had tried many medicines. Another witness said that the man could not be helped by medicine, 'even though he had a very experienced physician' (p. 238, *obwohl er einen sehr erfahrenen Arzt hatte*). Unfortunately, the notaries did not record the consequences for the man's mobility and general health with regard to his legs.

MII 6

A girl became blind aged 3, and remained so until she was 12, when the miracle occurred.

MII 7

A girl was blind in one eye for three years, and was healed when her parents prepared to take her to the tomb. [This miracle was originally rejected by the commission, but on a second hearing it seems the 'words of the witnesses were more obvious than at the first examination' (p. 238, *die Worte der Zeugen waren einleuchtender als bei der ersten Überprüfung*).]

MII 8

A girl had been unable to walk or stand from birth, and she had a hump on her back. After making a vow, she was gradually straightened up. Then her father carried her on his back to the tomb on which she was laid, after which she was taken to the hospital. There she gained the ability to walk and her hump disappeared.

MII 9

A man, who had been lame for almost three years, came to the tomb on crutches, where he was healed, and then threw away his crutches.

MII 10/11

Two boys from the same village were placed in a cart and taken to the tomb. One was 5 years old and had a crippled back and crippled legs, the other was 4 years old and also had crippled legs. Both returned home cured.

MII 12

A girl suffering from boils at the back of her head and between her shoulders.

[The notaries recorded that she was healed at home after a second visit to the tomb in the space of some six months, pointing out that this happened without taking any corporeal medicine at all. There is also interesting information about the transportation of sick or impaired people: the said girl was first taken to the tomb in a small box or chest 'since she could not be transported any other way' (p. 241, *weil sie nicht anders transportiert werden konnte*), and a year later, presumably since the girl had grown larger, she was carried in a different contraption 'which the porters of diverse goods use' (p. 241, *die die Träger verschiedener Güter benutzen*).]

MII 13

Cure of possessed girl.

MII 14

A 2-year-old boy who had been blind since birth, 'even though he had handsome eyes' (p. 242, *obwohl er schöne Augen hatte*), and was cured on a fourth visit to the tomb.

MII 15

A farm labourer (*Ackerknecht*) thought one night that he was being woken up by a cat and lashed out with his right hand to hit the cat, only to find he had lost the ability to make use of his hand. His hand remained crippled for two months. He was cured on a third visit to the tomb after he encountered an old man, who assured him he would be healed.

MII 16

A woman who had been blind in one eye for two years was healed immediately at the tomb.

MII 17

Resuscitation of a man hanged at the gallows.

MII 18

A man arrested as a thief was hanged but survived because the rope broke.

MII 19

A 7-year-old boy had a shaking arm, which made his hand useless, and his head was inclined towards his left shoulder so that he could not upright himself, nor stand up unaided, furthermore he could not use his left leg. After twelve weeks like this he was healed once he had been taken to the tomb.

MII 20

A 5-year-old boy had been placed on a horse and had fallen off, breaking his right arm above the elbow in such a way that the bone of his arm protruded through the flesh. After the boy lay like this for six weeks, his mother was admonished to call a physician; she refused, saying she would never call a physician, but would trust only the merits of St Elisabeth. She took her son to the tomb, and on returning home she put the boy in a bath, where suddenly the protruding bone, about the length of a finger, fell off and the flesh grew back on the arm again, so that within the hour the boy was able to use his arm for eating again.

MII 21

Resuscitation of a drowned one-and-a-half-year-old boy.

MII 22

A 10-year-old girl was blind for twenty-two weeks, regaining her sight after being placed on the tomb of St Elisabeth.

MII 23

A girl now 10 years old had had her right hand so swollen for two years that she could make no use of it. She was healed within a fortnight after a second visit to the tomb.

MII 24

A monastic lay brother who was on milling duty accidentally had his hand caught by the millstone and crushed so badly that the flesh was removed both on the inner and the outer parts of his hand, his bones were smashed and his nerves were ground up. The remains of his crushed hand were bent and crippled so that he could no longer stretch out his hand. Some weeks later he had a vision in which St Elisabeth appeared to him and he woke up cured. The miller, one of the witnesses, testified that he thought it impossible that the lay brother could ever make any use of his hand 'according to the course of nature' (p. 251, *nach dem Lauf der Natur*).

Notes and references

1 Introduction

1 Cited in C. Barnes, G. Mercer and T. Shakespeare, *Exploring Disability: A Sociological Introduction*, Cambridge: Polity, 1999, p. 7.

2 At the time when the British Council of Organisations of Disabled People (BCODP) was formed, the same terminology was also adopted by the Disabled People's International (DPI) in Europe in 1994. Disability studies academics and disability activists prefer to avoid the phrase 'people with disabilities', as it implies that a person's impairment defines the identity of the individual, a stance which blurs the crucial distinction between impairment and disability.

3 I will be using 'they' even in the singular, and am aware that this might irritate strict grammarians, whom I would like to point towards Ann Bodine's essay on singular 'they', which argues that prior to the nineteenth century and its prescriptive grammarians, the use of singular 'they' was widespread and accepted in both written and spoken English, the prescription coming about mainly through social motivation yet unable to stifle the usage; motivated equally socially I prefer to return to historical precedent and use the gender-indefinite pronoun. Cf. Ann Bodine, 'Androcentrism in prescriptive grammar: singular "they," sex-indefinite "he," and "he or she,"' *Language in Society*, 4, 1975, reprinted in: D. Cameron (ed.), *The Feminist Critique of Language: A Reader*, London and New York: Routledge, 1990, pp. 166–86.

4 Cf. D. Brothwell and A. T. Sandison (eds), *Diseases in Antiquity*, Springfield, MA: C. C. Thomas, 1967, which examines all kinds of pathologies from skeletal evidence with a wide-ranging geographical and historical scope.

5 Skeletons of severely arthritic dinosaurs, to name but one example, have been discovered.

6 P. H. N. Wood, *International Classification of Impairments, Disabilities and Handicaps: A Manual of Classifications Relating to the Consequences of Disease*, Geneva: World Health Organization, 1980.

7 Ibid., pp. 27–9. This is so far the only internationally accepted attempt at defining what disability is; it distinguishes impairment (the loss of a normal function of a bodily part), disability (a restriction resulting from impairment) and handicap (the disadvantage for an individual resulting from impairment or disability); these definitions are very much in the vein of the medical model and have therefore been heavily criticised by the disability movement.

8 University of Reading, Postgraduate Registration Form, Notes for guidance, 1994.

9 In this context it is worth quoting a modern person's own words with regard to perceptions of disease and visibility. A French speech therapist, aged 24 in 1960, who was an informant for a study on illness and self, said: 'As long as I don't see the external damages caused by the disease, I am not scared, but as soon as I see the damages...one disease, for example, that would scare me would be leprosy, because it would eat up

parts of one's own body' (C. Herzlich and J. Pierret, *Illness and Self in Society*, transl. E. Forster, Baltimore, MD: Johns Hopkins University Press, 1987, p. 41).

10 Martin F. Norden, *The Cinema of Isolation: A History of Physical Disability in the Movies*, New Brunswick, NJ: Rutgers University Press 1994, p. xi note 5 (p. 325): 'As far as the majority of Hollywood film-makers are concerned, they [epilepsy and cerebral palsy] remain "invisible" disabling circumstances.'

11 Sharon Dale Stone, 'The myth of bodily perfection', *Disability and Society*, 10(4), 1995, p. 417.

12 Epilepsy is sometimes referred to as *gutta caducus* (in thirteenth- and fourteenth-century English manuscripts), so that even though *gutta* mostly refers to the more specific gout, *gutta* can also mean an ailment in general. Cf. R. E. Latham, *Revised Medieval Latin Word-List from British and Irish Sources*, London: British Academy, 1965, s.v. 'gutt/a'.

13 J. Norri, *Names of Sickness in English, 1400–1550: An Exploration of the Lexical Field*, Helsinki: Academia Scientiarium Fennica, 1992, p. 87. Cf. also Hans Kurath (ed.) and Sherman M. Kuhn (associate ed.), *Middle English Dictionary*, Ann Arbor, MI: University of Michigan Press, 1954, s.v. *disese* and *siknes(se)*. '*Disese*' can mean 'bodily infirmity or disability; sickness, illness, disease; also, a malady or ailment'.

14 Susan Edgington, 'Medical care in the hospital of St John in Jerusalem', in: H. Nicholson (ed.), *The Military Orders Volume 2: Welfare and Warfare*, Aldershot: Ashgate, 1998, p. 32.

15 Neubert, Dieter and Günther Cloerkes, *Behinderung und Behinderte in verschiedenen Kulturen. Eine vergleichende Analyse ethnologischer Studien*, 2nd edn, Heidelberg: Edition Schindele, 1994, p. 38.

16 On leprosy cf. Peter Richards, *The Medieval Leper and his Northern Heirs*, Cambridge: D. S. Brewer, 1977, a general introduction to the topic; as is Françoise Bériac, *Histoire des lépreux au moyen age: une société d'exclus*, Paris: Editions Imago, 1988; F.-O. Touati, *Maladie et société au Moyen Âge. La lèpre, les lépreux et les léproseries dans la province ecclésiastique de Sens jusqu'au milieu du XIVe siècle*, Brussels: De Boeck Université, 1998, who investigated changing attitudes to leprosy over time based on one specific geographical location; S. N. Brody, *The Disease of the Soul: Leprosy in Medieval Literature*, Ithaca, NY: Cornell University Press, 1974, especially of interest with regard to the notion of moral defilement of lepers; M. W. Dols, 'The leper in medieval Islamic society', *Speculum*, 58(4), 1983, pp. 891–916, for a non-Western angle; L. Demaitre, 'The relevance of futility: Jordanus de Turre (fl. 1313–35) on the treatment of leprosy', *Bulletin of the History of Medicine*, 70, 1996, pp. 25–61; Thomas J. Garbáty, 'The Summoner's occupational disease', *Medical History*, 7, 1963, pp. 348–58, for medieval and modern medical views; and Gerard Lee, *Leper Hospitals in Medieval Ireland*, Dublin: Four Courts Press, 1996, on regional institutions.

17 Michel Foucault, with *Madness and Civilization*, first British edition London: Tavistock Publications, 1967; G. Rosen, *Madness in Society*, Chicago, IL and London: University of Chicago Press, 1968; B. Clarke, *Mental Disorder in Earlier Britain*, Cardiff: University of Wales Press, 1975; M. W. Dols, *Majnun: The Madman in Medieval Islamic Society*, Oxford: Oxford University Press, 1992.

18 Owsei Temkin, *The Falling Sickness: A History of Epilepsy from the Greeks to the Beginnings of Modern Neurology*, 2nd rev. edn, Baltimore, MD and London: Johns Hopkins University Press, 1971.

19 Cf. G. Williams, 'Representing disability: some questions of phenomenology and politics', in: C. Barnes and G. Mercer (eds), *Exploring the Divide: Illness and Disability*, Leeds: Disability Press, 1996.

20 On the topic of old age in the Middle Ages one may consult, for example, Georges Minois *History of Old Age: From Antiquity to the Renaissance*, transl. S. H. Tenison, Cambridge, MA and Oxford: Polity, 1989; also Joel T. Rosenthal, *Old Age in Late Medieval England*, Philadelphia, PA: University of Pennsylvania Press, 1996; and more recently Shulamith Shahar, *Growing Old in the Middle Ages: 'Winter Clothes Us in Shadow*

and Pain', London and New York: Routledge, 1997. Especially Shahar deals with the theme of old people as one of the diverse marginal groups, such as women, the poor, the sick and the impaired (cf. idem, pp. 2–3). Her book also discusses the various notions of old age in the Middle Ages, the outward appearance of the old body and its fragility, aspects of the (ideal and real) behaviour of the aged, the experience of old age amongst different social groups (e.g. amongst the clergy, nobility, urban society and the peasantry), and charitable organisations and old age. The question of age distribution has been addressed by J. C. Russell, who tried to answer the question of 'How Many of the Population Were Aged?' in a paper published in Michael M. Sheehan (ed.), *Aging and the Aged in Medieval Europe (Papers in Medieval Studies 11)*, Toronto: Pontifical Institute of Medieval Studies, 1990, pp. 119–27. Russell reckoned that for England in the period between the later thirteenth century and the fifteenth century roughly 8–9 per cent of the adult population could be described as 'elderly' (ibid., p. 124).

21 Cited by David Brindle, 'Study shows disabled prejudice', *Guardian*, 26 May 1998. The charity's research found that half of all people surveyed had no regular contact with anybody with a disability; more than 1 in 5 admitted feeling awkward in the presence of a disabled person; almost 1 in 3 agreed with the statement 'some people assume that a person in a wheelchair cannot be intelligent'; and a similar proportion said disabled people should not expect to be able to use public transport. Of the disabled people interviewed about their experiences, one person said: 'Since I've become ill, all my friends have disappeared. People don't want to know.' (This story is uncannily similar to the experience of a medieval disabled person as told in a collection of miracle accounts: a formerly social and jovial man loses all his friends after he became blind, since they do not wish to be near him. The story is related here in Appendix J XVIII, and is discussed in Chapter 5.3.)

22 Alison Daniels, 'Airline apology for bad form', *Guardian*, 30 July 1997.

23 Or even disability as defined by its apparent visibility to animals: a group of five mentally disabled adults were refused entry to a zoo on the Isle of Wight because, as the zoo's manager said '[t]he adults were severely mentally disabled and I was very concerned they may harm the animals. One even had a fit . . . and was trying to bite.' Human prejudices and sensitivities are extended to animals in that the animals are perceived as liable to get 'disturbed' at the sight of the mentally disabled; at the same time the disabled persons are grouped with animals in the emphasis on biting as aberrant (adult human) behaviour. Cf. Hannah Pool, 'Zoo barred disabled "to spare the animals,"' *Guardian*, 6 July 1996.

24 Campaigning groups such as Mencap and the Down's Syndrome Association oppose the operation, drawing attention instead to the aim of trying to have society accept the features of Down's syndrome. A Mencap spokeswoman commented: 'It is understandable that parents of children with Down's syndrome want the best for their sons and daughters. It is appalling that some parents are forced to consider plastic surgery because of the very open prejudices of society towards anyone who looks different.' 'Cosmetic surgery for Down's children', *Guardian*, 5 June 1997.

25 In this context it is interesting to note that many of the medieval supplicants in the miracle narratives who were orthopaedically impaired were described in the sources as moving along by crawling (see Chapter 5.3).

26 Quoted in Peter Lennon, '100 years of solitude', *Guardian*, 26 May 1999.

27 Amy M. Hamburger, 'The cripple and his place in the community', *The Annals of the American Academy of Political and Social Science*, 77, no. 166, 1918, p. 39, cited by Norden, *The Cinema of Isolation*, p. xii.

28 Herzlich and Pierret, *Illness and Self in Society*, p. 85.

29 Rosebud T. Solis-Cohen, 'The exclusion of aliens from the United States for physical defects', *Bulletin of the History of Medicine*, 21, 1947, p. 33.

30 Ibid., pp. 46–7. In general, any conditions 'of a more or less permanent character tending to call for institutional care or treatment' and 'all cases of diseased, deformed,

or crippled children who will require unusual care during childhood, and who are likely to be physically defective if they live to maturity' were barred according to the regulations of 1910.

31 Phil Greer, *Disability Times*, February 1999, cited in *Guardian*, 6 February 1999.

32 Maureen Paton, 'Hear me out', *Guardian*, 18 August 1998.

33 Cf. the seminal essay by Umberto Eco on concepts of the Middle Ages in popular and academic culture in contemporary Western society, 'Dreaming of the Middle Ages', in *Travels in Hyperreality*, transl. W. Weaver, London: Picador, 1987, pp. 61–72.

34 C. Frayling, *Strange Landscape: A Journey through the Middle Ages*, London: BBC Books, 1995, p. 14.

35 American academic Paul J. Gans in a posting to the on-line discussion group <soc.history.medieval>, 18 February 1999. It is interesting to note that even a historian as respected as Jacques Le Goff can dismiss medieval disability in a single sentence, and can state categorically: 'Sin manifested itself in the form of physical deformity and disease' (Jacques Le Goff, *The Medieval Imagination*, transl. A. Goldhammer, Chicago, IL and London: University of Chicago Press, 1988, p. 84). Regrettably and all too frequently this statement is taken as the starting point, because of the scholarly stature of Le Goff, for discussions of sin, illness and deformity. This very sentence is cited on the opening page of the essay by Judith Byrne, 'Sickness as a medium of wrath in scripture and its reflection in the medieval and modern world', in: Michael Brown and Stephen H. Harrison (eds), *The Medieval World and the Modern Mind*, Dublin: Four Courts Press, 2000, pp. 57–73, and sets the tone for an otherwise useful selection of references to biblical and *exempla* texts.

36 M. L. Evans, 'Deaf and dumb in Ancient Greece', in: L. J. Davis (ed.), *The Disability Studies Reader*, New York and London: Routledge, 1997, p. 29.

37 Ibid.

38 Emic: of, relating to, or involving analysis of linguistic or behavioural phenomena in terms of the internal structural or functional elements of a particular system, cf. *Merriam-Webster's Collegiate Dictionary*, Springfield, MA: 2004, Online. Available http://www.m-w.com (accessed 30 September 2004).

39 Etic: of, relating to, or having linguistic or behavioural characteristics considered without regard to their structural significance, cf. *Merriam-Webster's Collegiate Dictionary*, <www.m-w.com>.

40 See Neubert and Cloerkes, *Behinderung und Behinderte*, p. 20.

2 The theoretical framework of disability

1 C. T. Wood, 'The doctor's dilemma: sin, salvation, and the menstrual cycle in medieval thought', *Speculum*, 56, 1981, p. 710.

2 P. Abberley, 'Policing cripples: social theory and physical handicap', unpubl. paper, Bristol Polytechnic, 1985, p. 9, cited in Brendan J. Gleeson, *Second Nature? The Socio-Spatial Production of Disability*, unpubl. PhD thesis, Melbourne, 1993, p. 92.

3 Cf. Neubert, Dieter and Cloerkes, Günther, *Behinderung und Behinderte in verschiedenen Kulturen. Eine vergleichende Analyse ethnologischer Studien*, 2nd edn, Heidelberg: Edition Schindele, 1994, p. 10 for a list of some recent literature. With regards to ethnology, these authors point out that once the assured territory of European historiography has been abandoned, most statements concerning disability in other cultures lack a solid foundation and belong more to the realm of speculation than reliable insight ('Sobald dabei der gesicherte Boden der europäischen Geschichtsschreibung verlassen wird, entbehren solche Aussagen einer soliden Grundlage und sind der Spekulation näher als zuverlässigen Erkenntnissen' (ibid.). I regard it as important to qualify this criticism, and even sharpen the critique, by pointing out that one only needs to leave the 'assured territory' of *modern* European history to find previous epochs rife with speculation about reactions to disability.

4 See also Neubert and Cloerkes, *Behinderung und Behinderte*, p. 96 on the presence of 'extreme reactions' (exposure, neglect, downright killing of disabled people) not just in 'primitive' cultures but also in modern Western societies. Additionally, the special status (shaman, medicine person, prophet etc.) sometimes accorded to impaired people in non-European cultures is also notably absent in modern Western society.

5 Seth Koven, 'Remembering and dismemberment: crippled children, wounded soldiers, and the great war in Great Britain', *American Historical Review*, 99, no. 4, 1994, pp. 1167–202.

6 Deborah Cohen, *The War Come Home: Disabled Veterans in Britain and Germany, 1914–1939*, Berkeley, Los Angeles, CA and London: University of California Press, 2001.

7 Fredrick Watson, *Civilization and the Cripple*, London: John Bale, Sons & Danielson, 1930.

8 Watson, *Civilization and the Cripple*, 1930, pp. 3–4: 'Was it possible in fever-stricken townships, threatened with ceaseless conflict and all its allies of famine and disease, that there was room for the sickly and incapacitated?'

9 Ibid., p. 5.

10 H. N. Haggard, *The Lame, the Halt and the Blind: Vital Role of Medicine in the History of Civilization*, London: Heinemann, 1932.

11 George Henderson and Willie V. Bryan, *Psychosocial Aspects of Disability*, Springfield, MA: 1984, pp. 4–5, cited in: Martin F. Norden, *The Cinema of Isolation: A History of Physical Disability in the Movies*, New Brunswick, NJ: Rutgers University Press, 1994, p. 7.

12 E. M. Bick, *A Source Book of Orthopaedics*, New York, 1968, cited by David Le Vay, *The History of Orthopaedics: An Account of the Study and Practice of Orthopaedics from the Earliest Times to the Modern Era*, Cornforth and Park Ridge: Parthenon, 1990, p. 44.

13 Deborah Marks, *Disability: Controversial Debates and Psychosocial Perspectives*, London and New York: Routledge, 1999, p. 28.

14 Hans Würtz, *Zerbrecht die Krücken. Krüppel-Probleme der Menschheit. Schicksalsstiefkinder aller Zeiten und Völker in Wort und Bild*, Leipzig: Leopold Voss, 1932.

15 The contents give a 'Verzeichnis bekannter Gebrechlicher und Ensteller' Würtz, *Zerbrecht die Krücken*, p. 5.

16 'Der Krüppel und seine Probleme', Würtz, *Zerbrecht die Krücken*, pp. 7–73.

17 'Lern- und Kernsprüche für Krüppel', Würtz, *Zerbrecht die Krücken*, pp. 393f.

18 'Der Mensch im Körperbehinderten ist nur seelisch und geistig zu heilen, zu 'entkrüppeln', Würtz, *Zerbrecht die Krücken*, p. 3.

19 C. Safilios-Rothschild, *The Sociology and Social Psychology of Disability and Rehabilitiation*, New York, 1970, cited by Brendon J. Gleeson, *Second Nature? The Socio-Spatical Production of Disability*, unpubl. PhD thesis, Melbourne, 1993. p. 96.

20 G. Melvyn Howe, *People, Environment, Disease and Death: A Medical Geography of Britain through the Ages*, Cardiff: University of Wales Press, 1997. The author throughout takes a 'Dark Age' view of the Middle Ages, as both the earlier and the later Middle Ages are for him totally backward medically, and everything is unhygienic and filthy. It appears the main source for the medieval period in Howe's recent work is in fact a rather antiquated publication by C. Creighton, *A History of Epidemics in Britain*, originally published in 1894, then re-published in a 2nd edn with additions by D. E. C. Eversley, E. A. Underwood and L. Ovenall, London: Cass, 1965.

21 This section in Howe's book mainly consists of a quote from C. H. Talbot, *Medicine in Medieval England*, London: Oldbourne, 1967.

22 L. Giuliani, 'Die seligen Krüppel. Zur Deutung von Mißgestalten in der hellenistischen Kleinkunst', *Archäologischer Anzeiger*, 1987, pp. 701–21.

23 V. Dasen, *Dwarfs in Ancient Egypt and Greece*, Oxford: Clarendon, 1993.

24 R. Garland, *The Eye of the Beholder*, London: Duckworth, 1995.

25 Ibid., p. 178.

26 Ibid.

27 Beth Cohen (ed.), *Not the Classical Ideal*, Leiden: Brill, 2000.

28 Daniel Ogden, *The Crooked Kings of Ancient Greece*, London: Duckworth, 1997.
29 N. Vlahogiannis, 'Disabling bodies', in: Dominic Montserrat (ed.), *Changing Bodies, Changing Meanings: Studies on the Human Body in Antiquity*, London and New York: Routledge, 1997, pp. 13–36.
30 M. L. Evans, 'Deaf and dumb in Ancient Greece', in: L. J. Davis (ed.), *The Disability Studies Reader*, New York and London: Routledge, 1997.
31 M. Michler, 'Die Krüppelleiden in "De morbo sacro" und "De articulis," '*Sudhoffs Archiv*, 45, 1961, pp. 303–28.
32 Ibid., p. 306.
33 Ibid., pp. 307–9.
34 The notion of τερασ (monster, prodigy) of earlier texts is accorded a place within the Hippocratic scheme of the regular human φυσισ (physis, physical shape or appearance) [Michler, 'Die Krüppelleiden', p. 311]. The texts give aetiological explanations of how these impairments may develop congenitally, and advise that treatment earlier in life has more chance of success than later treatment.
35 F. Haj, *Disability in Antiquity*, New York: Philosophical Library, 1970. The title is a misnomer, as the book actually deals with disability in the Near East during the Middle Ages and not 'antiquity' as is commonly understood.
36 J. Renger, 'Kranke, Krüppel, Debile – eine Randgruppe im Alten Orient?', in: Volker and Haas (eds), *Außenseiter und Randgruppen. Beiträge zu einer Sozialgeschichte des Alten Orients* Xenia. Konstanzer althistorische Vorträge und Forschungen, Heft 32, Konstanz: Universitätsverlag, 1992, pp. 113–26.
37 M. Miles, 'Disability in an eastern religious context: historical perspectives', *Disability and Society*, 10(1), 1995, pp. 49–69.
38 Henri-Jacques Stiker, *A History of Disability*, transl W. Sayers, Ann Arbor, MI: University of Michigan Press, 1999, p. 66.
39 Ibid.
40 Ibid., p. 72.
41 Ibid., p. 78.
42 Ibid., p. 83.
43 Ibid., pp. 83–4.
44 Ibid., p. 67. Stiker refers to Jean Delumeau, *La peur en occident, XIVe–XVIIIe siècles. Une cité assiégée*, Paris: Fayard, 1978.
45 Stiker, *A History of Disability*, p. 68.
46 Ibid., p. 85.
47 Ibid., p. 87.
48 Ibid., p. 77.
49 Ibid., pp. 87–8.
50 Ibid., p. 88.
51 W. Jaeger, *Die Heilung des Blinden in der Kunst*, 2nd edn, Sigmaringen: Jan Thorbeke Verlag, 1976.
52 K. F. Schlegel (ed.), *Der Körperbehinderte in Mythologie und Kunst*, Stuttgart and New York: Thieme, 1983.
53 W. Fandrey, *Krüppel, Idioten, Irre. Zur Sozialgeschichte behinderter Menschen in Deutschland*, Stuttgart: Silberburg-Verlag, 1990.
54 A. Hölter, *Die Invaliden. Die vergessene Geschichte der Kriegskrüppel in der europäischen Literatur bis zum 19. Jahrhundert*, Stuttgart and Weimar: Metzler, 1995.
55 K. E. Müller, *Der Krüppel. Ethnologia passionis humanae*, Munich: C. H. Beck, 1996.
56 Besides over-emphasising the disabled as a quasi sub-group of the poor in the Middle Ages, Stiker also alludes to the usual received ideas about the disabled as fools, following secondary sources only. Stiker, *A History of Disability*, p. 70.
57 Works by Michel Foucault relevant to these themes include *Madness and Civilization: A History of Insanity in the Age of Reason*, London: Tavistock, 1967; *The Order of Things: An Archaeology of the Human Sciences*, London: Tavistock, 1970; *The Birth of the Clinic*,

London: Tavistock, 1973, and *The History of Sexuality*, 3 vols, Harmondsworth: Penguin, 1984 and later.

58 Most importantly Bynum's book *Holy Feast and Holy Fast: The Religious Significance of Food to Medieval Women*, Berkeley, Los Angeles, CA and London: University of California Press, 1987.

59 Caroline Walker Bynum, 'The Female Body and Religious Practice in the Later Middle Ages', in: Michel Feher (ed.), *Fragments for a History of the Human Body, Part One*, New York: Zone Books, 1989, pp. 161–219.

60 Ibid., p. 162.

61 This concept and the critique of it are discussed by R. J. Evans, *In Defence of History*, London: Granta, 1997, pp. 184–5.

62 Elizabeth Deeds Ermarth, *Sequel to History: Postmodernism and the Crisis of Historical Time*, Princeton, NJ: Princeton University Press, 1992.

63 Evans, *In Defence of History*, p. 185.

64 On historiography in the Middle Ages cf. C. Holdsworth and T. P. Wiseman (eds), *The Inheritance of Historiography 350–900*, Exeter: University of Exeter, 1986, and P. Magdalino (ed.), *The Perception of the Past in Twelfth-Century Europe*, London and Rio Grande: Hambledon Press, 1992.

65 Otto of Freising, *The Two Cities*, C. C. Mierow transl. A. P. Evans and C. Knapp (eds), New York: Columbia University Press, 1966, p. 89.

66 Isidore of Seville: 'Sed comici privatorum hominum praedicant acta; tragici vero res publicas et regum historias. Item tragicorum argumenta ex rebus luctuosis sunt: comicorum ex rebus laetis.' *Isidori Hispalensis Episcopi Etymologiarum sive Originum* (ed.) W. M. Lindsay, 2 vols, Oxford: Clarendon, 1911, 1, Book VIII. vii. 6–7.

67 Prof Joachim Knape, Tübingen University, 'Historia: A medieval concept of knowledge?' presented at Leeds International Medieval Congress, July 1998.

68 Union of the Physically Impaired Against Segregation, *Fundamental Principles of Disability*, London, 1976, pp. 3–4, cited in: C. Barnes, G. Mercer and T. Shakespeare, *Exploring Disability: A Sociological Introduction*, Cambridge: Polity, 1999, p. 28.

69 J. C. Riley, 'Sickness in an early modern workplace', *Continuity and Change*, 2(3), 1987, pp. 363–85.

70 W. Hughes and K. Paterson, 'The social model of disability and the disappearing body: towards a sociology of impairment', *Disability and Society*, 12(3), 1997, p. 326.

71 See, Chapter 1.2, and Mike Oliver, *The Politics of Disablement*, Basingstoke: Macmillan, 1990.

72 Rob Imrie, 'Ableist geographies, disablist spaces: towards a reconstruction of Golledge's "Geography and the disabled,"' *Transactions of the Institute of British Geographers*, N. S., 21(2), 1996, p. 397.

73 Ibid.

74 Ann Shearer, *Disability: Whose Handicap?*, Oxford: Blackwell, 1981.

75 Originally published as: Erving Goffman, *Stigma: Notes on the Management of Spoiled Identity*, Englewood Cliffs, NJ, Prentice-Hall, 1963. Also the study on stigma as a concept by P. Hunt (ed.), *Stigma, the Experience of Disability*, London: Chapman, 1966.

76 Goffman, *Stigma: Notes on the Management of Spoiled Identity*, London: Penguin, 1968, reprinted 1990, pp. 14–15.

77 Ibid., p. 12.

78 I believe that since it is impossible to look at another person 'objectively', but only always subjectively from within one's social and cultural conditioning, a person would have solely a 'virtual' identity in Goffman's construct.

79 Goffman, *Stigma*, p. 65.

80 Ibid., p. 68.

81 René Girard, *The Scapegoat*, transl. Y. Freccero, London: Athlone Press, 1986, p. 18.

82 Ibid.

83 Ibid.

84 Gleeson, *Second Nature?*, p. 89, terms Goffman's theories the most 'notorious' exposition of the interactionist viewpoint.

85 P. Abberley, 'Disabled people – 3 theories of disability', *Occasional Papers in Sociology*, no. 10, Bristol Polytechnic, 1991, p. 11; cf. P. Abberley, 'The concept of oppression and the development of a social theory of disability', *Disability, Handicap and Society*, 2, no. 1, 1987.

86 Oliver, *The Politics of Disablement*, and Oliver, *Understanding Disability: From Theory to Practice*, Basingstoke: Macmillan, 1995. Stigma theory is not completely dead, however: Michael J. Hughes, *The Consequences of Facial Disfigurement*, Aldershot: Ashgate, 1998, still discusses the Goffmanesque notion of 'spoiled identity' and looks at the sociology of stigma.

87 Reginald R. Golledge, 'Geography and the Disabled: a survey with special reference to the vision impaired and blind populations', *Transactions of the Institue of British Geographers*, N. S., 18, 1993, p. 63.

88 Gleeson, 'A geography for disabled people?', *Transactions of the Institute of British Geographers*, N. S., 21(2), 1996, pp. 388–96. Gleeson argues that according to Golledge, the social experience of disability can only be explained as a pre-ordained ('natural') consequence of physical difference.

89 Inspired by the work of Foucault, there has been a surge of interest in bodies, both historical and contemporary. For the medieval period, notable examples include the volume edited by Sarah Kay and Miri Rubin, *Framing Medieval Bodies*, Manchester and New York: Manchester University Press, 1994, which amongst others discusses the aged body (article by S. Shahar), gender (R. Gilchrist), and the bodily 'other' with particular reference to hermaphroditism (M. Rubin); the collection of essays by Peter Biller and A. J. Minnis (eds), *Medieval Theology and the Natural Body* (York Studies in Medieval Theology 1) York: York Medieval Press, 1997, which treats the body from the point of view of medieval religious notions; and the symbolism and social context of late medieval and early modern bodies in Klaus Schreiner and Norbert Schnitzler (eds), *Gepeinigt, begehrt vergessen: Symbolik und Sozialbezug des Körpers im späteten Mittelalter und in der frühen Neuzeit*, Munich: Wilhelm Fink Verlag, 1992, which covers such diverse topics as the theological, anthropological and semantic notions of bodies, stigmatisation of the body, bodies as symbols and metaphors, corporal movement and gestures, and the reception and depiction of bodies in imagery. However, none of these scholarly treatments of medieval bodies have explicitly addressed the issues surrounding physically impaired bodies. To understand impaired bodies, in the medieval or any other historical period, we would have to follow the Lacanian insight that a person inhabits 'multiple subject–positions', meaning that we cannot speak of *the* medieval body, or even *the* medieval female, old, or impaired, body, but rather we would need to see groups and individuals as inhabiting a 'series of positions informed by a variety of discourses' (Miri Rubin, 'Medieval Bodies: Why Now, and How?', in: Miri Rubin (ed.), *The Work of Jacques Le Goff and the Challenges of Medieval History*, Woodbridge: Boydell, 1997, p. 217).

90 The late Rex Stainton Rogers, and Nick Lee – Department of Psychology, Reading University, personal communication.

91 Gleeson, *Second Nature?*, p. 32.

92 Hughes and Paterson, 'The social model of disability and the disapperaing body', p. 334.

93 Vic Finkelstein, *Attitudes and Disabled People*, Geneva: World Health Organization, 1980.

94 Gleeson, *Second Nature?*, and Gleeson, 'A geography for disabled people?', also Golledge, 'Geography and the disabled', and Imrie, 'Ableist geographies, disablist spaces'.

95 Gleeson, *Second Nature?*, dissertation abstract.

96 It is debatable whether 'feudalism' is still a valid construct with regard to medieval modes of production or political organisation. See the seminal article by

Elizabeth A. R. Brown, 'The tyranny of a construct: feudalism and historians of Medieval Europe', originally published in the *American Historical Review*, 79, 1974, pp. 1063–88, reprinted in: Lester K. Little and Barbara H. Rosenwein (eds), *Debating the Middle Ages*, Malden and Oxford: Blackwell, 1998, pp. 148–69; also the work of Susan Reynolds, ed. *Fiefs and Vassals: The Medieval Evidence Reinterpreted*, Oxford: Oxford University Press, 1994.

97 Gleeson, *Second Nature?*, dissertation abstract, pp. 151–2.

98 Ibid., p. 156.

99 Gleeson, 'A geography for disabled people?', pp. 387–96. This article was supported by Rob Imrie, 'Ableist geographies, disablist spaces'. Both articles were challenged and responded to by Reginald G. Golledge, 'A response to Gleeson and Imrie', *Transactions of the Institute of British Geographers*, N. S., 21(2), 1996, pp. 403–11.

100 Gleeson, 'Disability Studies: a historical materialist view', *Disability and Society*, 12(2), 1997, pp. 179–202.

101 Gleeson, *Second Nature?*, dissertation abstract.

102 Jacques Le Goff, 'The framework of time and space', in his *Medieval Civilization*, Oxford: Blackwell, 1988; also E. P. Thompson, 'Time, work-discipline, and industrial capitalism', in: M. W. Flinn and T. C. Snout (eds), *Essays in Social History*, Oxford: Clarendon, 1974.

103 The ecclesiastical calendar is in a sense the only calendar in the Middle Ages, and the imposition of ordered time on the inmates of monastic institutions, in the form of the various services and monastic hours, is the closest thing in this period to a kind of pre-capitalist structuration of time, of fixing and partitioning time according to set rules.

104 Gleeson, *Second Nature?*, p. 161. Also Gleeson, 'A geography for disabled people?', pp. 391–2, where he repeats the theory from his thesis, that the capacities of impaired people were devalued with the development of capitalism, when the worth of individual labour was appraised in terms of average productivity standards, so that 'slower', 'weaker' or more inflexible workers were devalued in terms of their potential for paid work; the spatial issue of the removal of the site of production from home to a separate workplace was further disabling.

105 Oliver, *The Politics of Disablement*, p. 27.

106 J. Sheer and N. Groce, 'Impairment as a human constant: cross-cultural and historical perspectives on variation', *Journal of Social Studies*, 44(1), 1988, p. 30.

107 Ibid., p. 26.

108 Oliver, *The Politics of Disablement*, p. 27.

109 Colin Barnes, 'Theories of disability and the origins of the oppression of disabled people in western society', in: L. Barton (ed.), *Disability and Society: Emerging Issues and Insights*, London: Longman, 1996, p. 47.

110 Cf. Mary Douglas, *Purity and Danger: An Analysis of Concepts of Pollution and Taboo*, London: Routledge & Kegan Paul, 1966.

111 Barnes, 'Theories of disability', p. 43.

112 Cited in: Barnes, 'Theories of disability', p. 49. Perhaps Tom Shakespeare was influenced by the Freudian notion of a symbolic dimension ascribed to disability, namely in that the fear of becoming disabled supposedly equates to the fear of castration. As Sigmund Freud wrote in his article 'The Uncanny' (1919), '[a] study of dreams, phantasies and myths has taught us that anxiety about one's eyes, the fear of going blind, is often enough a substitute for the dread of being castrated.' (*The Standard Edition of the Complete Works of Sigmund Freud, vol. 17 (1917–19): An Infantile Neurosis and Other Works*, ed. James Strachey, London, 1955, p. 231, cited in: Martin F. Norden, *The Cinema of Isolation: A History of Physical Disability in the Movies*, New Brunswick, NJ: Rutgers University Press, 1994, p. 6.)

113 Barnes, 'Theories of disability', p. 49.

114 Ibid., p. 50.

115 Cf. Dieter Neubert and Günther Cloerkes, *Behinderung und Behinderte in verschiedenen Kulturen. Eine vergleichende Analyse ethnologischer Studien*, 2nd edn, Heidelberg, 1994,

pp. 10–11 for a discussion of just this issue. Neubert and Cloerkes point out the contradiction between apparently assured knowledge about disability and actual lack of research, which is especially noticeable in the realm of the intercultural and historic variety of reactions to disability and the disabled ('Der Widerspruch zwischen angeblich gesichertem Erkenntnisstand und tatsächlichem Forschungsrückstand wird besonders deutlich im Bereich der interkulturellen und historischen Variabilität von Reaktionen auf Behinderung und Behinderte.' [Neubert and Cloerkes, p. 10]).

116 Laura Lee Downs, 'If "Woman" is just an empty category, why am I afraid to walk alone at night? Identity politics meets the postmodern subject', *Comparative Studies in Society and History*, 35, 1993, p. 416, cited in Evans, *In Defence of History*, p. 211.

117 See my criticism of Gleeson above.

118 Sheer and Groce, 'Impairment as a human constant', p. 23.

119 Ibid., p. 24.

120 Gleeson, 'Disability Studies: a historical materialist view', p. 185.

121 See also the historiographical section in Chapter 2.1. As Elizabeth Bredberg put it, '[i]nevitably, these histories present a history of unabated progress, from the misery and neglect of ancient history to the enlightened and effective treatment available in the present' (E. Bredberg, 'Writing Disability History: problems, perspectives and sources', *Disability and Society*, 14(2), 1999, pp. 190–1).

122 Ibid., p. 192.

123 Foucault did not realise that the *Stultifera Navis* was a literary metaphor, not an actual practice of responding to insane persons, and also failed to understand the difference between the late medieval concepts of 'folly' and 'madness': the ship is for fools, not mad people. Cf. Bredberg, 'Writing Disability History', p. 195, and W. B. Maher and B. Maher, 'The ship of fools: *Stultifera Navis* or *Ignis Fatuus?*', *American Psychologist*, 37(7), 1982, pp. 756–61.

124 Bredberg, 'Writing Disability History', p. 199.

125 See for example Aaron I. A. Gurevich, *Historical Anthropology of the Middle Ages*, ed. Jana Howlett, Cambridge: Polity, 1992.

126 R. A. Scott, 'The construction of conceptions of stigma by professional experts', in: D. M. Boswell and J. M. Wingrove (eds), *The Handicapped Person in the Community: A Reader and Sourcebook*, London: Tavistock Publications, 1974, pp. 109–10.

127 Shearer, *Disability: Whose Handicap?*, p. 8.

128 Neubert and Cloerkes, *Behinderung und Behinderte*.

129 Ibid., p. 11.

130 Ibid., p. 88.

131 Ibid., 'Es kann deshalb von einer Tendenz zur Variabilität der sozialen Reaktion auf Behinderte gesprochen werden.'

132 Ibid., p. 89.

133 Ibid., p. 90.

134 C. Herzlich and J. Pierret, *Illness and Self in Society*, transl. E. Forster, Baltimore, MD: Johns Hopkins University Press, 1987, p. xi.

135 Ibid., p. xvi.

136 Ibid., p. 118.

137 Benedicte Ingstad and Susan Reynolds Whyte (eds), *Disability and Culture*, Berkeley, Los Angeles, CA and London: University of California Press, 1995.

138 Susan Reynolds Whyte and Benedicte Ingstad, 'Disability and culture: an overview', in: Ingstad and Whyte (eds), *Disability and Culture*, pp. 14–15.

139 Ibid., p. 17.

140 'Je zentraler diese Werte jedoch für das gesellschaftliche Wertsystem sind... und je größer die Abweichung ist, desto massiver wird die Bedrohung empfunden.' S. Karstedt, 'Soziale Randgruppen und soziologische Theorie', in: M. Brusten and J. Hohmeier (eds), *Stigmatisierung, Band 1. Zur Produktion gesellschaftlicher Randgruppen*, Neuwied/Darmstadt, 1975, p. 183, cited in Neubert and Cloerkes, *Behinderung und Behinderte*, p. 15.

141 Robert Murphy, *The Body Silent*, London: Phoenix House, 1987, pp. 131–2.
142 Barnes, 'Theories of disability', p. 51.
143 Stiker, *A History of Disability*, p. 69. But a few lines later, Stiker turns his concept of liminality on its head. Alluding to the geographical-metaphorical location at the fringes of the known world of the 'monstrous' (as in the monstrous races) in medieval thought, Stiker believes that the 'monstrous' disabled pose a challenge: 'The disabled, the "monsters" immanent in our society and not on its borders, heighten our fears, because *they are already there* [*sic*].' Here, for Stiker, the disabled themselves are not liminal through their contrasting localisation with what he sees as the truly liminal monsters.
144 Ivan Illich, *Limits to Medicine. Medical Nemesis: The Expropriation of Health*, Harmondsworth: Penguin, 1977, p. 124.
145 Neubert and Cloerkes, *Behinderung und Behinderte*, p. 92. See also ibid., pp. 32–3, for the different ethnological models that could correspond to 'impairment' and 'disability'.
146 Ibid., p. 92.
147 Cf. ibid., p. 93: 'Es geht um nicht weniger als den Unterschied zwischen der Einschätzung eines "Sachverhalts" und der Einschätzung eines "Menschen". Bei der Einschätzung eines Menschen ist eben nicht nur dessen körperlicher, geistiger oder psychischer Zustand von Bedeutung, sondern auch seine sozialen Beziehungen und vieles andere mehr.'
148 Rubin, 'Medieval bodies', p. 209.
149 Ibid., p. 217.
150 Barnes, 'Theories of disability', p. 51.
151 Neubert and Cloerkes, *Behinderung und Behinderte*, p. 14.

3 Medieval theoretical concepts of the (impaired) body

 1 On the theme of the body in theology, both medieval and modern, see Lawrence E. Sullivan, review article, 'Body works: knowledge of the body in the study of religion', *History of Religions*, 30(1), 1990, pp. 88–99; Antoine Vergote, 'The body as understood in contemporary thought and Biblical categories', *Philosophy Today*, 35, 1991, pp. 93–105; James B. Nelson, *Body Theology*, Louisville: Westminster, 1992; and James F. Keenan, 'Current theology note: Christian perspectives on the human body', *Theological Studies*, 55, 1994, pp. 30–246.
 2 On disability in Judaic thought, see Lynn Holden, *Forms of Deformity* (Journal for Study of the Old Testament Supplement Series 131), Sheffield: Sheffield Academic Press, 1991, a revised doctoral thesis with a rather repetitive motif-index of bodily abnormality, deformity and disability taken from Jewish literature, commentary and legend up to the twelfth century; also see Judith Z. Abrams, *Judaism and Disability: Portrayals in Ancient Texts from the Tanach through the Bavli*, Washington, DC: Gallaudet University Press, 1998 for a general survey; an older but very useful publication is Julius Preuss, *Biblisch-Talmudische Medizin. Beiträge zur Geschichte der Heilkunde und der Kultur überhaupt*, originally publ. 1911, reprint Wiesbaden: Fourier-Verlag, 1992.
 3 C. J. Brim, *Medicine in the Bible*, New York: Froben, 1936, pp. 19–20.
 4 A strange episode, which has prompted various interpretations. In the older view, exemplified by James Hastings (ed.), *A Dictionary of the Bible*, 2 vols, Edinburgh: T. & T. Clark, 1900, p. 329, the issue of interpretation is effectively brushed aside on a textual basis, suggesting that 'this curious passage appears to be corrupt'. A more recent commentator, F. Davidson (ed.), *The New Bible Commentary*, 2nd edn, London: Intervarsity Fellowship, 1954, tried to explain it so: the Jebusites are taunting David by boasting that even their blind and lame people are strong enough to hold out against him, which angers David, so that he wants to show the Jebusites that they are in fact themselves the 'blind' and 'lame'; the last sentence refers to the words of David being used in a kind of proverbial fashion, making a mocking reference to over-confidence.

5 Medieval illustrations to this psalm often show a figure, in front of a building, who is hit by arrows and covered with sores (Psalms 38:2: 'quoniam sagittae tuae infixae sunt mihi'). See also Heinz Meyer, 'Metaphern des Psaltertextes in den Illustrationen des Stuttgarter Bilderpsalters', in: C. Meier and U. Ruberg (eds), *Text und Bild. Aspekte des Zusammenwirkens zweier Künste in Mittelalter und früher Neuzeit*, Wiesbaden: L. Reichert Verlag, 1980, p. 185.

6 A. Ohry and E. Dolev, 'Disabilities and handicapped people in the Bible', *Koroth*, 8 (5–6), 1982, p. 63.

7 Hastings, *A Dictionary of the Bible*, 2, s.v. 'medicine', p. 330, added up the occurrences of blindness, as in the words 'blind' or 'blindness', in the Bible, and tried to distinguish between literal and metaphorical sense. Blindness occurs 87 times in total (35 times in the Old Testament and 52 times in the New), of which 41 times it is used in a metaphorical sense, with 39 references to a literal lack of sight. In the New Testament alone, 36 references are made to literal and 16 to metaphorical blindness.

8 Deuteronomy 17:1 stipulates against the offering up of any animal in sacrifice that has a 'blemish' (see also Leviticus 22:22, where blind, broken or maimed animals are mentioned), while Deuteronomy 23:1 forbids a man who is 'wounded in the stones' or 'hath his privy member cut off' from entering 'into the congregation of the Lord'.

9 Deuteronomy 28:29.

10 Deuteronomy 28:35.

11 Deuteronomy 28:61.

12 Leviticus 19:9–10, repeated at 23:22. Compare this with medieval English agricultural by-laws, which reserve the right to glean while harvesting is still taking place to the infirm, the old and people otherwise unable to partake in harvesting. On the subject of gleaning, see W. O. Ault, 'Open-field husbandry and the village community, a study of agrarian bye-laws in medieval England', *Transactions of the American Philosophical Society*, 55, part 7, 1965, and Ault, *Open-Field Farming in Medieval England: A Study of Village By-Laws*, London: Allen & Unwin, 1972.

13 Leviticus 19:14.

14 Leviticus 21:17–20.

15 Moses prohibits membership of the priesthood to those who are blind, lame, have strange noses, or have strange limbs. Vienna, Österreichische Nationalbibliothek, *Bible of King Wenceslas*, Codex Vindobonensis 2759, fol. 121r, dated to *c*.1400.

16 Bernard Orchard, Edmund F. Sutcliffe, Reginald C. Fuller and Ralph Russell (eds), *A Catholic Commentary on Holy Scripture*, London: Nelson, 1953, p. 241.

17 A. Donaldson (transl.), *The Apostolical Constitutions*, 17, Ante-Nicene Christian Library, Edinburgh: no publisher, 1880, section 8, paragraphs 77–9, p. 267.

18 See Elizabeth Bredberg, 'Writing disability history: problems, perspectives and sources', *Disability and Society*, 14(2), 1999, p. 193.

19 Cf. Emil Friedberg (ed.), *Corpus iuris canonici*, 2 vols, Leipzig: Tauchnitz, 1879–81, 2, cols 144–6.

20 Ruth Mellinkoff, *Outcasts: Signs of Otherness in Northern European Art of the Late Middle Ages*, 2 vols, Berkeley, Los Angeles, CA and Oxford: University of California Press, 1993, 1, p. 114.

21 On a digressory note, it is worth pointing out that the issue of impaired people in holy orders is still not satisfactorily resolved in the modern Catholic Church. In 1995 the Vatican 'provoked fury by issuing a decree banning men who suffer from an allergy to gluten from becoming priests' (Madeleine Bunting, 'Wafer allergy bars priests', *Guardian*, 10 October 1995). The Vatican insisted on communion wafers containing gluten as the only suitable kind of wafers; gluten can trigger the debilitating coeliac disease.

22 A. Cobban, *English University Life in the Middle Ages*, London: UCL Press, 1999, p. 19. Cf. Queen's Commissioners (ed.), *Statutes of the Colleges of Oxford*, 3 vols, Oxford and London: no publisher, 1853, I, ch. 7, p. 7.

23 Cobban, *English University Life*, p. 19. Cf. J. M. Fletcher, 'The teaching of arts at Oxford, 1400–1520', *Paedagogica Historica*, 7, 1967, p. 443.

24 Cobban, *English University Life*, p. 19. Cf. R. C. Schwinges, 'Admission', in: H. de Ridder-Symoens (ed.), *Universities in the Middle Ages, vol. 1: A History of the University in Europe*, Cambridge: Cambridge University Press, 1992, p. 172.

25 John 9:2–3.

26 *Codex aureus epternacensis*, fol. 53v, made at Echternach, *c*.1030, now Nuremberg, Germanisches Nationalmuseum, illustrating John 9:1–7.

27 The wall painting is now in New York, Metropolitan Museum of Art.

28 John 9:39–41. The Pharisees ask if they also are blind (in the metaphorical sense) and Jesus replies if they were blind (innocent) they would be without sin, but since they say they see (they only think they understand), their sin remains with them. Wheareas quite a few of the other healing miracles are related in more than one gospel, this particular miracle can only be found in John.

29 Jesus 'brach [...] mit der Vorstellung, daß Krankheit die Folge von Sünde sei; angesichts des Blindgeborenen heißt es: 'Weder er noch seine Eltern haben gesündigt [John 9:3]; ebensowenig waren ihm Kranke unrein und deswegen unberührbar' (Arnold Angenendt, *Geschichte der Religiosität im Mittelalter*, Darmstadt: Wissenschaftliche Buchgesellschaft, 1997, p. 130).

30 Mark 2:2–12, Luke 5:18–25 and Matthew 9:2–7.

31 Now in the Louvre in Paris.

32 Oxford, Bodleian Library, cover of MS Douce 176.

33 Now at Darmstadt, Hessische Landesbibliothek, HS. 1640.

34 London, British Library, MS Royal 20.B.IV, fol. 61v, dating from the early fifteenth century.

35 W. von Siebenthal, *Krankheit als Folge von Sünde. Eine medizinhistorische Untersuchung*, Hannover: Schmorl und von Seefeld, 1950, p. 42. However, Hastings, *A Dictionary of the Bible*, 2, s.v. 'medicine', p. 326, had tried to play down such a causal link: 'the conjecture that the paralysis was a judgment on him for immorality, on account of our Lord's having prefaced his cure by declaring the forgiveness of his sins, [is a] deduction [...] not warranted by the very slender data from which [it is] drawn'.

36 Siebenthal, *Krankheit als Folge von Sünde*, p. 43.

37 A young boy (Mark 9:17–29), and the Gadarene madman (Mark 5:2–19 and Luke 8:27–36)

38 Mark 7:32–36.

39 Mark 8:22–25.

40 Mark 10:46–52, Bartimaeus is healed because of his faith; at Matthew 20:30–34 the same episode is told with two unnamed beggars, and this time even faith is not an issue to their healing.

41 John 5:2–9.

42 One of the wooden ceiling panels shows the miracle at Bethesda (John 5:4), depicting an angel with a crippled person and others surrounding the pool.

43 Acts 5:15–16.

44 Masaccio's fresco, from the first half of the fifteenth century, is in the Brancacci chapel of Santa Maria del Carmine, Florence.

45 Acts 8:5–8.

46 Acts 14:8–10.

47 Acts 3:1–10.

48 In the north transept of the upper church of San Francesco.

49 In the Brancacci chapel, Santa Maria del Carmine.

50 R. W. Mackelprang and R. O. Salsgiver, 'People with disabilities and social work: historical and contemporary issues', *Social Work: Journal of the National Association of Social Workers*, 41(1), 1996, p. 8.

51 Mackelprang and Salsgiver, 'People with disabilities and social work', p. 8. The authors rely for most of their material on other social studies texts, rather than on any works dealing with medieval history, or history of medicine; most of the statements

on medieval disabled people appear to have been drawn from H. Livneh, 'On the origins of negative attitudes toward people with disabilities', *Rehabilitation Literature*, 43, 1982, pp. 338–47, and H. Livneh, 'Disability and monstrosity: further comments', *Rehabilitation Literature*, 41, 1980, pp. 280–3.

52 Shari Thurer, 'Disability and monstrosity: a look at literary distortions of handicapping conditions', *Rehabilitation Literature*, 41, 1980, p. 14.

53 P. K. Longmore, 'Uncovering the hidden history of people with disabilities', *Reviews in American History*, 15, 1987, p. 355.

54 Nancy Weinberg and Carol Sebian, 'The Bible and disability', *Rehabilitation Counselling Bulletin*, 23(4), 1980, p. 273, cited in Martin F. Norden, *The Cinema of Isolation: A History of Physical Disability in the Movies*, New Brunswick, NJ: Rutgers University Press, 1994, p. 7.

55 Mark Geller of University College London has studied ancient Babylonian medical texts, and presented some of his findings in a paper 'Anatomy of Babylonian Medicine', presented as part of a seminar series on magic and medicine in the Department of Classics, University of Reading, February 1999.

56 James 5:15.

57 Frederick S. Paxton, *Christianizing Death: The Creation of a Ritual Process in Early Medieval Europe*, Ithaca, NY and London: Cornell University Press, 1990, p. 32.

58 Ibid., p. 28. The threat is at John 5:14, after Christ has healed the infirm man at the pool of Bethesda: 'Behold, thou art made whole: sin no more, lest a worse thing come unto thee.'

59 Paxton, *Christianizing Death*, p. 28.

60 Ibid. pp. 49–51.

61 *Le liber ordinum en usage dans l'église wisigothique et mozarabe d'Espagne du cinquième au onzième siècle* (ed.) Mario Férotin, Monumenta ecclesiae liturgica 5, Paris, 1904, p. 72, cited in: Paxton, *Christianizing Death*, pp. 72–3, with the Latin text given at p. 73 note 101.

62 Paxton, *Christianizing Death*, p. 73.

63 Ibid., pp. 78–82.

64 Ibid., p. 82.

65 Ibid., p. 154.

66 The Latin reads: 'et peccata remittuntur et consequenter corporalis salus restuitur'; in *Monumenta Germaniae Historica, Concilia aevi Karolini DCCCXLIII–DCCCLIX* (ed.) W. Hartmann, Hanover, 1984, 3. 223, c. viii, cited in Paxton, *Christianizing Death*, p. 164 and Latin at p. 165 note 6.

67 Paxton, *Christianizing Death*, p. 165.

68 Ibid., pp. 207–8.

69 Shulamith Shahar, *Childhood in the Middle Ages*, transl. C. Galai, London and New York: Routledge, 1992, p. ix.

70 Mark 8:22–6.

71 Bede, *In Marc.*, *Corpus Christianorum Series Latina*, Turnhout: Brepols, 1953, 120, pp. 534–5; see William D. McCready, *Miracles and the Venerable Bede*, Toronto: Pontifical Institute of Medieval Studies, 1994, p. 23.

72 Bede, *In Marc*, pp. 455–6.

73 McCready, *Miracles and the Venerable Bede*, p. 26.

74 On the second *vita*, see P. Courcelle, *Recherches sur saint Ambroise: 'vies' anciennes, culture, iconographie*, Paris: Etudes augustiniennes, 1973.

75 On medieval hagiography there exists a rich literature, which is beyond the focus of this volume, but of which some general modern works include Jacques Dubois and J.-L. Demaitre, *Sources et méthodes de l'hagiographie médiévale*, Paris: Éditions du Cerf, 1993; Thomas Head (ed.), *Medieval Hagiography: An Anthology*, New York and London: Routledge, 2000, which gives over thirty texts in translation from late antiquity to the fifteenth century; a more specific geographic focus is provided by Thomas Head, *Hagiography and the Cult of Saints: The Diocese of Orléans, 800–1200*,

Cambridge: Cambridge University Press, 1990, while hagiography is presented from the angle of political economy and the visual topography of sainthood by B. Abou-el-Haj, *The Medieval Cult of Saints: Formations and Transformations*, Cambridge: Cambridge University Press, 1994.

76 Information on *passioni*, *vitae*, and the two lives of St Ambrose is from Clare Pilsworth, 'Medicine, hagiography and manuscripts in Italy, *c*.800–*c*.1000', *Social History of Medicine*, 13(2), 2000, pp. 253–64.

77 Another titulus of the *Decretales* of Pope Gregory IX, titulus XX in Liber I, *de corpore vitiatis ordinandis vel non*, concerns impediments to the ordination of priests in cases of physical impairment. Cap. I states the case of a priest who lacked parts of his fingers but could still be ordained, provided that he could celebrate solemnly without scandal (*quin ipse sine scandalo possit solenniter celebrare*); while cap. II deals with the visual impairment of a cleric from the see of Canterbury who was nevertheless permitted to be promoted to the episcopate (*in promotione tua ex multa dispensatione procedat*); cap. III concerns those clerics who were 'eunuchs', either by accident or from birth (*eunuchus, si per insidias hominum factus, vel ita natus sit*) but could also be ordained; cap. VI provided for dispensation for an abbot with mutilated hands (*Mutilatus manu, si promotus fuerit in abbatem*); and cap. VII concerned the monk Thomas of Brixen, who in his childhood had suffered an accident involving injury to his right thumb (*in annis puerilibus esset constitutus, quaedam barra ferrea super dextrae suae pollicem fortuito casu cadens*) but could still be ordained as a priest. Cf. Friedberg, *Corpus Iuris Canonicis*, 2, cols 144–6.

78 Cited in Darrel W. Amundsen, *Medicine, Society, and Faith in the Ancient and Medieval Worlds*, Baltimore, MD and London: Johns Hopkins University Press, 1996, p. 266.

79 Cf. Rudolph Allers, 'Microcosmos: from anaximandros to paracelsus', *Traditio*, 2, 1944, pp. 319–407.

80 Michael Goodich, *From Birth to Old Age: The Human Life Cycle in Medieval Thought, 1250–1350*, Lanham, MD and London: University Press of America, 1989, p. 65.

81 'Sicut in corpore omnia membra regit sanitas, sic in anima omnes motus componit puritas, et sicut aegritudo corruptio est sanitatis, sic corruptio privatio est puritas. Sicut vero vita sine sanitate et cum insanabili languore est longa protractio deficientis naturae, sic propositum religionis sine puritate umbra sine veritate, species sine pulchritudine, membra sine vegetatione, ut itaque cadaver exangue et emortuum est corpus sine anima, sic religio sine munditia. Virtus virtutum, vita membrorum, sanitas complexionum est religio sine maculo [James 1:27] propositum bonum cum sanctimonia.' Cited in Goodich, *From Birth to Old Age*, p. 30 note 21. Peter of Celle was a friend of John of Salisbury, and Peter's treatise *De puritate anime* was left unfinished. However, of the existing parts, the second part of the treatise deals with 'those elements of corruption in Christians' lives which impede their progress toward heavenly purity' (*Peter of Celle: Selected Works*, ed. and transl. Hugh Feiss, Kalamazoo, MI: Cistercian Publications, 1987, p. 14). The main modern edition of Peter of Celle's work is to be found in Jean Leclercq, *La Spiritualité du Pierre de Celle*, Paris: J. Vrin, 1946, with *De puritate anime* at pp. 190–1.

82 See the discussion of these concepts in Heinrich Schipperges, *Die Kranken im Mittelalter*, Munich: C. H. Beck, 3rd edn, 1993, p. 37.

83 An illness can be viewed as an ontological deficit. For reasons associated with this notion, medieval surgical practice apparently refrained from direct substitution or reconstruction of prosthetic body parts, restricted instead to conservation of what corporeal matter was there, or to restoration of such matter. See Schipperges, *Die Kranken im Mittelalter*, p. 169.

84 'Krankheit wird auch als Strafe für persönliche Schuld aufgefaßt, dies aber äußerst vorsichtig und nie verallgemeinernd' (Schipperges, *Die Kranken im Mittelalter*, p. 20).

85 *Ancrene Wisse: Guide for Anchoresses*, transl. and intro. Hugh White, London: Penguin Books, 1993, p. 88.

86 On the topic of holy anorexia see the studies by Caroline Walker Bynum, *Holy Feast and Holy Fast: The Religious Significance of Food to Medieval Women*, Berkeley, Los Angeles, CA and London: University of California Press, 1987, and Walter Vandereycken and Ron Van Deth, *From Fasting Saints to Anorexic Girls: The History of Self-Starvation*, London: Athlone Press, rpt. 1996. Ailred's condition is described in F. M. Powicke (transl. and ed.), *The Life of Ailred of Rievaulx, by Walter Daniel*, London: Nelson, 1964, pp. 39–41.

87 The *vita* of Alpais of Cudot describes her condition in gruesome detail: due to permanent weakness she lay on her bed for almost a year; her chest, shoulders, kidneys and all viscera were so haggard and puss-filled, that her body stank so much that not just bystanders but her own mother and brothers shrank back even though filial compassion filled them; for food her impoverished mother tossed her some bread as one would a dog, which she was unable to catch with her hands due to the rotting of her flesh from her arms; and her brothers asked her mother to refrain from giving her food so that she might die of starvation ('Von dauernder Schwäche befallen, lag sie ungefähr ein ganzes Jahr auf einem harten und groben Bett…Ihre Brust und Schultern, Nieren und alle Eingeweide, bis in den Leib hinein dürr und eitrig, jagten den sie Betrachtenden sollchen Abscheu ein und ließen einen solchen Gestank aufsteigen, dass sogar ihre Mutter…und ihre Brüder ihr näher zu kommen zurückschreckten, obschon sie aus geschwisterlicher Liebe mit ihren Schmerzen Mitleid hatten…Und da die Mutter arm war und nichts anderes hatte, was sie ihr hätte geben konnen, warf sie ihr wie einem Hund hier und da ein Stück Gerstenbrot hin. Das konnte sie aber weder mit der Hand fangen noch zum Mund führen, da ihre Hände schon ausgedörrt waren und von der starken Fäulnis des Fleisches von den Armen getrennt und geschieden…Auch war sie ihren Brüdern so zuwieder und lästig, dass sie ihre Mutter baten, sie solle aufhören, ihr Essen zu geben, sodass sie so hungers sterbe.'). *Vita I, 2*, E. Stein (ed.), *Leben und Visionen der Alpais von Cudot*, Tübingen, 1995, p. 122, cited in P. Dinzelbacher, *Europa im Hochmittelalter 1050–1250. Eine Kultur- und Mentalitätsgeschichte*, Darmstadt: Primus Verlag, 2003, p. 96. Dinzelbacher surmises that the treatment of Alpais by her mother and her brothers was a kind of passive euthanasia, and also thinks that Alpais suffered from leprosy.

88 Caroline Walker Bynum, *Fragmentation and Redemption: Essays on Gender and the Human Body in Medieval Religion*, New York: Zone Books, 1992, p. 188.

89 Ibid., p. 189.

90 Ibid., citing Elsbet Stagel, *Das Leben der Schwestern zu Töss beschrieben von Elsbet Stagel* (ed.) Ferdinand Vetter, Deutsche Texte des Mittelalters, 6, Berlin, 1906, p. 37.

91 Ibid., pp. 188–9.

92 Cf. the collection of essay in Sharon Farmer and Barbara H. Rosenwein (eds), *Monks and Nuns, Saints and Outcasts: Religion in Medieval Society*, Ithaca, NY and London: Cornell University Press, 2000, especially the articles by Sharon Farmer ('The Beggar's Body') and Catherine Peyroux ('The Leper's Kiss').

93 Umberto Eco, *On Beauty*, transl. A. McEwen, London: Secker & Warburg, 2004, p. 133.

94 Bonaventure of Bagnoregio, *Commentary on the Book of Sentences*, I, 31, 2, cited by Eco, *On Beauty*, pp. 132–3.

95 John Gibb and William Montgomery (eds), *The Confessions of Augustine*, New York: Arno Press, 1979, *Confessionum liber* VII, v. 7, pp. 172–4.

96 P. Michel, *Formosa deformitas. Bewältigungsformen des Hässlichen in mittelalterlicher Literatur*, Bonn: Bouvier, 1976, pp. 33–9.

97 Augustine, *De natura boni*, 14. See Michel, *Formosa deformitas*, p. 44. On the ape as the satanic inversion of the human, the corrupt human or as the ugly foil to human beauty, see H. W. Janson, *Apes and Ape Lore in the Middle Ages and the Renaissance* (Studies of the Warburg Institute vol. 20), London: Warburg Institute, 1952. On the ugliness of apes see also Manfred Bambeck, ' "Malin comme un singe" oder Physiognomik und Sprache', *Archiv für Kulturgeschichte*, 62, 1979, pp. 292–316.

98 Augustine, *De vera religione*, XL, 75, *Corpus Christianorum. Series Latina*, Turnhout: Brepols, 1954, 32, p. 236: 'Sed adest diuina prouidentia, quae hanc ostendat et non malam propter tam manifesta uestigia primorum numerorum, in quibus sapientiae dei non est numerus, et extremam tamen esse miscens ei dolores et morbos et distortiones membrorum et tenebras coloris et animorum simultates ac dissensiones, ut ex his admoneamur incommutabile aliquid esse quaerendum.' The German translation of the Latin reads: 'Die Vorsehung zeigt, daß die Schönheit der Körperwelt die niederste Schönheit ist, denn sie gesellt ihr Schmerzen bei und Krankheiten, Verkrümmung der Glieder und Trübung der Farbe..., um uns dadurch zu ermahnen, ein Unwandelbares zu suchen.' See Michel, *Formosa deformitas*, p. 51.

99 William of Auvergne, *Tractatus de bono et malo*, cited by Eco, *On Beauty*, p. 132.

100 Bonaventure of Bagnoregion, *Itinerarium mentis in Deum*, II, 7, cited by Eco, *On Beauty*, p. 62.

101 Eco, *On Beauty*, p. 85.

102 Ibid., pp. 143–5.

103 Ibid., p. 147. The Middle Ages may have been 'fascinated by composite monsters...as well as by corporal transformations' (Jeffrey J. Cohen, *Medieval Identity Machines* (Medieval Cultures 35), Minneapolis, MN: University of Minnesota Press, 2003, p. xviii) but fascination does not invariably imply a positive valuation. The Middle Ages, and even more so modern scholars, can talk and theorise *ad tedium* about monstrosity, difference, or otherness, and be fascinated perhaps precisely because of the perceived difference to normative phenomena, yet still happily continue(d) to apply negative value judgements to physical difference.

104 John Scotus Erigena, *De divisione Naturae*, V, cited by Eco, *On Beauty*, p. 85.

105 Alexander of Hales, *Summa Halesiana*, II, cited by Eco, *On Beauty*, p. 149.

106 Thomas Aquinas, *Summa Theologiae*, I, 39, 8, cited by Eco, *On Beauty*, p. 88.

107 Umberto Eco, *The Aesthetics of Thomas Aquinas*, London: Radius, 1988, p. 126.

108 'Si vero accipiantur membra, ut manus et pes et huiusmodi, earum dispositio naturae conveniens, est pulchritudo.' See Thomas Aquinas, *Summa Theologia*, I–II, 54, Ic. Cited by Eco, *The Aesthetics of Thomas Aquinas*, p. 127.

109 'Anima enim coniuncta corpori, eius complexiones imitatur secundum amentiam vel docilitatem, et alia huiusmodi...', Thomas Aquinas, *De veritate*, 26, 10c. Cited by Eco, *The Aesthetics of Thomas Aquinas*, p. 128.

110 'In corpore humano potest esse deformitas dupliciter; uno modo ex defectu alicuius membri, sicut mutilatos turpes dicimus; deest enim eis debita proportio ad totum', Thomas Aquinas, *Commentarium in Quatuor Sententiarum P. Lombardi Libros*, 44, 3, Ia, C. Cited by Eco, *The Aesthetics of Thomas Aquinas*, p. 100 and note 88 (p. 249).

111 Eco, *The Aesthetics of Thomas Aquinas*, p. 100.

112 Ulrich probably studied under Albertus Magnus. His main work *De summo bono*, which was written between 1265 and 1274, is an attempt to systematise the philosophical and theological thoughts of Albertus Magnus, although only six of the eight planned books were completed due to Ulrich's premature death. The sources Ulrich used were Augustine, Pseudo-Dionysius (Dionysius the Areopagite), Aristotle, and the texts and commentaries of his esteemed teacher Albertus Magnus; to a degree, Ulrich also depended on Thomas Aquinas' commentary on the *Sentences* (cf. R. Auty (ed.), *Lexikon des Mittelalters*, 9 vols, Munich: Artemis Verlag, 1997–9, 8, cols 1202–3). *De summo bono*, Book I, has been edited by J. Daguillon (Bibl. Thom. 12), no place of publication, 1930, 14*–29*, which also includes a *tabula quaestionum* of the entire work; a study of Ulrich's philosophical and theological concepts is available by F.-B. Stammkötter, *Die philosophische Tugendlehre bei Albert dem Großen und Ulrich von Straßburg*, Dissertation Bochum University, 1996.

113 Michel, *Formosa deformitas*, p. 54.

114 John of Salisbury, *Policraticus of the Frivolities of Countiers and the Footprints of Philosophers* (Cambridge Texts in the History of Political Thought), Book V, ch. 2, ed. and transl. Cary J. Nederman, Cambridge: Cambridge University Press, 1990, p. 67.

115 Miri Rubin, *Corpus Christi: The Eucharist in Late Medieval Culture*, Cambridge: Cambridge University Press, 1991, p. 270.

116 See the discussion of the body's 'offices' in Marie-Christine Pouchelle, *The Body and Surgery in the Middle Ages*, transl. R. Morris, Cambridge: Polity, 1990, p. 118.

117 Ibid., p. 118.

118 Valentin Groebner, *Defaced: The Visual Culture of Violence in the Late Middle Ages*, New York: Zone Books, 2004, p. 12. For a study of disfigurement and ugliness from a multi-disciplinary approach see Ursula Hoyning-Süess and Christine Amrein (eds), *Entstellung und Häßlichkeit. Beiträge aus philosophischer, medizinischer, literatur- und kunsthistorischer sowie aus sonderpädagogischer Sicht* (Beiträge zur Heil- und Sonderpädagogik 17), Bern: Haupt Verlag, 1995.

119 J. P. Migne, ed., 'Deus non requirit corporis decorem, sed animae pulchritudinem', *Patrologia Latina*, Paris: Garnier, 184, 1857–1939, cols 1293f. See Michel, *Formosa deformitas*, pp. 83–6. Thomas, born in the middle of the twelfth century, was a monk at the Cistercian abbey of Froidmont (founded 1134), Oise, north of Paris; he addressed some of his works to the Cistercian nuns, as in the text *Liber* or *Tractatus de modo beni vivendi ad sororem* from which the above quote stems (though that same text is only attributed to Thomas and there is no conclusive evidence for his authorship). He is best known for his *vita* of Thomas Becket, composed between 1214 and 1224.

120 Song of Solomon 1:5: 'I am black, but comely'.

121 Michel, *Formosa deformitas*, pp. 87–8.

122 Isaiah 53:2–3: 'he hath no form nor comeliness; and when we shall see him, there is no beauty that we should desire him. He is despised and rejected of men; a man of sorrows, and acquainted with grief: and we hid as it were our faces from him; he was despised, and we esteemed him not'. See also Michel, *Formosa deformitas*, p. 17.

123 Michel, *Formosa deformitas*, p. 17. See also Roswitha Klinck, 'Die lateinische Etymologie des Mittelalters', *Medium Aevum*, 17, 1970, pp. 29–80.

124 Matthew of Vendôme, *Ars versificatoria*, I, 38 ff., see Michel, *Formosa deformitas*, pp. 62–3.

125 Michel, *Formosa deformitas*, pp. 62–3.

126 See Roy A. Wisbey, 'Wunder des Ostens in der Wiener Genesis und in Wolframs Parzival', in: Johnson, Steinhoff and Wisbey (eds), *Studien zur frühmittelhochdeutschen Literatur. Cambridger Colloquium 1971*, Berlin: E. Schmidt, 1974, pp. 180–214, and Wisley, 'Die Darstellung des Häßlichen im Hoch- und Spätmittelalter', in: W. Harms and L. P. Johnson (eds), *Deutsche Literatur des späten Mittelalters. Hamburger Colloquium 1973*, Berlin: E. Schmidt, 1975, pp. 9–34.

127 See also the section dealing with aetiologies of congenital impairment in Chapter 4.2, for a further discussion of the medieval idea that the monstrous races were the product of the ingestion of forbidden food.

128 Michel, *Formosa deformitas*, pp. 62–3. The interbreeding of angels and women is found at Genesis 6:4.

129 Jan Ziolkowski, 'Avatars of ugliness in medieval literature', *The Modern Language Review*, 79, 1984, pp. 1–20. See also Beate Schmolke-Hasselmann, '"Camuse chose": die Häßlichkeit als ästhetisches und menschliches Problem in der altfranzösischen Literatur', in: Albert Zimmermann (ed.), *Die Mächte des Guten und Bösen*, Berlin and New York: De Gruyter, 1976, pp. 442–52, and Barbara Seitz, *Die Darstellung häßlicher Menschen in mittelhochdeutscher erzählender Literatur von der 'Wiener Genesis' bis zum Ausgang des 13. Jahrhunderts*, PhD dissertation, Tübingen University, 1967.

130 Wisbey, 'Die Darstellung des Häßlichen', pp. 9–34.

131 Ibid., p. 19. In *Yvain*, lines 307ff., besides having a crooked back, this literary 'monster' is also described as black, of giant stature, with a large head, his hair sticking out in tufts, ears like those of an elephant, a flat face with teeth like those of a wild boar, and a chin that merges into his chest.

132 Wisbey, 'Die Darstellung des Häßlichen', p. 20.

133 Wisbey, 'Die Darstellung des Häßlichen', pp. 28–9.

134 Particularly the literary figure of the peasant is stereotypically the ugly physical 'other' to the beautiful noble, cf. the article by Danielle Buschinger, 'L'homme laid dans la littérature médiévale allemande un example: le *ackerkneht* dans la *Couronne* de Heinrich von dem Türlin (1230)', in: Centre Universitaire d'Etudes et de Recherches Médiévales d'Aix (eds), *Le beau et le laid au Moyen Âge* (Senefiance 43), Aix-en-Provence: CUER MA, 2000, pp. 57–65.

135 See Elizabeth C. Evans, 'Physiognomics in the Ancient World', *Transactions of the American Philosophical Society*, new series, 59(5), 1969, pp. 5–105. In the fables of Aesop, physical features of people are made fun of, cf. John Henderson (transl.), *Aesop's Human Zoo: Roman Stories about Our Bodies*, Chicago, IL: University of Chicago Press, 2004.

136 Albertus Magnus, *De animalibus*, I–ii–2, see Lynn Thorndike, *A History of Magic and Experimental Science*, 2, New York and London: Columbia University Press, 1923, p. 575.

137 Albertus Magnus, *Summa de creaturis*, II.7.1, see N. H. Stenek, 'Albert on the Psychology of Sense Perception', in: J. A. Weisheipl (ed.), *Albertus Magnus and the Sciences*, Toronto: Pontifical Institute of Medieval Studies, 1980, pp. 266–7. Pietro d'Abano (*c.*1250–1316) had also thought of the body in terms of a mirror of the soul in his *Compilatio phisiognomiae* written at Paris in 1295, cf. Wolfram Prinz, 'Die Physiognomie', in: Wolfram Prinz and Iris Marzik, *Die Storia oder die Kunst des Erzählens in der italienischen Malerei und Plastik des späten Mittelalters und der Frührenaissance 1260–1460*, Mainz: Philipp von Zabern, 2000, I, pp. 480–1. On physiognomic thought in the thirteenth century see W. Sauerländer, '*Phsionomica est doctrina salutis*. Über Physiognomik und Porträt im Jahrhundert Ludwigs des Heiligen', in: M. Büchsel and P. Schmidt (eds), *Das Porträt vor der Erfindung des Porträts*, Mainz: Philipp von Zabern, 2003, pp. 108–9, 111.

138 Mellinkoff, *Outcasts*, Vol. 1: Text, p. 115. The original French is cited by J. Huizinga, *The Waning of the Middle Ages*, transl. F. Hopman, Harmondsworth: Penguin, 1976, p. 34: 'Que homs de membre contrefais/ Est en sa pensée meffais,-/ Plains de pechiez et plains de vices.'

139 On the link between astrology and physiognomy see T. S. Barton, *Power and Knowledge: Astrology, Physiognomics, and Medicine*, Ann Arbor, MI: University of Michigan Press, 1994. On medieval physiognomy in general, cf. K. Schönfeldt, *Die Temperamentenlehre in deutschsprachigen Handschriften des 15. Jahrhunderts*, no place of publication, 1962; also W. Ginsberg, *The Cast of Character: The Representation of Personality in Ancient and Medieval Literature*, Toronto: University of Toronto Press, 1983, and Joseph Ziegler, 'Text and context: on the rise of physiognomic thought in the later Middle Ages', in: Itzak Hen (ed.), *Essays on Medieval Law, Liturgy and Literature in Honour of Amnon Linder*, Turnhout: Brepols, 2001, pp. 159–82.

140 Melissa Percival, *The Appearance of Character: Physiognomy and Facial Expression in Eighteenth-Century France*, London and Leeds: W. S. Maney & Son, 1999, p. 13, where the author discusses the development of physiognomical theories prior to the Enlightenment. Medieval physiognomics originated in the pseudo-Aristotelian *Physiognomonica* (ibid., p. 2) and dealt with the relation of character to physical appearance, with some treatises also available in the vernacular (cf. *Lexikon des Mittelalters*, 6, Munich: Artemis Verlag, 1993, col. 2117, s.v. 'Physiognomik'). In medieval physiognomy, the four humour theory was expanded to include character traits as seen to be derived from bodily constitution, the structure of the face, and from facial and corporal expressions. The interpretation of such signs also followed the scheme established by medical texts, discussing them *a capite ad calcem*. In the late fifteenth and then the sixteenth centuries a link was made between physiognomy, the study of lines on a person's forehead and chiromancy (that is, palmistry), as well as with astrology. As humans were a microcosm of the universe, the macrocosm, so the face and/or the hands were a microcosm of the human body as a whole. In this way the study of

the signs inherent in the human body became linked with the study of the signs of the universe, for example, with astrology.

141 *Le compost et calendrier des bergiers*, Paris, 1493.

142 Cited by Mellinkoff, *Outcasts*, Vol. 1: Text, pp. 116–17. Also G. Marchant, *The Kalendar and Compost of Shepherds*, intro. G. C. Heseltine, London: P. Davies, 1931, p. 152. *The Kalendar of Sheepehards (c.1585)*, facsimile ed. with intro. by S. K. Heninger, jr, NewYork: Scholar's Facsimiles and Reprints, 1979, cap. 42, p. 171, uses almost exactly the same words, except that reference is made to 'default' of the feet, not the forehead, as in Heseltine's edition. It is not quite clear what Marchant means by 'naturally' impaired persons who are to be avoided; perhaps he means the congenitally impaired, or perhaps all disabled people (including those whose impairment was acquired in later life), since they are all 'defective' in their natural members.

143 On this subject cf. Fritz Neubert, 'Die volkstümlichen Anschauungen über Physiognomik in Frankreich bis zum Ausgang des Mittelalters', *Romanische Forschungen*, 29, 1911, pp. 557–679, who also mentions how different ethnic groups were treated according to physiognomy, and how extremes of size (dwarfs and giants), old age, and people with hunchbacks were rated according to physiognomics.

144 'in vultu deformitates oculorum, faciei, vel gestuum contrahere horribiles ad inspiciendum alijs hominibus', Johannes Nider, *Formicarium*, Douai, 1602, ii.9, pp. 155–6, cited by Dyan Elliott, 'The physiology of rapture and female spirituality', in: Peter Biller and A. J. Minnis (eds), *Medieval Theology and the Natural Body* (York Studies in Medieval Theology 1), York: York Medieval Press, 1997, p. 156. The story of a 13-year-old novice who was demonically possessed is also told by Nider, who said that the symptoms included raptures and a miraculous knowledge of Latin. After being exorcised, however, in this case matters were made worse, since 'the boy was again a rustic as before but with a difference: his face took on an unwonted and horrible aspect and such a doltish expression that it was unclear that he could attain the degree of literacy required for the priesthood'. *Formicarium*, iii.1, pp. 183–4, cited by Elliott, 'The physiology of rapture and female spirituality', p. 156.

145 The *Lumen animae* was probably compiled no later than the early fourteenth century, and the passages attributed to Theophilus cannot actually be found in *De diversibus artibus*. See Thorndike, *A History of Magic and Experimental Science*, 3, p. 554.

146 Mellinkoff, *Outcasts*.

147 Ibid., I, p. li.

148 Psalms 16:10.

149 Acts 2:32.

150 A. Angenendt, ' "In meinem Fleisch werde ich Gott sehen." Bernward und die Reliquien', in exhibition catalogue, *Bernward von Hildesheim und das Zeitalter der Ottonen*, M. Brandt and A. Eggebrecht (eds), 1, Hildesheim and Mainz: Philipp von Zabern, 1993, p. 362. On the theme of perfect bodies after the resurrection see R. Heinzmann, *Die Unsterblichkeit der Seele und die Auferstehung des Leibes. Eine problemgeschichtliche Untersuchung der frühscholastischen Sentenzen- und Summenliteratur von Anselm von Laon bis Wilhelm von Auxerre* (Beiträge zur Geschichte der Philosophie und Theologie des Mittelalters. Texte und Untersuchungen, 40.3), Münster: Aschendorff, 1965, and H. J. Weber, *Die Lehre von der Auferstehung der Toten in den Haupttraktaten der scholastischen Theologie von Alexander von Hales zu Duns Skotus* (Freiburger Theologische Studien), Freiburg: Herder, 1973.

151 Cited in: Robert Hughes, *Heaven and Hell in Western Art*, London: Weidenfeld & Nicolson, 1968, p. 109. I am grateful to Emma Rogers for this reference. Cf. also James Gollnick, *Flesh as Transformation Symbol in the Theology of Anselm of Canterbury: Historical and Transpersonal Perspectives* (Texts and Studies in Religion 22), Lewiston and Queenston: Edwin Mellen Press, 1985.

152 See exhibition catalogue, *Bernward von Hildesheim und das Zeitalter der Ottonen*, with illustration of the Ottonian *Treve Apocalypse*, now at Trier, Stadbibliothek, Hs. 31, fol. 67r.

153 Now Stiftsbibliothek Melk, MS 1903 (olim 1833), fol. 109v.

154 A modern German translation of the text in *Lucidarius* reads: 'Angenommen, ein Wolf frisst einen Menschen, und den Wolf ein Bär, und den Bären ein Löwe, wie kann aus denen allen der Mensch auferstehen? – Was Menschenfleisch war, das ersteht auf, was dem Tier angehörte, das bleibt [tot]. Der es geschaffen hat, der kann es wohl unterscheiden. Sie erstehen alle so auf, dass ihnen kein Haar fehlt... Wie ein Hafner, der aus zerbrochenem Ton ein neues Gefäß schafft, so tut Gott: er macht wieder einen schönen Menschen, dem es an nichts gebricht.' Cited by Peter Dinzelbacher, *Europa im Hochmittelalter 1050–1250. Eine Kultur- und Mentalitätsgeschichte*, Darmstadt: Primus Verlag, 2003, p. 57.

155 Augustine, *Concerning the City of God against the Pagans*, 22.16, transl. H. Bettenson, London: Penguin, 1972, rpt. 1984, p. 1056.

156 Ibid.

157 Ibid., 22.17, p. 1057. It is interesting to note that at this point Augustine is discussing whether women are resurrected with a female body or not, and has to go to great lengths to emphasise that 'a woman's sex is not a defect; it is natural'.

158 See Caroline Walker Bynum, *The Resurrection of the Body in Western Christianity, 200–1336*, New York: Columbia University Press, 1995, p. 11.

159 Augustine, *City of God*, 22.19, p. 1062.

160 See Bynum, *The Resurrection of the Body*, p. 77.

161 Tertullian, *On the Resurrection of the Flesh*, 57, cited in: Jeffrey Burton Russell, *A History of Heaven: The Singing Silence*, Princeton, NJ: Princeton University Press, 1997, p. 68.

162 'In illa enim resurrectionis gloria erit corpus nostrum subtile quidem per effectum spiritalis potentiae, sed palpabile per ueritatem naturae.' Gregory the Great, Liber XIV, LVI, 72 (19,26), *Moralia in Iob*, Libri XI–XXII, *Corpus Christianorum Series Latina*, vol. CXLIII, Turnhout: Brepols, 1979, p. 743. Gregory stated that a person would rise again surrounded by their skin, so that through this all doubt in the true resurrection would be removed ('Et rursum circumdabor pelle mea. Dum aperte pellis dicitur, omnis dubitatio uerae resurrectionis aufertur'). Furthermore, in eternity there would be no corporal corruption ('in aeterna incorruptione regnabit', LVI, 72, p. 744). Gregory explicitly clarified that all resurrected people would rise again in their flesh ('Confiteor quia omnes in hac carne resurgemus', LVI, 74, p. 745). Also paraphrased in Russell, *A History of Heaven*, p. 95.

163 Otto of Freising, *The Two Cities*, C. C. Mierow (transl.), A. P. Evans and C. Knapp (eds), New York: Columbia University Press, 1966, pp. 469–70.

164 Ibid., p. 470.

165 Augustine, *City of God*, 22.19, pp. 1060–2.

166 Otto of Freising, *The Two Cities*, pp. 470–1. On the status of monstrosities as human or not, see Augustine, *City of God*, 16.8, pp. 661–4.

167 Augustine, *Enchiridion*, 87, cited in: Amundsen, *Medicine, Society, and Faith*, p. 65.

168 J. B. Friedman, *The Monstrous Races in Medieval Art and Thought*, Cambridge, MA: Harvard University Press, 1981, pp. 108–21 discusses the etymology, and the cultural and theological meaning, of 'monsters'. On Augustinian notions of monsters, Friedman states that these were essentially seen as violations of nature which were produced deliberately by God to show divine superiority and command over the laws of nature. Monsters, in other words, were seen to exist in demonstration of God's will. By the high and later Middle Ages, the essential humanity of 'monsters' had become accepted, as Friedman demonstrates through citations from canon and civil lawyers (pp. 179–81) of the period; the main criterion as to whether a severely deformed or 'monstrous' child was acknowledged as human appeared to be whether it was born with a head (which could then be baptised). The civil lawyers of the medieval period gave intellectual support to the notion of a formal humanity as a starting point for any discussion of human worth within the scheme of the universe (Friedman, p. 180). More recently there are discussion of monsters and the monstrous by David Williams,

Deformed Discourse: The Function of the Monster in Mediaeval Thought and Literature, Exeter: University of Exeter Press, 1996, and the collection of essays edited by Bettina Bildhauer and Robert Mills, *The Monstrous Middle Ages*, Cardiff: University of Wales Press, 2003. For a postmodern analysis of the medieval notion of the monstrous, with particular emphasis on giants and concepts of masculinity in medieval literature, see Jeffrey Jerome Cohen, *Of Giants: Sex, Monsters, and the Middle Ages* (Medieval Cultures 17), Minneapolis, MN: University of Minnesota Press, 1999. The subject of menstruation and monstrous birth has been discussed by Peggy McCracken, *The Curse of Eve, The Wound of the Hero: Blood, Gender, and Medieval Literature*, Philadelphia, PA: University of Pennsylvania Press, 2003. Further work is needed with regard to monstrosity and physical impairment in the Middle Ages, and any such investigations are beyond the scope of this present book.

169 Peter Lombard, *Sentences*, Book 4, distinction 44, chapters 1–3, see Bynum, *The Resurrection of the Body*, pp. 123–4.

170 Russell, *A History of Heaven*, pp. 119–20.

171 Cited in Bynum, *The Resurrection of the Body*, p. 168.

172 See ibid., p. 254.

173 See ibid., pp. 145–6, and John Scotus Erigena, *Periphyseon*, Book 5, chapters 22–3 in *Patrologia Latina*, 122, col. 898–907 on the disintegration of the body.

174 Caroline Walker Bynum, 'Warum das ganze Theater mit dem Körper? Die Sicht einer Mediävistin', *Historische Anthropologie*, IV, 1, 1996, pp. 1–33.

175 Unlike among Gnostics, who divided the human being into philosophic constituents made up of soma, psyche and pneuma, in ascending order of spirituality.

176 Russell, *A History of Heaven*, p. 44.

177 Or 'discord' of body and soul, in the sense that body and soul struggle with each other for supremacy, though one could still regard both not as disunited elements, but more like two sides of the same coin; on the dialogue between spiritual and carnal sides see Douglas Moffat (ed. and transl.), *The Old English Soul and Body*, Woodbridge, NJ: D. S. Brewer, 1990. For a more general discussion of body and soul, see Piero Boitani and A. Torti (eds), *The Body and the Soul in Medieval Literature: J. A. W. Bennett Memorial Lectures, Tenth Series 1998*, Woodbridge, NJ: D. S. Brewer, 1999.

178 Hildegard of Bingen, *On Natural Philosophy and Medicine: Selections from Cause et Cure*, (transl. and ed.) Margret Berger, Cambridge: D. S. Brewer, 1999, p. 48.

179 Ibid., These sentiments form part of Hildegard's discussion of the conception and 'ensoulment' of the foetus in the womb.

180 See Miri Rubin, *Corpus Christi*, p. 30 for a discussion of these notions.

181 William of Auvergne, *De Universo*, I, 13, in: Angenendt, *Geschichte der Religiosität im Mittelalter*, p. 258. A printed edition of William of Auvergne's *De universo* is in *Guilielmi Alverni opera omnia*, François Hotot (ed.), 1, 2, Paris, 1674; a discussion of the ideas of William of Auvergne can be found in Richard Heinzmann, 'Zur Anthropologie des Wilhelm von Auvergne (gest. 1249)', *Münchener Theologische Zeitschrift*, 16, 1965, pp. 27–36. On bodily resurrection and the soul see also Richard Heinzmann, 'Die Unsterblichkeit der Seele und die Auferstehung des Leibes', *Beiträge zur Geschichte der Philosophie des Mittelalters*, 40(3), 1965, and Hermann J. Weber, *Die Lehre von der Auferstehung der Toten in den Haupttraktaten der scholastischen Theologie* (Freiburger Theologische Studien 91), Freiburg: Herder, 1973.

182 Aquinas, *De 1 Corinth.*, cap. 15, lect. 2, in: S. E. Fretté, (ed.), *Opera Omnia*, vol. 21, Paris, 1876, pp. 33–4: '... anima ... non est totus homo, et anima mea non est ego', cited in: Bynum, 'Warum das ganze Theater mit dem Körper?', p. 21. Cf. *Summa contra Gentiles*, lib. 4, cap. 70, and *Summa Theologia* Ia, q. 75, art. 4; in both these passages Aquinas is quite adamant that the soul is only part of the person, just as a hand or foot is only a part of the body. For a discusion of Aquinas's psychological theories, see Anthony Kenny, *Aquinas on Mind*, London: Routledge, 1994. The perfect restitution of impaired persons, maimed bodies, bodies destroyed by wild animals etc. is mentioned by

Aquinas in *Summa Theologica*, suppl. QQ. 78, art. 3, 5, 5: 2876–7, and QQ. 79, art. 1–2, 5: 2877–81; these passages are referred to by Fernando Vidal, 'Brains, bodies, selves and science: anthropologies of identity and the resurrection of the body', *Critical Inquiry*, 28, 2002, pp. 930–74.

183 'Das gelebte Leben wird mit seinem Erfahrungspotential verewigt; nicht eine gesichtslose Seele tritt ins Jenseits ein, sondern die von ihrem eigenen Weltleben geprägte...' (Angenendt, *Geschichte der Religiosität im Mittelalter*, p. 724).

184 Bynum, 'Warum das ganze Theater mit dem Körper?', pp. 20–1.

185 Bynum, *The Resurrection of the Body*, p. 11.

186 On *exempla* see the annotated handbook of some 5400 instructive medieval stories, arranged alphabetically, together with another lengthy index of smaller topics, by Frederic C. Tubach, *Index Exemplorum: A Handbook of Medieval Religious Tales*, Helsinki: Suomalainen Tiedeakatemia, 1969. Also Joseph A. Mosher, *The Exemplum in the Early Religious and Didactic Literature of England*, New York: Columbia University Press, 1911: J.-T. Welter, *L'exemplu dans la littérature religieuse et didactique du moyen âge*, no place of publication, 1927; C. Bremont, Jacques Le Goff and Jean-Claude Schmitt, *L'exemplum*, Turnhout: Brepols, 1982; and W. Haug and B. Wachinger (eds), *Exempel und Exempelsammlungen*, Tübingen: Niemeyer, 1991. An overview of medieval *exempla* is provided by *Lexikon des Mittelalters*, 4, Munich: Artemis Verlag, 1989, cols. 162–5, s.v. 'Exempel, exemplum'. In the Latin literature of the Middle Ages, *exempla* become widespread from the twelfth century onwards, as recommended by *artes praedicandi* manuals on preaching, for example by Guibert of Nogent, gaining increasing popularity after the twelfth century, with many collections of *exempla*, tales, fables and morally edifying stories being produced. One could cite here for instance the *Golden Legend* of Jacobus de Voragine as one such collection from the thirteenth century (cf. Jacobus de Voragine, *The Golden Legend: Readings on the Saints*, ed. and transl. W. G. Ryan, 2 vols, Princeton, NJ: Princeton University Press, 1993).

187 G. R. Owst, *Literature and Pulpit in Medieval England: A Neglected Chapter in the History of English Letters and of the English People*, Oxford: Blackwell, 2nd edn, 1966, p. 186.

188 Owst (ibid., pp. 186–209) lists examples from sermons in English manuscripts that deal with all sorts of such subjects, from astronomy, geography, human biology, to animals and birds. Although in Owst's collection of sermons there is only one direct mention of the resurrection of the body, including that of the body as whole, intact and non-disabled, one may assume that if all kinds of other, equally abstruse subjects, like eclipses of the sun (p. 190) are deemed suitable by medieval authors for inclusion in sermons, then there is no reason to suppose that other sermons, not listed by Owst, may not have touched more on the physical resurrection.

189 British Library, MS Royal 18 B. XXIII, fol. 89 verso, cited in Owst, *Literature and Pulpit in Medieval England*, p. 524. Owst did not date this manuscript, however, more recently, H. L. Spencer, *English Preaching in the Late Middle Ages*, Oxford: Clarendon, 1993, also discussing this particular manuscript states that it contains sermons in Latin and English and stems from the fifteenth century (p. 222). Owst also mentions that the 'ioyes of paradyis' are extolled upon in *Old English Homilies of the Twelfth Century*, ed. R. Morris, *Early English Text Society*, original series 53, pp. 230–2, and by John Bromyard, in his *Summa predicantium*, s.v. 'Gaudium', furthermore by Dan Michel, *Ayenbite of Inwyt*, ed. Richard Morris, *Early English Text Society*, original series 23, 1866, new edn, Pamela Gradon, reissue 1965 p. 75, and by Richard Rolle, *The Pricke of Conscience*.

190 *Everyman and Medieval Miracle Plays* (ed.) A. C. Cawley, London and Melbourne: Dent, new edn, and rpt. 1977, p. 194, lines 97–100. The York cycle is preserved in a fifteenth-century manuscript, see Dent, p. xi.

191 Bynum, *The Resurrection of the Body*, pp. 265–6. See Albertus Magnus, *De resurrectione*, tract. 3, q. 1, p. 305 in: Wilhelm Kübel, 'Die Lehre von der Auferstehung der Toten nach Albertus Magnus', in *Studia Albertina: Festschrift für Bernhard Geyer zum 70. Geburtstage*

(ed.) Heinrich Ostlender (Beiträge zur Geschichte der Philosophie des Mittelalters Supplementband 4), Münster: Aschendorff, 1952; Aquinas, *Supplementum* to the *Summa Theologiae*, q. 93, art. 3, pp. 225–6 and q. 96, art. 13, pp. 239–40 in: *Sancti Thomae Aquinatis doctoris angelici opera omnia iussu impensaque Leonis XIII p.m. edita*, 12, Rome: Ex Typographia Polyglotta, 1906.

192 On the theme of sexual differences which were believed, in the thought of the Church father Jerome, for example, to still remain at the Resurrection, see Peter Brown, *The Body and Society: Men, Women and Sexual Renunciation in Early Christianity*, London: Columbia University Press, 1989, pp. 382–4.

193 The identity of Jews according to medieval theology and canon law was seen primarily in terms of their religion, cf. Peter Biller, 'Views of Jews from Paris around 1300: Christian or "Scientific"?', in: D. Wood (ed.), *Christianity and Judaism* (Studies in Church History 29), Oxford: Blackwell, 1992, p. 190. With regard to physical characteristics, Jews were believed to differ from Christians in that they suffered from 'flux' (like a menstruating woman), both male and female, so that flux was regarded as a specific Jewish *infirmitas* (Peter Biller, pp. 192f.).

194 Bernard Hamilton, 'The Cathars and Christian Perfection', in: Peter Biller and Barrie Dobson (eds), *The Medieval Church: Universities, Heresy, and the Religious Life. Essays in Honour of Gordon Leff*, Woodbridge, NJ: Boydell Press, 1999, p. 13, states that the Cathars believed that, having received the *consolamentum*, after death their souls were freed from a cycle of reincarnation, to be reunited with their bodies in the 'Land of the Living'. Bernard Hamilton furthermore points out that according to Cathar belief, the Good God 'could not be asked for any kind of material aid – protection from pain, or illness, or even persecution – because he had no authority over the physical world, which was entirely subject to the God of Evil'. One group of Cathars, the Albanenses, apparently even denied that Christ can have performed miracles of corporeal healing (ibid., p. 21 and note 76). I am indebted to Prof Malcolm Barber for drawing my attention to this article.

195 To the best of my knowledge no one has ever looked at this question before.

4 Impairment in medieval medicine and natural philosophy

1 Cf. C. Barnes and G. Mercer (eds), *Exploring the Divide: Illness and Disability*, Leeds: Disability Press, 1996.

2 On the subject of medical schools and universities, see also a brief listing of medical teaching institutions, together with a short description of the textbooks used and the curriculum studied at select universities in F. H. Garrison, *History of Medicine*, Philadelphia, PA and London: W. B. Saunders, 2nd edn, 1929, pp. 174–5. A much more succinct example of what medical subjects and texts were studied is given for Bologna in 1405, in K. Park, *Doctors and Medicine in Early Renaissance Florence*, Princeton, NJ: Princeton University Press, 1985, pp. 245–8.

3 L. García-Ballester, 'Introduction: Practical medicine from Salerno to the Black Death', in: L. García-Ballester, R. French, J. Arrizabalaga and A. Cunningham (eds), *Practical Medicine from Salerno to the Black Death*, Cambridge: Cambridge University Press, 1994, p. 5.

4 M. R. McVaugh, *Medicine Before the Plague: Practitioners and Their Patients in the Crown of Aragon 1285–1345*, Cambridge: Cambridge University Press, 1993, p. 3. Medicalisation is not an anachronistic term to use with regard to the medieval period, as McVaugh insists, since medieval medicine is not just 'quaint or foolish or in some sense fundamentally "other"' from modern medicine (ibid.).

5 Darrel W. Amundsen, *Medicine, Society, and Faith in the Ancient and Medieval Worlds*, Baltimore, MD and London: Johns Hopkins University Press, 1996, pp. 1–2.

6 Cf. Karl Hauck, 'Gott als arzt. eine exemplarische skizze mit text- und bildzeugnissen aus drei verschiedenen religionen zu phänomenen und gebärden der heilung', in: C. Meier and U. Ruberg (eds), *Text und Bild. Aspekte des Zusammenwirkens zweier Künste in*

Mittelalter und früher Neuzeit, Wiesbaden: L. Reichert Verlag, 1980. Hauck uses the gold bracteates (gold coins) found in Scandinavia as evidence for the widespread diffusion of the pictorial tradition of healing hands, that is the laying-on of hands by the deity in a thaumaturgic act. On the theme of Christ as *soter*, see also Martin Honecker, 'Christus medicus', in: Peter Wunderli (ed.), *Der kranke Mensch in Mittelalter und Renaissance* (Studia humaniora. Düsseldorfer Studien zu Mittelalter und Renaissance. Band 5), Düsseldorf: Droste Verlag, 1986, pp. 27–43.

7 Cited in Amundsen, *Medicine, Society, and Faith*, p. 266.
8 This interpretation is based on evidence form Southern France, Italy and Aragon, cf. McVaugh, *Medicine Before the Plague*, p. 171.
9 The confusion in the secondary literature and the quagmire of scholarly opinion have been superbly deconstructed and analysed by Darrel W. Amundsen, 'Medieval canon law on medical and surgical practice by the clergy', in: Amundsen (ed.), *Medicine, Society, and Faith*, pp. 222–47, including an extensive bibliography concerning this issue.
10 This implies the concept of *neutralitas*. See also Heinrich Schipperges, *Der Garten der Gesundheit. Medizin im Mittelalter*, Munich and Zurich: Artemis Verlag, 1985, pp. 62–3, on health and illness as polarised extremes along a spectrum. In a follow-up study of medicine in the Middle Ages, Schipperges repeats his view of *neutralitas* as a transitional territory where the poor, the weak, beggars, the blind, orphans, widows, cripples, pilgrims and the exiled are located in medieval society (Heinrich Schipperges, *Die Kranken im Mittelalter*, Munich: C. H. Beck, 3rd edn, 1993, p. 20).
11 Avicenna, *Canon*, Book I, fen 2, cf. Nancy G. Siraisi, *Medieval and Early Renaissance Medicine: An Introduction to Knowledge and Practice*, Chicago, IL and London: University of Chicago Press, 1990, p. 120.
12 Cf. Siraisi, *Medieval and Early Renaissance Medicine*, p. 120. Another theoretical model was suggested in a brief text, the *Isagoge Iohannicii*, which was a translation of the Arabic *Masa'il fit – tibb*. This text, by Iohannicius, became one of the standard introductory textbooks for students of Salernitan medicine in the twelfth century. Medicine is here organised into theory and practice, and the theoretical part of the text divides ill-health into natural, non-natural and contra-natural conditions. 'Non-natural' conditions referred to ill-health brought about by environmental factors, in other words by outside influences on the body, while 'contra-natural' referred to pathological conditions (cf. John H. Baldwin, *The Language of Sex: Five Voices from Northern France around 1200*, Chicago, IL and London: University of Chicago Press, 1994, p. 12 and pp. 14–15). Congenital impairment, according to this scheme, would best fit into the category of 'contra-natural', while acquired impairment is more difficult to position in one category alone.
13 Isidore of Seville, *Etymologiarum*, Book IV, 1.1, in 'Isidore of seville: the medical writings', trans. with intro. and commentary William D. Sharpe, *Transactions of the American Philosophical Society*, new series 54(2), 1964, p. 55.
14 *Micrologus*, cited by C. H Talbot, *Medicine in Medieval England*, London: 1967, pp. 59–60.
15 Ibid.
16 R. Mellinkoff, *Outcasts: Signs of Otherness in Northern European Art of the Late Middle Ages*, 2 vols, Berkeley, Los Angeles, CA and Oxford: University of California Press, 1993, I: Text, p. 115 note 11, citing D. Bax, *Hieronymus Bosch: His Picture – Writing Deciphered*, Rotterdam: A. A. Balkema, 1979, p. 67 note 76.
17 'The first case is when Þe sekenesse is simpliche or by itself vncurable as lepre. The secounde, when Þe sekenesse is curable of itself, it is neuerÞelatter incurable in an vnbuxom pacient oÞer nouȝt myghti to suffre Þe payne, as Þe cancre in a particuler membre. The Þridde is when Þe cure of Þat sekenes schulde engendre a worse sekenesse, as an olde mormale (i. dede apple) oÞer olde emoraydes ihelede.' Guy de Chauliac, Preface, *The Cyrurgie of Guy de Chauliac*, ed. M. S. Ogden, *Early English Text Society*, no. 265, 1971, p. 3.

18 Ronald C. Finucane, *Miracles and Pilgrims: Popular Beliefs in Medieval England*, Basingstoke: Macmillan, new edn, 1995, p. 66.

19 'Die Abgrenzung zwischen Behinderung und Krankheit ist unscharf.' Dieter Neubert and Günther Cloerkes, *Behinderung und Behinderte in verschiedenen Kulturen. Eine vergleichende Analyse ethnologischer Studien*, Heidelberg: Edition Schindele, 2nd edn, 1994, p. 33.

20 Cf. Neubert and Cloerkes, *Behinderung und Behinderte*, pp. 33–4.

21 Jean-Noël Biraben, 'Das medizinische Denken und die Krankheiten in Europa', in: Mirko D. Grmek (ed.), *Die Geschichte des medizinischen Denkens. Antike und Mittelalter*, transl. C. Fiedler and S. Dietrich. Munich: C. H. Beck, 1996, p. 390. Ergotism poisoning was particularly prevalent in western Europe during the ninth to early eleventh centuries, reaching a climax in the eleventh century, when many people were left crippled by the effects of poisoning (ibid., p. 391). However, possibly environmental changes (less conducive to fungal growth in rye) and certainly dietary changes (more consumption of wheat) during the high and later Middle Ages led to a retreat of ergotism (ibid., p. 398), so that we have to look for other causes of mobility impairment during the later period.

22 'Spiritum infirmitatis [Luke 13:11] spiritum uentum dicit, quia multae infirmitates in corpore ex [corrupto are ueniunt]', *Supplementary Commentary on Genesis, Exodus and the Gospels*, 28, in Bernard Bischoff and Michael Lapidge, *Biblical Commentaries from the Canterbury School of Theodore and Hadrian* (Cambridge Studies in Anglo-Saxon England 10), Cambridge: Cambridge University Press, 1994, p. 394 (Latin) and p. 395 (transl.). The manuscript is in Milan, Biblioteca Ambrosiana, M. 79 sup.

23 J. Henderson, 'The Black Death in Florence: medical and communal responses', in S. Bassett (ed.), *Death in Towns: Urban Responses to the Dying and the Dead, 100–1600*, Leicester: Leicester University Press, 1992, pp. 139–41. Another fourteenth-century notion was that disease could be spread through the eyes of the sick.

24 Henri de Mondeville, *Chirurgie*, cited in Marie-Christine Pouchelle, *The Body and Surgery in the Middle Ages*, transl. Cambridge: 1990, p. 55. Mondeville continued by describing the three ways the 'common' people had of regarding causeless diseases:

    1   The surgeon is unable to treat them, unless he specializes in curing diseases which are caused by spells, and no others.

    2   Such illness is due solely to the misfortune of the sufferer.

    3   It comes from glorious and almighty God, that it was he who sent it, and that thus surgeons can do no good, because they cannot oppose God. Moreover, it is commonly believed that God and the disease would rise up against the surgeon if he undertook to tend the patient (ibid.).

25 Galen's (then surviving) work was translated from Greek into Latin by Pietro d'Abano (d. 1316) and Nicola da Reggio (d. 1350). A printed edition of Galen can be found in: *Galenus Opera* (ed.) C. Kühn, 20 vols, Leipzig, 1821–33. Texts belonging to the Hippocratic corpus had been Latinised early on, for example, Isidore of Seville in the early seventh century already had access to such Latin versions, cf. 'Isidore of Seville: The medical writings', p. 12. On the availability of Latin translations of Hippocrates, see H. E. Sigerist, 'The Latin medical literature of the early middle ages', *Journal of the History of Medicine*, 13, 1958, p. 133.

26 Soranus, active in the early second century, that is approximately contemporary with Galen's birth, had already written about the correct procedure for swaddling and massaging infants to prevent deformations of the still soft bones (*Soranus' Gynecology*, transl. Owsei Temkin, Baltimore, MD and London: Johns Hopkins University Press, orig. pbl. 1956, rpt. 1991, Book II, ix 'How to swaddle', pp. 84–6, and Book II, xvi 'On the bath and massage of the newborn', pp. 105–6).

27 Galen, *De morborum causis*, 7, cited in Christine Hummel, *Das Kind und seine Krankheiten in der griechischen Medizin. Von Aretaios bis Johannes Aktuarios (1. bis 14. Jahrhundert)*,

Frankfurt: Peter Lang, 1999, p. 275. Again, Soranus had already drawn attention to the problems associated with walking and standing too early: if the infant stands up too early 'the legs may become distorted in the region of the thighs' (*Soranus' Gynecology*, Book II, xx 'How one should make the infant sit up and endeavor to walk', p. 115).

28 Galen, *In Hippocratis librum de officina medici commentarii*, I 22, cited in Hummel, *Das Kind und seine Krankheiten*, p. 278.

29 Galen, *In Hippocratis de articulis librum commentarii*, IV, 4, cited in Hummel, *Das Kind und seine Krankheiten*, pp. 278–9. Galen further discussed the correct procedure for the bandaging of bones in children (*In Hippocratis de articulis librum commentarii IV*, Book I, cap. 1) and also mentioned that dislocation of the tibia was apparently frequent in children (*In Hippocratis librum de officina medici commentarii*, III 32), cf. Hummel, pp. 27–40.

30 Galen, *In Hippocratis de articulis librum commentarii*, III 6, cited in Hummel, *Das Kind und seine Krankheiten*, pp. 275–7. Galen also described the case history of a deformed boy (*De sanitate tuenda libri IV*, Book I, cap. 10), cf. Hummel, pp. 27–40.

31 For an overview of ancient medical theories of congenital impairment cf. Christian G. Bien, *Erklärungen zur Entstehung von Mißbildungen im physiologischen und medizinischen Schrifttum der Antike* (Sudhoffs Archiv Beihefte 38), Stuttgart: Franz Steiner Verlag, 1997, and for an easily accessible introduction to the subject Angelika Dierichs, *Von der Götter Geburt und der Frauen Niederkunft* (Kulturgeschichte der antiken Welt Band 82), Mainz: Philipp von Zabern, 2002.

32 Leonides's aetiology and prognosis on hydrocephalus is referred to by Aetios of Amida (around 525, he was physician to the emperor Justinian).

33 Hummel, *Das Kind und seine Krankheiten*, pp. 176–7.

34 Aretaios, *On acute and chronic diseases*, III 7, 1–2; this work is now only extant in fragments. Cf. Hummel, *Das Kind und seine Krankheiten*, pp. 272–3.

35 Aretaios, *On acute and chronic diseases*, III 7, 5. Cf. Hummel, *Das Kind und seine Krankheiten*, pp. 272–3.

36 Aretaios, *On acute and chronic diseases*, III 7, 8. Cf. Hummel, *Das Kind und seine Krankheiten*, pp. 272–3.

37 *Celeres Passiones*, III 5, 48. Cf. Hummel, *Das Kind und seine Krankheiten*, p. 170.

38 *Celeres Passiones*, III 5, 50. Cf. Hummel, *Das Kind und seine Krankheiten*, p. 170.

39 Galen, *De locis affectis*, IV.4, see Bischoff and Lapidge, *Biblical Commentaries*, pp. 521–2.

40 Galen, *Comm. in librum Hippocratis de humoribus*, I.1, see Bischoff and Lapidge, *Biblical Commentaries*, pp. 521–2.

41 Paul of Aegina, *Epitome*, III.23, see Bischoff and Lapidge, *Biblical Commentaries*, pp. 521–2.

42 Alexander of Tralles, *De medicina*, III.1, see Bischoff and Lapidge, *Biblical Commentaries*, pp. 521–2.

43 *Second Commentary on the Gospels*, 73 [on Mark 7:32]: 'Deaf and dumb. Some commentators say that these illnesses come from an evil spirit; physicians, however, do not think in these terms, but say that they arise from contracted and dormant veins.' (Surdum et mutum. Dicunt aliqui tractores illas infirmitates a daemonio esse; medici autem non sic opinantur, sed de uenis contractis et dormientibus aiunt euenisse.) Cited in Bischoff and Lapidge, *Biblical Commentaries*, p. 408 (Latin) and p. 409 (transl.). The text, extant in an eleventh-century manuscript (Milan, Biblioteca Ambrosiana, M. 79 sup.), was probably composed in the mid-seventh to the mid-eighth century, therefore during the time when Theodore of Tarsus (d. 690) was archbishop of Canterbury. Through Theodore, knowledge of Greek writings, including that of medical texts, may well have reached Anglo-Saxon England. Bischoff and Lapidge, however, have been unable to identify the medical textual source for the idea that contracted veins cause deafness, which still needs to be established (Bischoff and Lapidge, pp. 521–2).

44 Meletius, *De natura hominis*, J.-P. Migne (ed.), in: *Patrologia graeco-latina*, Paris: Garnier, 1857, 64, cols 1075–1310. In his text (cap. XI, *de voce*) Meletius also discusses obstructions to vocal activity:

> Vocis vero impedimenta (quo incommodo premi non nullis accidit) hoc quidem pacto fieri solent. Cum enim membranae, quae a thorace procedentes ad spinam usque tendunt, pectus obturatum reddiderint, sic ut in in thorace geminos fieri ventriculos acccidat, inter ipsos pulmo medius consistere cernitur. Hi itaque duo ventriculi sic invicem sejuncti sunt, ut, a dextra in laevam, ac a laeva vicissim ad dextram permutari nequeant. Itaque humorem quemdam, ex immodico frigore, seu ex nimio calore provenientem, in ipsos quos asseruimus ventriculos quandoque profluere, eosque obturatos reddere contingit, qua ex causa vocis impedimenta ac eloquii provenire compertum habemus. Si autem alterum ex ventriculis obturari acciderit, imperfecta dimidiataque vox sequitur. utroque vero patiente, tota penitus vox intercipitur.
>
> (*De natura hominis*, col. 1202)

45 Ynez Violé O'Neill, *Speech and Speech Disorders in Western Thought Before 1600* (Contributions in Medical History, Number 3), Westport, CT and London: Greenwood Press, 1980, p. 101.

46 S. Rubin, *Medieval English Medicine*, New York: Barnes & Noble, 1974, p. 198, citing chapter LVII of Bartolomeus Anglicus, *De proprietatibus rerum*.

47 Ibid.

48 Ibid., p. 199, citing chapter LVII of Bartolomeus Anglicus, *De proprietatibus rerum*. It seems Bartolomaeus Anglicus distinguished between what we now term osteo-arthritis and between rheumatoid arthritis, here describing the symptoms of the rheumatoid version.

49 Ibid., p. 206. Guy de Chauliac cited Galen ('Gylded men haue noght ye podacre') in his discussion of gout, Book VI, doctrine 1, ch. 1, *The Cyrurgie of Guy de Chauliac*, p. 363.

50 Book VI, doctrine 1, ch. 1, *The Cyrurgie of Guy de Chauliac*, pp. 362–4.

51 Regarding the dating, S. de Renzi, who edited Salernitan texts (*Collectio Salernitana*, 5 vols, Naples, 1852–9), had placed the *Practica* in the twelfth century, while Lynn Thorndike (*A History of Magic and Experimental Science*, New York and London: Columbia University Press, I, 2nd printing with corrections, 1929, p. 738) reckoned it could not have been that early on textual grounds.

52 Thorndike, *A History of Magic and Experimental Science*, I, pp. 738–9. Thorndike cited a contemporary expert, who asserted this in fact represented 'the typical history of a case of Bell's palsy occurring after a 'chill' (ibid., p. 739 note 1).

53 John of Gaddesden, *Rosa Anglica*, ed. W. Wulff, *Irish Texts Society*, 35, 1929, cited in Rubin, *Medieval English Medicine*, pp. 206–7.

54 John of Gaddesden, *Rosa Anglica* (ed.) Wulff, p. 249, cited in Rubin, *Medieval English Medicine*, p. 207. Also, if young people suffered from a fever and produced green urine, then they would become affected by paralysis or cramp, too.

55 'Of Þe crampe. Aueroys vnderstood by Þe crampe schortynge of Þe membres or soche a hastynesse Þat Þay may noght be bowed ne spred abroad. For in Þe crampe Þe wirchynge is loste, as in Þe pallesye, but Þere is chaungynge.' Book III, doctrine 1, ch. 1, *The Cyrurgie of Guy de Chauliac*, p. 199.

56 'Of Þe pallesie. The pallesie foloweÞ also woundes and smytynges, moste of Þe hede and of alle Þe bakke...The pallesye forsoÞe is mollificacioun of Þe synowes wiÞ priuacioun of felynge and of movynge ofte tymes, As Þe crampe was hardenesse wiÞ euel and wiÞ chaunged mouynge....As Þe appoplexye is softenes of al Þe body, so is Þe pallesye of an half parte, somtyme forsoÞe of Þe ri3t side and somtyme of Þe lefte side and somtyme forsoÞe of one partye, as of Þe foote or of Þe hande. And Þerfore take Þat dyuysioun of Þe vnyuersal or particuler crampe in Þe pallesie. Þe vnyuersal

is of al the side and particuler of one membre' (Book III, doctrine 1, ch. 1, *The Cyrurgie of Guy de Chauliac*, pp. 202–3).

57 '... if Þere come noyeng to Þe nuke and to Þe synowes Þat comen Þerof, Þai lede to Þe pallesye of Þe handes if it be of Þe ouer lynkes, of Þe feete if it be of Þe nether lynkes.' Book V, doctrine 1, ch. 3, *The Cyrurgie of Guy de Chauliac*, p. 344.

58 William of St Thierry, *De natura corporis et animae libro duo*, lib. II, *Patrologia Latina* (ed.) J.-P. Migne, Paris: Garnier, 1857–1939, 180, cols 713–14, see also O'Neill, *Speech and Speech Disorders*, p. 130.

59 O'Neill, *Speech and Speech Disorders*, p. 134. A similar explanation for speech disorders can be found in the works of William of Conches, except that he emphasises the humoral impact (see next paragraph).

60 'Þogh wlaffynge may come of Þe crampe, of vlceres and ofte tyme of oÞer passiouns of Þe tonge, neuerÞelatter it cometh of Þe pallesye and of moystures dronken in in Þe synowes and in Þe brawnes and vnder Þe tonge. Whose cause and tokenes forsoÞe ben as of Þe commune pallesye, and Þerwith comeÞ fluxe of spotil withoute wille, ne Þay may not speke forth right ne schewe... in childerne when Þat Þay come to ado-lescence (I. to 3ong manis age), ben ful ofte tymes amendede, as Avicen saith.' Book VI, doctrine 2, ch. 2, part 5 [given erroneously as 4], (*The Cyrurgie of Guy de Chauliac*, pp. 481–2).

61 'stopping of hir snewis Þorou3/ corrupte humours Þat maken Þe tonge laxe, and fallen into a palesye.' *Healing and Society in Medieval England: A Middle English Translation of the Pharmaceutical Writings of Gilbertus Anglicus* (ed.) Faye M. Getz, WI: University of Wisconsin Press, 1991, p. 97 [fol. 139].

62 Isidore of Seville, *Etymologiarum*, Book IV, 7.25, in 'Isidore of Seville: The Medical Writings', p. 59. Sharpe noted that *corporis inpensatio* 'suggests an extensive disorder interfering with sensation, coordination, and other bodily functions' (ibid.).

63 'Gicht: Wenn nun das Schaumige und Lauwarme, jetzt also der Livor des Feuchten und Trockenen, ihr Maß überschritten haben, so daß der Schaum hochsteigt und siechendem Wasser gleich einen Rauch macht und das Lauwarme sich in Tropfen auflöst, dann beugen diese Säfte im Wirbel ihrer Widersprüche den Nacken des Menschen, krümmen seinen Rücken und machen ihn gänzlich gichtbrüchig, bis er von diesem Leiden erlöst wird; gleichwohl kann er ein hohes Alter erreichen.' W. Wilhelmy, 'Hildegards natur- und heilkundliches Schrifttum' in: H.-J. Kotzur (ed.), *Hildegard von Bingen 1098–1179*, Mainz: Philipp von Zabern, 1998, p. 288, citing Hildegard of Bingen, *Causae et curae*.

64 'Livors' were those humours which were dependent on the other two dominant humours, according to the complexion of an individual.

65 'Lähmung: Wenn das Feuchte und das Lauwarme, hier den Livor des Trockenen und Schaumigen bildend, wie ein gefährlicher Windstoß über ihre Grenzen hinaus-gewirbelt werden, dann werden sie wie in eine Erschütterung der Winde gebracht und bringen gefährlich klingende Geräusche hervor wie ein Donnergetöse. Und jenes Geräusch tönt durch die Gefäße und das Mark sowie in den Schläfen eines solchen Menschen; daher wird bei solchem Leiden der Mensch gelähmt und im ganzen Körper kraftlos.' Wilhelmy, 'Hildegards natur- und heilkundliches Schrifttum', p. 288, citing Hildegard of Bingen, *Causae et curae*.

66 'Dies dauert so lange, bis die genannten Livores sich verzogen haben und wieder in die rechte Bahn zurückgekehrt sind. Aber mit Gottes Erlaubnis kann solch einer doch recht lange leben., Ibid., p. 288, citing Hildegard of Bingen, *Causae et curae*.

67 'Queritur quare quedam membra vel partes aliquorum non ex nativitate sed ex tem-pore graciliores vel grossiores debito efficiuntur?... Unde quamplura emergunt incommoda ut ydropisis ex multa humiditate et pauco calore, paralysis ex humore et multa frigiditate, similiter et passio scialgica, et artetica, et mania, et melancolia, et litargia, et multe alie passiones. Accidit autem tumor aliquoti <e> s exterius ex con-quassatione, vel ex ictu, vel vulnere, vel stricta et forti ligatione.' Question B 120,

The Prose Salernitan Questions: Edited from a Bodleian Manuscript (Auct. F. 3.10) (Auctores Britannici Medii Aevi V), ed. Brian Lawn, London: British Academy, 1979, pp. 56–7.

68 Nancy G. Siraisi, *Taddeo Alderotti and His Pupils: Two Generations of Italian Medical Learning*, Princeton, NJ: Princeton University Press, 1981, p. 288.

69 Ibid.

70 O'Neill, *Speech and Speech Disorders*, pp. 128–9. William of Conches echoed some of the notions of brain function hinted at by Meletius, but William's ideas appear more precise and thought out.

71 The passage reads in full:

> Queritur de quodam balbutiente qui cum stringeretur per manum amittebat loquelam, similiter si super eum manus ponatur? R. Balbutiens duobus fit modis, fit lubricate nervorum et debilitate eorum. Quidam enim nervi sunt in linguam lingue alligati et ysophago, ut que sapiunt lingue sapiunt stomaco et que displiceant lingue displicent stomaco. Unde cum aliquem rem insipidam sumit que stomaco displicet, provocatur ad nauseam cum quo contingit multam humiditatem abundare, ex qua humiditate ipsi nervi lingue lubrici efficiuntur, unde fit loquele impedimentum. Debilitate hoc modo contingit; humiditas a cerebro fluens veniens ad ipsos nervos debilitat, quibus debilitatis succedit balbutiens. Notandum est quod omnes nervi principium habent a cerebro. Quidam illo mediante cum quo manus vel pes contingebatur, quia nervi ledebantur et cerebrum, quo leso et debilitato humiditas nimium defluens a cerebro quam non potuit retinere, lubricando nervos loquelam impedit ne fiat. Vel potest ad intentionem anime. Dum enim quis dolet, tota anime intentio illuc dirigitur et aliarum actionum non reminiscitur quod in illo esse non potuit. Dum enim nervi distringerentur, quia dolor aderat anima illius totam suam intentionem in illo dirigebat, unde loqui non recordabatur.
>
> (Question B 85, *The Prose Salernitan Questions*, pp. 40–1)

72 O'Neill, *Speech and Speech Disorders*, pp. 179–80.

73 'Quare omnes muti surdi sunt? Responsio. Nervi qui veniunt ad linguam in sua origine continui sunt nervis qui veniunt ad aures. Si ergo contingat aliquem humorem opilare nervos lingue circa principia, opilantur et illi qui veniunt ad aures, unde simul fit mutus et surdus' (Question Ba 12, *The Prose Salernitan Questions*, p. 163).

74 'Quare omnis cecus bene audit, et quare mutus a nativitate est surdus? Solutio. Bene audit cecus quia spiritus animalis qui debebat transire ad oculos, ad aures convertitur, unde bene audit. Mutus est surdus quia non oportet nervos multum movere ad formandum vocem semivocalem, unde humiditas eam copulans redundat ad aures et obturat, unde efficitur surdus' (Question R 9, *The Prose Salernitan Questions*, p. 343).

75 The full text of this passage reads:

> Quidam cecidit et ita concussatus est quod spatio duarum horarum visum amisit et auditum ex parte. Dum iacuit audivit, sed quando stetit, vel sedit, vel ambulavit, nichil audivit. Responsio. In casu illo conquassatum est cerebrum et fantastica cellula conturbata. Opticus nervus obtusus radium visibilis spiritus ad exteriora non misit. Surdus factus est propter tim<panorum> conquassationem et audibilium nervorum debilitationem. Audivit quando auditur quia fumositate ad superiora ascendente, pervii fuerunt audibiles nervi spiritibus et patuit instrumentum auditus. Corpore enim existente super latus, discurrunt spiritus per singula membra. Quando autem stat vel sedet, cessat auditus propter fumositatem stomachi cessantem.
>
> (Question Ba 28, *The Prose Salernitan Questions*, p. 168)

76 Aristotle, *Generation of Animals*, where the reason is given of the similarity in the nature of semen and the brain; see Danielle Jacquart and Claude Thomasset, *Sexuality and Medicine in the Middle Ages*, transl. M. Adamson, Cambridge: Polity, 1988, p. 56.

77 *Causae et curae*, Book II, see Joan Cadden, *Meanings of Sex Difference in the Middle Ages: Medicine, Science, and Culture*, Cambridge: Cambridge University Press, 1993, p. 87.

Hildegard then later (in Book IV of *Causae et curae*) provided a recipe for curing men and women who had sustained various eye disorders, not necessarily blindness, due to an excessive libido.

78 Albertus Magnus, *Questions on Animals*, cited in Jacquart and Thomasset, *Sexuality and Medicine in the Middle Ages*, pp. 55–6.

79 Cited in Jacquart and Thomasset, *Sexuality and Medicine in the Middle Ages*, p. 56. Jacquart and Thomasset intriguingly speculate that blindness and other eye disorders may in fact have had a connection with sexual intercourse, in that certain sexually transmitted diseases, notably *chlamydia trachomatis*, can cause ocular disorders. In support of their theory they claim that 'the frequency of ocular infections in the Middle Ages clearly indicates the presence of the trachoma. ... The constant association we have encountered between diseases of the eyes and sexuality is then easy to understand' (ibid., p. 181).

80 *Regimen vitae*, Traktat I, 'von der mynne', lines 12–15, in: *Das Regimen Sanitatis Konrads von Eichstätt: Quellen – Texte – Wirkungsgeschichte* (Sudhoffs Archiv Beihefte 35), ed. Christa Hagenmeyer, Stuttgart: Franz Steiner, 1995, p. 204. The Latin version (*Regimen sanitatis*, Traktat I, 4.2, lines 13–16, Hagenmeyer p. 83) reads: 'Scias propterea, quod ex dimissione coitus, secundum quod <ponit> Avicenna predicto capitulo, accidit corpori tenebrositas visus et vertigo et gravitas capitis et apostemata, sed coitus temperatus eos sanat.'

81 *Regimen vitae*, Traktat I, 'von der mynne', lines 29–31: 'Sy macht faul alles pluot unnd machet pidmen an den henden und hindert das gehoeren und das sehen und benympt dem leib alle seine krafft...und machet auch schier alt...', *Das Regimen Sanitatis Konrads von Eichstätt*, p. 204. The Latin version (*Regimen sanitatis*, Traktat I, 4.2, lines 28–31, Hagenmeyer p. 83) reads: 'Dicunt enim [Avicenna + Almansor], quod coitus distemperatus et multus et frequens nervis infert nocumentum magnum, quia tremorem <facit>, auditum oculosque fortiter ledit, corporis virtutes destruit corpusque corrumpit ac debilitat atque senescere cito facit...'.

82 See Appendix F 1.1.

83 '[A]poplexie is a sekenes Þat com[eÞ o]f stopping of Þe principal pla[cis Þat b]en in a mannes brayn Þrow [sum co]rrupte humour. And Þis [sikenes b]ynemeÞ a mannnes wit/ and his felyng for Þe tyme and al maner meving wiÞouteforÞe, saaf only breÞing. ...The more sleeÞ a man Þe first day, for it is incurable. The meen sleeÞ a man withyn Þre daies, or ellis turneÞ into a palesie; Þe lasse withyn vii daies, or turneÞ into palesie. And Þis sikenes comeÞ of moche flevme or of moche corrup blode Þat filliÞ Þe principal places of a mannes brayn. And if it be in so grete plente Þat it filliÞ al Þe brayn, Þen it makeÞ a man to leese his wittis, as his sy3te, his hering, his tasting, his smelling, and his meving also. Þis is Þe more apoplexie. But if Þe humour stoppe not but Þe hyn/dre place of Þe brayn Þer-as Þe senewes han her begynnyng, Þan it bynemeÞ not a mannes wittis, but his meving. And Þis is Þe lasse apoplexie' (Getz (ed.), *Gilbertus Anglicus*, pp. 27–8 [fols. 70v – 71v]).

84 Book II, xvii 'How and When to give the Newborn the Breast', *Soranus' Gynecology*, p. 110. Soranus' opinions on obstetrics and gynaecology were current throughout the medieval period up to the sixteenth century, made popular mainly through the Latin translation by Muscio of around 500; his popularity waned somewhat after the influx of Arabic medical texts and the rise of Galenic theories from the eleventh century onwards.

85 Est quidam qui a pectine inferius membra habet desiccata, et extenuata, et motu voluntario destituta, et fere omni sensu. Ad obligationes tamen bene se habet, ab operatione animalis virtutis nullo modo impeditur, sive spiritualis, sive naturalis. Responsio. Ex enfraxi patitur, unde cum propter opilationem sanguinis non habeat descensum ad inferiora, male nutriuntur et extenuantur. Inde motu destitutus est quia propter eandem opilationem spiritus non habet recursum per nervos motus operativos. Sensum ex parte habet quia non ita sunt opilati nervi sensibiles quin spiritus per eos aliquem habeat discursum (Question P 98, *The Prose Salernitan Questions*, p. 243).

86 Isidore of Seville, *Etymologiarum*, Book XI, 1.145, in ' Isidore of Seville: The Medical Writings', p. 48.

87 Caroline Walker Bynum, *Fragmentation and Redemption: Essays on Gender and the Human Body in Medieval Religion*, New York: Zone Books, 1992, pp. 226–7.

88 'Et quid dubitas sperma matris in conceptu esse cum videas filios similes matribus nasci infirmitatesque earum contrahere?' Question B 11, *The Prose Salernitan Questions*, p. 7.

89 See Jacquart and Thomasset, *Sexuality and Medicine in the Middle Ages*, p. 53. 'Weak' sperm in medieval thought, that is sperm produced in the left testicle, could also mean sperm that leads to the conception of a female foetus, the female being the 'weaker' gender (see Carole Rawcliffe, *Medicine and Society in Later Medieval England*, Stroud: Sutton, 1995, pp. 172–5 for a brief discussion of medieval theories of conception).

90 *On Generation*, 10, see Helen King, 'Making a man: becoming human in early Greek medicine', in: G. R. Dunstan (ed.), *The Human Embryo: Aristotle and the Arabic and European Traditions*, Exeter: University of Exeter Press, 1990, p. 14.

91 Päivi Pahta (ed.), *Medieval Embryology in the Vernacular: The Case of* De Spermate (Mémoires de la Société Néophilologique de Helsinki LIII), Helsinki: Société Néophilologique, 1998, p. 42.

92 'Cuidam puero nascenti defuerunt oculi et aures. Responsio. In qualitate spermatis potuit esse vitium, vel in matrice, vel in principio generationis, scilicet in virtute informativa.' Question Ba 95, *The Prose Salernitan Questions*, p. 186.

93 Albertus Magnus, *De animalibus*, XXI, 11–13, in: Claude Lecouteux, *Les nains et les elfes au moyen age*, Paris: Imago, 1988, p. 24. Albertus Magnus was an Aristotelian, so it is worth pointing out that Aristotle proposed two theories for the causes of dwarfism. According to one, the uterus was too small for the development of the embryo, and according to the other, the neonate did not receive enough nourishment for proper growth once born (*Problemata Theodora Gaza interprete*, X, 12, in: *Aristoteles Opera*, III, Berlin, 1831, pp. 432 ff., see Lecouteux, *Les nains*, p. 24).

94 'Upanishad of the Embryo', cited by Lakshmi Kapani, 'Notes on the garbha-upanishad', in: Michel Feher (ed.), *Fragments for a History of the Human Body*, part three, New York: Zone Books, 1989, p. 178. The word 'na-pumsaka', here translated as 'eunuch', literally means 'without virile character', which is sometimes translated to mean hermaphrodite, or one who possesses the characteristics of both sexes. The Vedic medical texts often linked malformations and infirmities to a lack or insufficiency of an organic element, for example, lack of the fire element in the case of blindness. In the medical texts, it was only perceived to be the fault of the parents when there was a serious problem with semen. The *Upanishad*, however, attributes physical deformity to a troubled spirit (*manas*), which means the parents' mental state determines a child's physical appearance. Doctors, conversely, considered bad 'karma' to be responsible for birth defects (cf. Kapani, 'Notes on the Garbha-Upanishad', pp. 186–7).

95 Hildegard of Bingen, *Scivias*, liber I, visio IV, *Patrologia Latina*, 197, cols 415–34. Also *Scivias* (Wisse die Wege), transl. and ed. W. Storch, Augsburg: Pattloch, 1997, p. 69:

> Du siehst auf der Erde auch Menschen, die in ihren Gefäßen Milch tragen und daraus Käse bereiten. Das sind Männer und Frauen auf Erden, die menschlichen Samen in ihrem Körper tragen, aus dem das Menschen-geschlecht, aus vielen Völkern bestehend, hervorgeht. Ein Teil davon ist dick und ergibt fetten Käse, weil der Same in seiner Kraft brauchbar, gut ausgereift und richtig gemischt, tüchtige Menschen erzeugt. ...Und ein anderer Teil ist dünn; aus ihm gerinnt magerer Käse. Dieser Same, in seiner Kraftlosigkeit unbrauchbar, halbreif und schlecht gemischt, erzeugt schwächliche Menschen. ...Doch aus einem Teil verdorbener Milch entsteht bitterer Käse, weil dieser Same, in kraftloser Mischung, leichtfertig hervor-gebracht und unnütz vermengt, mißgestaltete Menschen erzeugt.
>
> (This translation cited by W. Wilhelmy, 'Sexualität,
> Schwangerschaft und Geburt in den Schriften Hildegards von Bingen'
> in: H.-J. Kotzur (ed.), *Hildegard von Bingen 1098–1179*, Mainz:
> Philipp von Zabern, 1998, pp. 336–7.)

96 Cf. Cadden, *Meanings of Sex Difference in the Middle Ages*, p. 92.

97 Jacquart and Thomasset, *Sexuality and Medicine in the Middle Ages*, p. 54. To the objection of his disciple that consequently a person who had hands, feet or ears hacked off would nevertheless engender a healthy child, William replied that nature, because it avoids imperfection, substitutes a similar part of the missing body in the developing embryo (ibid.).

98 'Ad hoc quidem aliud habemus argumentum, videmus enim quod si pater aliquam infirmitatem incurabilem in aliquo suo membro obtineat ut ciragram vel podagram, filius in eodem membro similem incurrit infirmitatem, et hoc unde nisi quia in germine contraxit infirmitatis illius causam et originem' (Question B4, *The Prose Salernitan Questions*, p. 3).

99 'Queritur quare a ceco genitus oculis non careat. Similiter si aliquis truncatus manibus vel pedibus vel auribus vel naso coeat, puer qui inde nascitur non carebit istis membris?' (Question B 5, *The Prose Salernitan Questions*, p. 3).

100 'Natura imperfectionem fugiens unumquodque in suo genere perficere laborat. Materia igitur ex aliis membris contracta illud quod deest parenti in formatura perficit in partu. Membra nempe non sunt omnia dissimilia; quid igitur de ossibus aliorum membrorum contrahit in ossa manuum convertit, quid carne in carnem, quid nervis in nervos, et sic de aliis' (Question B 5, *The Prose Salernitan Questions*, p. 3).

101 'Moreouer Avicen saith þat akyes of ioyntes ben of some of tho sekenesses þat ben hadde by heritage, for-whie þe sperme (i. þe sede) of man is after þe complexioun of hym þat gendreth.' Book VI, doctrine 1, ch. 1, *The Cyrurgie of Guy de Chauliac*, p. 366.

102 See Pahta (ed.), *De spermate*, pp. 94–6. A Middle English translation was made in the second half of the fifteenth century, now extant in one manuscript copy, on which Pahta's edition is based.

103 The text explains that as the four humours affect changes in the body as a whole, similarly they also change the complexion of sperm, and provides a lengthy listing of the different physical complexions, quality of sperm and associated disorders, which are transmitted from parent to offspring (*De spermate*, lines 227–87, pp. 191–9).

104 Pahta (ed.), *De spermate*, p. 42.

105 '. . . palasy, stonyed and douteful of mynde, . . . in al armonyes and melodies grete ache of bones to hym' (*De spermate*, lines 284–6, pp. 197–9).

106 The Middle English version reads:

> That if concepcioun be in houris of blac coler, the fader and moder bien conceived in the same houris, and sperme be in the lift part, the mayden shal be malencolious naturaly, epilentic, paralitic and after that splenetic, quartanly, foolissh, dulle, shal be like to fader and moder, nor in any maner shal mow temper hir nature, whiche and thiese thynges toguyder suffrith.
>
> (*De spermate*, lines 480–86, p. 233)

107 The Middle English reads:

> Sumtyme forsoth of holle fader and holle moder we see a chield born halt, laame, or croked mowth or nose havyng, and so appierith a chield to have dyuers forme of fader and moder for the superfluite of humours or also sumtyme for the chaunge, for whi that power that the sperme hath in his place, the same nature it hath in the matrice. It happith that of the fader occupied with dyuers passiouns or of the moder drawith the chield toguyder with passiouns, sumtyme also of norisshyng of mylk.
>
> (Ibid., 214–22, p. 189)

108 Because in high medieval natural philosophy milk was believed to be menses that had been 'boiled' by the maternal body and thereby transmuted into milk, milk retained some of the dangers of menstrual fluid; mothers should therefore not feed their newborns with their own milk until several days after birth, when the mother's complexion had 'cooled down', according to Vincent of Beauvais (cf. William F. MacLehose,

'Nurturing danger: high medieval medicine and the problem(s) of the child', in: John Carmi Parsons and Bonnie Wheeler (eds), *Medieval Mothering*, New York and London: Garland, 1996, pp. 11–12).

109 Cited by Talbot, *Medicine in Medieval England*, p. 95. William had been surgeon to Simon de Montfort (d. 1218) during the Albigensian Crusade.

110 Leon Battista Alberti, *I libri della famiglia* = *The Family in Renaissance Florence*, transl. Renée Neu Watkins, Columbia: University of South Carolina Press, 1969, p. 121.

111 Ibid.

112 C. S. F. Burnett, 'The planets and the development of the embryo', in: G. R. Dunstan (ed.), *The Human Embryo: Aristotle and the Arabic and European Traditions*, Exeter: University of Exeter Press, 1990, p. 95.

113 See Burnett, 'The planets and the development of the embryo', p. 96. The notions first expressed by Constantinus Africanus were taken up by the Salernitan questions on medicine and natural philosophy in the late twelfth century, then were cited in a variant form in Hélinand of Froidmont's *Chronica* (written between 1210 and 1216), and were quoted in full by Vincent of Beauvais in the mid-thirteenth century in his *Speculum naturale*, and popularised through *De secretis mulierum*, a highly influential text attributed (falsely) during the Middle Ages to Albertus Magnus. The sources for Constantinus Africanus seem to have been Arabic medical texts (ibid., p. 100).

114 *De humana natura*, ' "De etate planetarum in embrione": In octavo Saturnus reiterata vice similiter infrigidando embrioni et matrici gravitatem infert: suaque siccitate humores extenuans embrioni nutrimentum parcius tribuit.' Text in Burnett, 'The planets and the development of the embryo', p. 101.

115 The Hippocratic texts had already noticed the differences in survival between seven-month and eight-month births, but had not linked this phenomenon to the planets (Burnett, 'The planets and the development of the embryo', p. 101).

116 'In septimo mense completa sunt omnia membra et secundum naturalem disposi-tionem ordinata. Unde si fetus in eo mense educatur, salubre est quia per naturalem fortitudinem atque matricis confortationem emittitur, unde vivax est et salubre. Si vero in octavo, malum et mortale' (Question B 118, *The Prose Salernitan Questions*, p. 54).

117 'Significatur enim quod aliquod retinaculum sit fractum, unde si emittitur non a nature fortitudine sed ab eius debilitate educatur, quare mortale est et si vivat tabidus vivit' (Question B 118, *The Prose Salernitan Questions*, p. 54).

118 'In octavo Saturnus iterata vice, qui infrigdando embryonem matrici gravitatem affert, suaque siccitate humores extenuans parvum nutrimentum ipsi fetui attribuitur, unde si tunc emittitur dierum vacuitatem sequitur' (Question B 118, *The Prose Salernitan Questions*, p. 55). A related Salernitan question (Question P 144, ibid., p. 259) in another manuscript (Cambridge, Peterhouse 178) was also concerned with planetary influence on the survival chances of the new-born:

> Queritur quare puer antequam totus compleatur, id est in fine sexti mensis, non nititur ad exeundum, et si forte contingeret quod exiret moreretur? Solutio. Si tunc exiret, cum non esset completus, moreretur. In septimo viveret si exiret quia completus esset. In octavo moritur quia nimis laboravit ad exitum, et ex nimio labore et debilitate moritur in octavo. In nono mense, etsi laboret in exeundo, tamen quia fortis est et multum requievit, bene vivit. … Et cum Luna habet vivificatoriam unam qualitatem, si exeat vivit. In octavo, quia Saturnus iterum dominatur, tunc puer moritur si exeat quoniam Saturnus mortificatorias habet qualitates.

119 Cf. *Blockbücher des Mittelalters. Bildfolgen als Lektüre*, Gutenberg Museum, Mainz: Philipp von Zabern, 1991, p. 199, catalogue entry 52.

120 Cf. Ibid., p. 202, catalogue entry 53.

121 The Middle English text reads: 'It happith bifore and sumtyme that the doughter is nat like non of hir parentis, and that is for the nature of the planetis. Sumtyme

a chield is born dum, without feete, without hede, without eyen, without heryng, *etc.* And therof I promitte me and afferme to yield reason, witnesse of Ipocras, that of al the substaunces of animate or souled bodies bien ligat, bounden, and joyned in planetis and signes, nexed to the iiij elementis …'. *De spermate*, lines 636–43, p. 251.

122 Ælfric, *The Homilies of the Anglo-Saxon Church: The Homilies of Ælfric*, ed. Benjamin Thorpe, 2 vols, London, 1844 and 1846, I, pp. 100–2, cited in: Karen Louise Jolly, *Popular Religion in Late Saxon England: Elf Charms in Context*, Chapel Hill, NC and London: University of North Carolina Press, 1996, p. 88.

123 Hildegard of Bingen, *On Natural Philosophy and Medicine: Selections from Cause et Cure*, transl. and ed. Margret Berger, Cambridge: D. S. Brewer, 1999, pp. 50–1.

124 Ibid., p. 82.

125 Ibid., p. 63.

126 Ibid.

127 Albertus Magnus, *Physica*, II, tr. 2, c. 17, cited by B. B. Price, 'The physical astronomy and astrology of Albertus Magnus', in: J. A. Weisheipl (ed.), *Albertus Magnus and the Sciences*, Toronto: Pontifical Institute of Medieval Studies, 1980, pp. 180–1.

128 Albertus Magnus, *De natura boni*, tr. 2, p. 3, c. 2, 2, 3, A, 1, 1 – Albertus is here following the ideas of Firmicus Maternus, *Matheseos*, IV, c1, n. 10 – cited by Price, 'The physical astronomy and astrology of Albertus Magnus', pp. 180–1.

129 Albertus Magnus, *Problemata determinata*, q. 35, cited by Price, 'The physical astronomy and astrology of Albertus Magnus', pp. 180–1.

130 Leviticus 15:19.

131 Leviticus 20:18.

132 Mary Douglas, *Purity and Danger: An* 1966, p. 61. On penance cf. McNeill and Gamer, *Medieval Handbooks of Penance*, New York: Columbia Unversity Press, 1938 (repr. 1990). Archbishop Theodore further said that women required a forty-day purgation after giving birth; this 'churching' persisted until modern times in some regions of Europe. However, Gregory the Great, in a letter of 597 to Augustine, recounted by Bede (*Ecclesiastical History of the English People*, transl. Leo Sherley-Price, London: Penguin, rev. ed. 1990, p. 84), had said that a woman must not be prohibited from entering a church during her menses (cf. Charles T. Wood, 'The doctors' dilemma: sin, salvation, and the menstrual cycle in medieval thought', *Speculum*, 56, 1981, p. 714). The official Church view during the high and later Middle Ages did not regard 'churching' as mandatory, cf. Peter Biller, 'Childbirth in the middle ages', *History Today*, 36(8), 1986, p. 48.

133 Jerome, *Commentary on Ezechiel*, 6.18. (cf. P. L. 25, 173), cited in J. T. Noonan, *Contraception: A History of Its Treatment by the Catholic Theologians and Canonists*, Cambridge, MA: Harvard University Press, 1966, p. 85. The common belief that children conceived during menstruation were born sickly, seropurulent (that is, pus-filled) or dead was, for example, also found in Pliny, *Historia naturalis*, 7.15.67.

134 Cf. Thorndike, *A History of Magic and Experimental Science*, I, pp. 400–3.

135 *The Recognitions*, IX, 9, cited by Thorndike, *A History of Magic and Experimental Science*, I, p. 414.

136 Gratian, *Decretum*, 1.56.10, reference in: John Boswell (ed.), *The Kindness of Strangers: The Abandonment of Children in Western Europe from Late Antiquity to the Renaissance*, New York: Pantheon Books, 1988, p. 338.

137 *De contemptu mundi sive de miseria conditionis humanae*, 1.5: 'Qui fertur esse tam detestabilis et immundus, ut ex ejus contactu fruges non germinent, arescant arbusta, moriantur herbae, amittant arbores foetus, et si canes inde comederint in rabiem efferantur. Concepti fetus vitium seminis contrahunt, ita ut leprosi et elephantici ex hac corruptione nascantur.' Cited in Dyan Elliott, *Fallen Bodies: Pollution, Sexuality and Demonology in the Middle Ages*, Philadelphia, PA: University of Pennsylvania Press, 1999, p. 116 and p. 233 note 49. Cf. *Patrologia Latina*, 217, col. 704.

138 Cf. William F. MacLehose, 'Nurturing Danger: High Medieval Medicine and the Problem(s) of the Child', in: John Carmi Parsons and Bonnie Wheeler (eds), *Medieval Mothering*, New York and London: Garland, 1996, pp. 8–9.

139 Raymond (*Summa* 4.2.6), Duns Scotus (*On the Sentences [Oxford Report]* 4.32), and Aquinas (*On the Sentences* 4.32.1.2.2), references in Noonan, *Contraception*, p. 282.

140 Dan Michel, *Ayenbite of Inwyt*, ed. Richard Morris, new ed. Pamela Gradon, *Early English Text Society*, o. s. 23, 1866, reissue 1965, pp. 223–4. For a discussion of menstruation as a cause of monstrous births in medieval literary texts see Peggy McCracken, *The Curse of Eve, The Wound of the Hero: Blood, Gender, and Medieval Literature*, Philadelphia, PA: University of Pennsylvania Press, 2003.

141 Albertus Magnus, *De animalibus*, 15, tractatus II, *de natura spermatis*, referenced in Wood, 'The doctors' dilemma', pp. 715–16.

142 See Wood, 'The doctors' dilemma', pp. 715–16.

143 In this context a statement by Thomas Aquinas makes sense. Aquinas discussed a decretal whereby a wife was obliged to have intercourse with her leprous husband, even though any resulting child would also have the disease. Aquinas responded (*On the Sentences* 4.32.1.1): 'Although the offspring is born infirm, yet it is better for it to be thus, than not to be at all.' As Noonan has remarked, the principle 'better to be than not to be' applied in this (admittedly narrow) case (Noonan, *Contraception*, p. 282). Accordingly, for Aquinas a deformed/impaired or diseased child was preferable to none at all. In general, though, the high medieval theologians and canonists took the view that 'it was better that a child not be conceived than that he be conceived with . . . physical deficiencies' (ibid., p. 283). On the concept of *horror vacui* in general, cf. E. Grant, 'Medieval explanations and interpretations of the dictum that "nature abhors a vacuum," ' *Traditio*, 29, 1973, pp. 327–56.

144 Helen Rodnite Lemay, 'Human sexuality in twelfth-through fifteenth-century scientific writings', in: Vern. L. Bullough and James Brundage (eds), *Sexual Practices and the Medieval Church*, Buffalo: Prometheus Books, 1982, p. 201

145 Ibid., p. 203. Cf. Commentary on *De secretis mulierum*, Venice, 1508, f.E6 v.

146 On this topic of the power of the maternal imagination to influence the physical appearance of the child cf. Marie-Hélène Huet, *Monstrous Imagination*, Cambridge, MA and London: Harvard University Press, 1993, which deals mainly with Renaissance and early modern notions of imagination, but discusses some of the earlier ideas as well. I will further discuss the concept of maternal imagination below.

147 Cf. James A. Brundage, *Law, Sex and Christian Society in Medieval Europe*, Chicago, IL: University of Chicago Press, 1987, pp. 451–2.

148 *De secretis mulierum*, Venice, 1508, f. E6 recto, see Helen Rodnite Lemay, 'Some thirteenth and fourteenth century lectures on female sexuality', *International Journal of Women's Studies*, 1(4), 1978, p. 397.

149 Robert of Flamborough, *Liber penitentialis* (Studies and Texts 18), ed. J.-J. Firth, Toronto: Pontifical Institute for Medieval Studies, 1971, cited by Boswell, *The Kindness of Strangers*, p. 338.

150 On issues of contraception cf. the seminal work by Noonan, *Contraception*; also J. M. Riddle, 'Oral contraceptives and early-term abortifacients during classical antiquity and the middle ages', *Past & Present*, 132, 1991, pp. 3–32; and P. P. A. Biller, 'Birth-control in the West in the thirteenth and early fourteenth centuries', *Past & Present*, 94, 1982, pp. 3–26. That medieval people were probably well aware of the 'safe periods' is backed up by the fact that already in the sixth century Aetius of Amida, a Byzantine court physician, recognised the existence of a less fertile, or infertile, period at the beginning and at the end of the menstrual cycle (cf. Bullough and Brundage, *Sexual Practices and the Medieval Church*, p. 16).

151 Berthold von Regensburg, *Vollständige Ausgabe Seiner Predigten*, ed. F. Pfeiffer, Vienna, 2 vols, 1862, I, pp. 322–4, cited by Boswell, *The Kindness of Strangers*, p. 338.

152 Berthold von Regensburg, *Vollständige Ausgabe Seiner Predigten*, ed. F. Pfeiffer, Vienna, 2 vols, 1862, I, pp. 323–8, cited by Mary M. McLaughlin, 'Survivors and surrogates: children and parents from the ninth to the thirteenth centuries', in: Lloyd De Mause (ed.), *The History of Childhood*, New York: Psychohistory Press, 1974, note 44.

153 Synodal de l'Ouest, 96: '... si in puerperio, quod prohibetur in lege, sive menstruis... ubi est etiam periculum corporale et patris pariter propter periculum elephantie et prolis, quia ex corrupto semine nascitur corruptus fetus et fere semper, ut asserunt fisici, vel gibbosus vel contractus', *Les Statuts synodaux français du XIIIe siècle*, ed. and transl. Odette Pontal, 2 vols, Paris, 1971, Collection de Documents Inédits sur l'Histoire de France. Section de Philologie et d'Histoire no. 9 + 15, cited in: Boswell, *The Kindness of Strangers*, pp. 338–9.

154 Cf. inter alia MS Bayerische Staatsbibliothek clm 18404 (s.XIV), fol. 128r., reference in Boswell, *The Kindness of Strangers*, p. 403.

155 On the topic of the new sexual codes which are embraced by early Christianity in the late-antique world, see Peter Brown, *The Body and Society: Men, Women and Sexual Renunciation in Early Christianity*, London: Columbia University Press, 1989, p. 439 and note 43, who mentions that Caesarius of Arles, *Sermon* 44.7, already pointed out that intercourse on Sundays begets lepers and epileptics.

156 Clarissa W. Atkinson, *The Oldest Vocation: Christian Motherhood in the Middle Ages*, Ithaca, NY and London: Cornell University Press, 1991, p. 91. Cf. Gregory of Tours, *Liber de virtutibus sancti Martini episcopi*, II. 24, in: Raymond Van Dam, *Saints and their Miracles in Late Antique Gaul*, Princeton, NJ: Princeton University Press, 1993, p. 240. The boy had been conceived 'on the night before a Sunday', as the mother confesses (ibid.).

157 Gregory of Tours, *Liber de virtutibus sancti Martini episcopi*, II. 24, in: Van Dam (ed.), *Saints and their Miracles in Late Antique Gaul*, p. 240.

158 Patricia Skinner, *Health and Medicine in Early Medieval Southern Italy*, Leiden, New York and Brill: 1997, p. 48.

159 Ibid., p. 49; cf. C. Klapisch, 'Attitudes devant l'enfant', *Annales de Démographie Historique*, 1973, p. 65.

160 Skinner, *Health and Medicine in Early Medieval Southern Italy*, p. 49. However, later Skinner does use onomastic evidence from southern Italy to point out that impaired children could survive to adulthood (ibid.).

161 Ibid., p. 48 note 36.

162 Gregory of Tours, *Liber de virtutibus sancti Martini episcopi*, II. 24, in: Van Dam, *Saints and their Miracles in Late Antique Gaul*, p. 240. This story is also discussed by Danièle Alexandre-Bidon and Didier Lett, *Children in the Middle Ages: Fifth–Fifteenth Centuries*, transl. J. Gladding, Notre Dame: University of Notre Dame Press, 1999, p. 12. In support of my reading of the text, that abandonment or infanticide was unthinkable for Gregory of Tours, see Boswell, *The Kindness of Strangers*, p. 212.

163 Very occasionally it was the person of the saint him or herself who was impaired, and who as a child had narrowly escaped infanticide. This happened in the case of St Odile, at the end of the ninth century, who had been born blind, and whose mother had to hide her for a year from her father, who tried to kill her (Alexandre-Bidon and Lett, *Children in the Middle Ages*, p. 17).

164 H. Herrmann, *Die Stellung unehelicher Kinder nach kanonischem Recht*, Amsterdam: Grüner, 1971, p. 37.

165 Brundage, *Law, Sex and Christian Society in Medieval Europe*, p. 156.

166 Ecclesiasticus 23:25, regarding the children of an adulterous woman: 'Her children shall not take root, and her branches shall bring forth no fruit' [Sirach 23:35 in Vulgata]. Adulterous procreation is also mentioned at Wisdom of Solomon 3:16: 'As for the children of adulterers, they shall not come to their perfection, and the seed of an unrighteous bed shall be rooted out', and Wisdom of Solomon 4:6: 'For children begotten of unlawful beds are witnesses of wickedness against their parents in their trial.'

167 Augustine, *De bono conjugali*, liber I, C. 16(18) (in *Patrologia Latina*, 40, col. 386) says that all human beings are honourable if they have no personal fault, error, sin or culpability, so that therefore good or bad children are not caused by the parentage of such children. In *Contra Faustum Manichaeum* (in *Patrologia Latina*, vol. 42, col. 440), Augustine states that parental sins are not to be transferred to their children. Again, in his text against the Donatists, *De baptismo contra Donatistas* (in *Patrologia Latina*, vol. 43, col. 122), Augustine writes that the status of the mother or her carnal relations are not decisive, but only the personal culpability of a child is a deciding factor for sin. Gregory the Great in a letter to bishop Columbus in Numidia (*Epistolarum lib. XII, epistola VIII ad Columbum Numidiae episcopum*, in *Patrologia Latina*, vol. 77, col. 1224) also says that it is personal culpability and not alien (i.e. illegitimate) heritage which make a person unsuitable for holding office in the Church. John Chrysostom, in his third homily on Matthew, equally does not blame children for the sins of their parents. And Jerome, in *Contra Joannem Hierosol. Admonitio* (in *Patrologia Latina*, 23, col. 389), says that being born adulterously is not the fault of the one born, but of the one begetting: 'Nasci de adulterio non est eius culpa, qui nascitur, sed illius, qui generat.' Cf. Herrmann, *Die Stellung unehelicher Kinder nach kanonischem Recht*, pp. 42–3.

168 Augustine, *De peccatorium meretis et remissione*, cap. 57 (XXIX), transl. Marcus Dodd, 2, *The Works of St Augustine*, Edinburgh, 1885, in: Vern L. Bullough (ed.), *Sexual Variance in Society and History*, New York, London, Sydney and Toronto: Wiley Interscience, 1976, p. 193.

169 Quoted by M. J. Tucker, 'The child as beginning and end: fifteenth and sixteenth century English childhood', in: Lloyd De Mause (ed.), *The History of Childhood*, p. 233. Cf. T. H. White (ed.), *The Bestiary*, New York: no publisher, 1965, p. 104. It is interesting to note that childhood itself can be seen as an impairment, in the context of the 'Ages of Man' theme, whereby infancy, the first age, is 'without wit, strength or cunning and may do nothing that profits' (Pynson's *The Kalendar of Shepherdes* of 1506, quoted in Tucker, 'The child as beginning and end', p. 230); here one may also note the emphasis on profit – in the light of Gleeson's theories mentioned (in Chapter 2.2 on modern disability theories) it is interesting to observe how notions of the profitableness of something or someone begin to creep in towards the end of the Middle Ages.

170 Quoted in Rawcliffe, *Medicine and Society in Later Medieval England*, p. 8. Cf. *Dives and Pauper*, ed. P. Heath Barnum, *Early English Text Society*, 275, 1976 and 280, 1980, 1, p. 129.

171 On negative attitudes to procreation and carnal lust as a consequence of Original Sin, see also Shulamith Shahar, *Childhood in the Middle Ages*, London and New York: Routledge, 1992, p. 14.

172 Shakespeare, *The Merchant of Venice*, III.V.1.

173 'The belief in the linkage between evil spirits and/or parental misconduct and the birth of a disabled newborn appears widespread. Present in preindustrial and later industrial Europe and America, it also occurs among the Hopi and the Ainu. In societies that view one's present state as a reflection of past deeds and transgressions, the life of a disabled child or adult may be made difficult, with sharply limited social and economic options' (Jessica Sheer and Nora Groce, 'Impairment as a human constant: cross-cultural and historical perspectives on variation', *Journal of Social Studies*, 44(1), 1988, p. 28).

174 *Bisclavret*, vv. 312–14 and *Yonec*, vv. 325–27, in: Baldwin (ed.), *The Language of Sex*, p. 220.

175 Book I, x, *Soranus' Gynecology*, pp. 37–8.

176 Ibid., p. 38.

177 One question asked why a child resembled the man whom the woman will have seen at the moment of conception, and the response revolved around the connection between the form of the sperm and the impact of the imagination: sperm took on the shape, 'the likeness of the thing', which the imagination had conceived of. Question W 7, *The Prose Salernitan Questions*, pp. 268–9:

> Quare fetus similis ei homini generatur quem in concipiendo mulier viderit presentem, vel meditando imaginata fuerit absentem? Responsio. Sperma, quod

fetus est materia, naturaliter habet se et apertum est ad singulas eiusdem speciei formas equaliter suscipiendas. Itaque cum a singulis membris corporis collectum cerebrum, naturali calore et spiritu impellente, ascendat, quadam proprietate eius rei de qua tunc anima fantasticabatur ibi inficitur. Cum qua sibi innata ad matricem accedens, natura operante, secundum proprietatem immutatur, et informatur, et in similitudinem rei prius ab anima concepte. Ex eo fetus generatur.

178 'Queritur si mulier pregnans a quarto mense in antea aliquid cum nimio desiderio appetat quod habere non possit, et ponat ibi manum in facie vel in alio membre, quare consimilis forma eius quod apppetit nascitur postea in simili membro pueri? R. Dum mater aliquid multum appetit, spiritus in fantastica cellula multum commovetur et per imaginationem similis forma representatur, unde spiritus in se formam suscipit. Si ergo mater manu comprimit aliquam partem, spiritus sibi retentus immutat humorem secundum se. Spiritus ergo et humores sic immutati demittuntur ad nutrimentum fetus, mutantur in essentiam partis similis ei cui impressa est manus. Unde et similis forma imprimitur illi parti, que impressa immutat locum secundum se, quare ei similis efficitur' (Question B35, *The Prose Salernitan Questions*, p. 19).

179 See M. Anthony Hewson, *Giles of Rome and the Medieval Theory of Conception: A Study of the* De formatione corporis humani in utero, London: Athlone Press, 1975, p. 193. 'Giles concludes that such cases are very rare' (ibid.).

180 Elliott, *Fallen Bodies*, pp. 38–9 and p. 186 note 20, where further such late medieval stories are cited.

181 *Reinfried von Braunschweig*, lines 19888 ff., ed. K. Bartsch, cited by Roy A. Wisbey, 'Die darstellung des häßlichen im hoch- und spätmittelalter', in: Wolfgang Harms and L. Peter Johnson (eds), *Deutsche Literatur des späten Mittelalters: Hamburger Colloquium 1973* (simultaneously published as *Publications of the Institute of Germanic Studies University of London*, vol. 22), Berlin: E. Schmidt, 1975, p. 27 note 63.

182 Genesis 30:2.

183 Genesis 30:39.

184 Genesis 30:41–42.

185 *In Secundum Librum Sententiarum*, Pt. II, Dist. xx, art. 1, see Hewson, *Giles of Rome*, p. 193 and p. 197 note 34.

186 Cited by M. L. Cameron, *Anglo-Saxon Medicine*, Cambridge: Cambridge University Press, 1993, p. 183. The original text is in MS British Library Cotton Tiberius A. iii, and an edited version of the original Old English can be found in T. O. Cockayne (ed.), *Leechdoms, Wortcunning and Starcraft of Early England*, 3 vols, *Rolls Series*, 1864–66, III, p. 144.

187 Vincent of Beauvais, *Speculum maius*, around 1250, cf. William F.MacLehose, 'Nurturing Danger: pp. 10–11.

188 'swâ sîner tohter keiniu truoc,/ vil dicke er des gein in gewuoc,/ den rât er selten gein in liez,/ viel würze er si mîden hiex/ die menschen vruht verkêrten/ unt sîn geslähte unêrten,/ 'anders denne got uns maz,/ dô er ze werke über mich gesaz,'/ ... etslîcher riet ir broeder lîp/ daz si diu werc volbrâhte,/ des ir herzen gir gedâhte./ sus wart verkêrt diu mennischeit' Wolfram von Eschenbach, *Parzival*, 10. 518, lines 15–29, transl. and ed. Wolfgang Spiewok, Stuttgart: Philipp Reclam, 2, 1981, p. 150.

189 Neubert and Cloerkes, *Behinderung und Behinderte*, p. 81.

190 For example, among the fellah peasantry of Egypt one finds the belief that disturbance to a pregnant woman's sleep could result in a physical effect on the foetus (e.g. being born with six fingers per hand); among the Yoruba of West Africa, organic agents such as the wrong or bad foods, the presence of insects or worms in the head, black or watery blood, bad smells etc. were put forward as explanations for illness and impairment (Ibid., p. 80). In this context, it is interesting to note that modern research has been able to establish a causal link between psychological stress in the mother and physical impairment in the foetus. 'Severe emotional stress during pregnancy

may cause malformations such as cleft palate, according to research published in [the] Lancet medical journal. Psychosocial stress affects the nervous system, hormone production, and the cardiovascular, metabolic and immune systems, say researchers' (Sarah Boseley, 'Cleft palates linked to pregnancy stress', *Guardian*, 8 September 2000).

191 'Mitleid mit Krüppeln und Personen, die an ekelhaften Uebeln laboriren, hat sich darauf zu beschränken: für deren angemessenen Aufenthalt in Siechenhäusern mit Gärten, die sie jedoch nie verlassen dürfen, zu sorgen. Der widrige Anblick solcher Unglücklichen muß dem öffentlichen Verkehr entzogen bleiben, denn der Eindruck auf Empfindsame, oder gar Schwangere, ist höchst bedenklich.' Cited in Eduard Seidler, 'Historische elemente des umgangs mit behinderung', in: U. Koch, G. Lucius-Hoene and R. Stegie (eds), *Handbuch der Rehabilitationspsychologie*, Berlin, Heidelberg, New York and London: Springer, 1988, p. 6.

192 On swaddling of infants, see also Shahar, *Childhood in the Middle Ages*, pp. 83–8, who mentions a few cases of impaired babies due to swaddling.

193 Quoted by Lloyd de Mause, 'The evolution of childhood', in: de Mause (ed,), *The History of Childhood*, p. 11.

194 Cited in Michael E. Goodich, *From Birth to Old Age: The Human Life Cycle in Medieval Thought, 1250–1350*, Lanham, MD and London: University Press of America, 1989, p. 88.

195 McLaughlin, 'Survivors and surrogates', p. 114. Palaeopathology has since shown us that midwives and incorrect swaddling may have been blamed quite needlessly: childhood polio (poliomyelitis or infantile paralysis) would often go unnoticed in children during the initial febrile phase at the onset of the disease, until the affected children were found to have a paralysed arm or leg, by which time a careless midwife could easily be blamed (cf. Calvin Wells, *Bones, Bodies and Disease*, London: Thames & Hudson, 1964, p. 92).

196 '... and rightith and strecchith out his lymes and bendith hem togedres with cradil bondis to kepe and saue the childe that he be not defasid with myscroked lymes.' *Sources for the History of Medicine in Late Medieval England*, transl. and ed. C. Rawcliffe, Kalamazoo, MI: Medieval Institute Publications, 1995, p. 108.

197 Jonas' 1540 translation into English of Eucharius Roesslin, *The Byrth of Mankynde*, cited by Tucker, 'The child as beginning and end', p. 241.

198 An alternative view of iatrogenesis is presented by Ivan Illich, who argues that the medical establishment itself is, in fact, a threat to health, in that greater medical 'progress' leads to a greater number of 'diseases' being regarded as such. Greater numbers of diseases which now require therapy also mean greater numbers of side-effects; more new diseases to be cured also lead to more medical intervention. 'Society has transferred to physicians the exclusive right to determine what constitutes sickness, who is or might become sick, and what shall be done to such people. Deviance is now 'legitimate' only when it merits and ultimately justifies medical interpretation and intervention' (Ivan Illich, *Limits to Medicine. Medical Nemesis: The Expropriation of Health*, Harmondsworth: Penguin, 1977, pp. 13–14).

199 Darrel W. Amundsen, 'Casuistry and professional obligations: the regulation of physicians by the court of conscience in the late middle ages', in: Amundsen (ed.), *Medicine, Society, and Faith in the Ancient and Medieval Worlds*, p. 255.

200 Cited in Faye Getz, *Medicine in the English Middle Ages*, Princeton, NJ: Princeton Unversity Press, 1998, p. 72, cf. *The Mirror of Justices*, ed. W. J. Whittaker, *Selden Society* 7, 1895, p. 137.

201 This was a case that came before the London Sheriff's Court of John Preston, cited in Getz, *Medicine in the English Middle Ages*, p. 72 and p. 130 note 46.

202 In 1422 or 1424, depending on whether you follow the discussion of the case in Gask or Talbot.

203 G. E. Gask (ed.), *Essays in the History of Medicine*, London: Butterworth & Co., 1950, pp. 101–2.

204 Cited from 'City records, plea and memoranda rolls, roll A 52, membrane 5', in: Gask (ed.), *Essays in the History of Medicine*, pp. 101–2.

205 Cited in Talbot, *Medicine in Medieval England*, p. 203. The full text of the case is printed in *Sources for the History of Medicine*, transl. and ed. Rawcliffe, pp. 28–9. Regarding this case, see also Michael T. Walton, 'The advisory jury and malpractice in Fifteenth Century London: the case of William Forest', *Journal of the History of Medicine*, 40, 1985, pp. 478–82.

206 The problems of self-regulatory bodies, like the British Medical Association today, dealing with 'customer' complaints were clearly already in evidence in the early fifteenth century.

207 McVaugh, *Medicine Before the Plague*, p. 209.

208 'mortalia sive mortis periculosa vel deterioracionis membrorum', cited in ibid., p. 212.

209 'que apparent esse facte cum baculo', cited in ibid., p. 212.

210 'ex eo quia non habet in capite nec in brachio aliqua effrectione ossi et habuit omnia bona signa in persona sua, quia non habet tumorem in capite nec sustinuit vomitum nec eciam stratimentum in persona sua, que essent signa periculosa. Quare dicit quod ipse est sine suspicione mortis vel debilitacionis et sic desuspitavit eundem', cited in ibid., p. 212. Regrettably, McVaugh does not indicate whether the source says anything about the outcome of the case, that is, whether the surgeon was right and the patient did make a full recovery.

211 Ibid., p. 213.

212 Ibid., p. 178.

213 This case is cited in Rawcliffe, *Medicine and Society in Later Medieval England*, p. 142. See also C. H. Talbot and E. A. Hammond, *The Medical Practitioners in Medieval England: A Biographical Register*, London: Wellcome Historical Medical Library, 1965, p. 128, who state that John Brown sued one John Dobson, the vicar of Melbourne, for £10, sometime between 1486 and 1493.

214 'Quare sompnus prohibetur post flebotomiam? Responsio. ... Vel spiritus animalis a capite ad instrumenta sensuum motum libere discernere non potest, quia humores qui sunt in motu opilarent nervos et facerent surditatem vel cecitatem.' Question P 13, *The Prose Salernitan Questions*, p. 211.

215 Celsus, *De medicina*, VII, 12, 4 transl. W. G. Spencer, London, 1938, cited in M. Eldridge, *A History of the Treatment of Speech Disorders*, Edinburgh and London: E. & S. Livingstone, 1968, p. 20. The Latin text is cited in H. Werner, *Geschichte des Taubstummenproblems bis ins 17. Jahrhundert*, Jena: Gustav Fischer, 1932, p. 27:

> Lingua vero quibusdam cum subjecta parte a primo natali die juncta est, qui ob id ne loqui quidem possunt. Horum extrema lingua vulsella prehenda est, sub eaque membrana incidenda, magna cum habita, ne venae, quae juxta sunt, violentur et profusione sanguine noceant.... Et plerique quidem, ubi consanuerunt, loquuntur.

216 O'Neill, *Speech and Speech Disorders*, p. 126.

217 Werner, *Geschichte des Taubstummenproblems*, p. 116.

218 P. Gravitt, *Charity and Children in Renaissance Florence: The Ospedale degli Innocenti, 1410–1536*, Ann Arbor, MI: University of Michigan Press, 1990, p. 194 note 30.

219 *Heilbronner Hebammensammlung*, § 21: 'Bei neugeborenen kindern dürfen sie sich ohne zustimmen des arztes nicht das Lösen der zunge annehmen, wodurch und wegen unverstand [sonst] großer schaden angerichtet wird', cited in P. Ketsch and A. Kuhn (eds), *Frauen im Mittelalter: Band 1. Frauenarbeit im Mittelalter. Quellen und Materialien*, Düsseldorf: Schwann, 1983, p. 283.

220 Quoted in Gravitt, *Charity and Children in Renaissance Florence*, p. 194.

221 See note 24 in this chapter.

222 One only needs to think here of the proscriptions regarding sexual intercourse advocated in the penitential of Robert of Flamborough (see note 149), and in

the preaching activity of Berthold of Regensburg (see notes 151 and 152) to see that such ideas must have filtered down all social hierarchies.

223 Henri de Mondeville, *Chirurgie*, cited in Pouchelle, *The Body and Surgery in the Middle Ages*, p. 46.

224 Thorndike, *A History of Magic and Experimental Science*, 3, pp. 246–7.

225 Ibid., pp. 362–3.

226 Two of the texts, the so-called *Leechbook of Bald*, and *Leechbook III*, that will be frequently alluded to here are found in a manuscript probably produced at Winchester around 950, now British Library, Royal MS 12.D.XVII, cf. Getz, *Medicine in the English Middle Ages*, p. 47.

227 Cf. *Leechdoms*, ed. Cockayne, 2, pp. 300–2.

228 Cameron, *Anglo-Saxon Medicine*, pp. 39–40.

229 Cf. *Leechbook III*, in *Leechdoms*, ed. Cockayne, 2, p. 342. The Old English text reads: Gif men sio heafodpanne beo gehlenced alege yone man upweard, drif ii stacan æt yam eaxlum, lege yonne bred yweores ofer ya fet, sleah yonne yriwa on mid slegebytle, hio gæy on riht sona.

230 British Library, MS Sloane 2839, fol. 11v–12r.

231 Cameron, *Anglo-Saxon Medicine*, p. 39.

232 Linda M. Paterson, 'Military surgery: knights, sergeants and Raimon of Avignon's version of the *Chirurgia* of Roger of Salerno (1180–1209)', in: C. Harper-Bill and R. Harvey (eds), *The Ideals and Practice of Medieval Knighthood II: Papers from the third Strawberry Hill conference 1986*, Woodbridge: Boydell, 1988, pp. 127–32.

233 Dublin, Trinity College, MS 158 *Colim* D.4.15, fols. 82r–93v, probably dating from the second quarter of the fifteenth century; the text in question is part of a larger section on medicine, which includes the mention of Galen, Asclepius and Hippocrates as authorities to back up what it says.

234 M. Benskin, 'For a wound in the head: a late medieval view of the brain', *Neuphilologische Mitteilungen*, 86(2), 1985, pp. 199–215.

235 Hummel, *Das Kind und seine Krankheiten*, p. 178.

236 Cf. Book II, doctrine 2, ch. 1, *The Cyrurgie of Guy de Chauliac*, p. 131. Guglielmo da Saliceto in his *Cyrurgia* had described a case of hydrocephalus in a child, which he had seen at a hospital in Cremona, but he said he had not employed any of the surgical techniques suggested by the authorities, because he regarded them as too dangerous (cf. Jole Agrimini and Chiara Crisciani, 'Wohltätigkeit und beistand in der mittelalterlichen christlichen kultur', in: Grmek (ed.), *Die Geschichte des medizinischen Denkens*, p. 207).

237 Vienna, Österreichische Nationalbibliothek, Codex Series Nova 2641, Book 2, fol.17r.

238 William of Malmesbury, *De gestis regum Anglorum*, liber V, § 403, ed. W. Stubbs, *Rolls Series* 90, 1887, 2, p. 479: 'apud Archas…crebris ictibus galea quassata cerebrum violatus'.

239 Orderic Vitalis, *Historia Ecclesiastica*, Book XII, 2, cf. *The Ecclesiastical History of Orderic Vitalis*, ed. M. Chibnall, Oxford: Clarendon, 6 vols, 1969–80.

240 Trepanned skulls are known from the archaeological record from prehistoric times onward, and are found in sites from both the Old World and the New. Charlotte Roberts and Keith Manchester, *The Archaeology of Disease*, Stroud: Allan Sutton, 2nd edn, 1995, pp. 93–4 briefly discuss evidence for successful trepanation from Peru, prehistoric France and later European sites, providing references to further literature on this subject.

241 D. De Moulin, *A History of Surgery with Emphasis on the Netherlands*, Dordrecht, Boston, MA and Lancaster: Nijhoff, 1988, p. 59. Could Geert have been subjected to a trepanation because of mental problems? Could he have been regarded as mentally unstable, or even possessed, before he became an acknowledged religious personality? Perhaps it is too modern an assumption to draw a link between a person's mental condition and strong religious fervour. Or did he just have insufferable headaches? All these conditions have been 'treated' with trepanation by different societies at different times.

242 Talbot, *Medicine in Medieval England*, pp. 96–7. Additionally, most of the fractures in arms, legs and collar bones found on the skeletal remains of the individuals buried at Øm had healed. Talbot calls this 'a remarkable tribute both to the surgical knowledge and practice of the monks and of their medical assistants' (ibid.).

243 London, British Library, Sloane 1975, fol. 93.

244 E. J. Kealey, *Medieval Medicus: A Social History of Anglo-Norman Medicine*, Baltimore, MD: Johns Hopkins University Press, 1981, p. 5.

245 'Ben esdeven per aventura, quant que tart,/ Que cavalliers es per so cap feritz de dart/ E per so nas, si que cel olls n'a ben regart,/ Per ses aureylas eissament et d'autra part.' Cited in Paterson, 'Military surgery', p. 132.

246 Now Vienna, Österreichische Nationalbibliothek, Codex Vindobonensis 93, fol. 91v.

247 A. Politzer, *A History of Otology*, transl. S. Milstein, C. Portnoff and A. Coleman from orig. German ed. of 1907, I, Phoenix, AZ: Columella Press, 1981, p. 21.

248 Ibid., p. 25.

249 Ibid., p. 27.

250 *Chirurgia magna*, doctr. III, tract. III, cap. 2: 'aures ad audiendum cum subtilibus vocibus incitare', cited in H. Feldmann, *Die geschichtliche Entwicklung der Hörprüfungsmethoden*, Stuttgart: G. Thieme, 1960, p. 2.

251 Politzer, *A History of Otology*, I, p. 30.

252 '...Þou shalt vndirstonde Þat olde sekenes of Þe eris, and namely defnes, ben vncurable...', Getz (ed.), *Gilbertus Anglicus*, p. 77 [fol. 118v].

253 'It is schewed by Avicen Þat a kyndely deefnesse of euery outake of Þe vttre stoppynge wiÞouteforth and Þat deefnesse Þat is vnkyndely, cronyk of two ȝere, and Þat Þat is of a cicatrisacioun (i. erre) or of an aposteme yhardenede is noght curede.' Book VI, doctrine 2, ch. 2, part 3, *The Cyrurgie of Guy de Chauliac*, p. 472.

254 Hildegard of Bingen, *Subtilitates (Subtleties of Diverse Creatures)*, VII, 4, cf. Thorndike, *A History of Magic and Experimental Science*, 2, p. 145.

255 'Wundarznei' refers to medical procedures dealing with wounds and fractures, as opposed to internal medicine.

256 Mentioned in Harry Kühnel (ed.), *Alltag im Spätmittelalter*, Graz, Vienna and Cologne: Edition Kaleidoskop, 1984, p. 87, which regrettably gives no further reference as to the source for Pfolspeundt's *Wundarznei*. On 'cosmetic' surgery in general, see also W. E. Kunstler, 'Aesthetic considerations in surgical operations from Antiquity to recent times', *Bulletin of the History of Medicine*, 12, 1942, pp. 27–69.

257 On Albucasis, see Schipperges, *Die Kranken im Mittelalter*, p. 162.

258 Cited by T. Anderson and A. R. Carter, 'An archaeological example of medieval trauma', *Journal of Palaeopathology*, 6, 1994, p. 149. Cf. M. F. Ashley Montagu, 'A fourth century reference to anaesthesia', *Bulletin of the History of Medicine*, 19, 1946, pp. 113–14. A manuscript known as the *Bamberg Antidotarium* of the ninth century also mentions anaesthetics, in the form of a 'soporific sponge', and later medical authors too, such as Theodoric, Gilbertus Anglicus, or Guy de Chauliac, made references to such a device (see Garrison, *History of Medicine*, p. 153). For the later medieval period, see L. E. Voigts and R. P. Hudson, 'A surgical anesthetic from late medieval England', in Sheila Campbell, Bert Hall and David Klausner (eds), *Health, Disease and Healing in Medieval Culture*, Basingstoke and London: Macmillan, 1992, pp. 43–56.

259 *Leechdoms*, ed. Cockayne, 2, p. 56. The Old English reads: 'Wið hærscearde: hwit cwudu gecnuwa swiðe smale, do æges Þæt hwite to 7 meng swa Þu dest teafor, onsnið mid seaxse, seowa mid seolce fæste, smire mid Þonne mid Þære sealfe utan 7 innan ær se seoloc rotige. Gif tosomne teo rece mid handa, smire eft sona.'

260 Cameron, *Anglo-Saxon Medicine*, p. 169. Apparently, 'no source has yet been found for this recipe; it would be interesting to know if Anglo-Saxon physicians had worked out these minutiae of treatment by themselves' (ibid.).

261 And in a recipe for sewing a ruptured abdomen, cf. *Leechdoms*, ed. Cockayne, 2, p. 358.

262 A jaundiced person is described as being the colour 'yellow as good silk', *Leechdoms*, ed. Cockayne, 2, p. 106.

263 Cameron, *Anglo-Saxon Medicine*, p. 103. Further links between the development of medicine with the development of commerce and trade routes can be found as linguistic evidence later in the medieval period: the 'apothecary' so commonly encountered in medieval medical professions derives from αποθηκαι the Byzantine term for local depots in the main harbours and at road termini, which comes into wide usage in thirteenth-century Italy, France and Germany, meaning 'druggist'. A lot of drugs needed for prescriptions were only available as imports from the East. 'The fact that the term for an import-export house came to be associated entirely with the meaning 'drug store' demonstrates emphatically the relation between trade and drugs during the early Middle Ages' (J. M. Riddle, 'Theory and practice in medieval medicine', *Viator*, 5, 1974, p. 168). In the ninth and tenth centuries imported ingredients were already utilised in medical recipes, as can be seen from texts of that period, and this shows that even at an early stage there was an import of foreign goods into Anglo-Saxon England. The names of Arabic plants occurring in the *Lacnunga* and the *Leechbook* further supports the implication that 'before the end of the tenth century newly imported Arab trade goods were so well known in England as to be used in the compounding of native remedies' (Cameron, *Anglo-Saxon Medicine*, p. 106).

264 Garrison, *History of Medicine*, p. 159.

265 Cameron, *Anglo-Saxon Medicine*, p. 27.

266 Bede, *Ecclesiastical History of the English People*, V.2, pp. 268–9. Bede mentions that as well as his speech impairment, the young man also had 'many scabs and scales' on his head so that no hair grew; before his cure he is described as being 'deformed, destitute, and dumb' (p. 269). It is interesting to note the association of destitution with impairment here, possibly as part of the topos of *infirmus* and *pauperus*, and the connection between these two categories (this theme will be discussed a little more in Chapter 5.3).

267 *Lacnunga*, CLIIa, cited in Valerie I. J. Flint, *The Rise of Magic in Early Medieval Europe*, Oxford: Oxford University Press, 1991, p. 287. Cf. J. H. G. Grattan and C. Singer, *Anglo-Saxon Magic and Medicine Illustrated Specially from the Semi-Pagan Text 'Lacnunga'*, Oxford: Wellcome Historical Medical Museum, 1952, pp. 180–1.

268 Guglielmo da Saliceto, *Cyrurgia* was printed, together with his *Summa conservationis et curationis*, in Venice, 1489 – his work was therefore still of interest some 200 years after it had originally been written, and was not relegated to the status of outmoded or redundant textbook.

269 Garrison, *History of Medicine*, p. 154.

270 Nancy G. Siraisi, 'How to write a Latin book on surgery: organising principles and authorial devices in Guglielmo da Saliceto and Dino del Garbo' in: L. García-Ballester, R. French, J. Arrizabalaga and A. Cunningham, *Practical Medicine from Salerno to the Black Death*, p. 103.

271 Unfortunately William of Saliceto neglects to inform his readers how old the patient was when the injury was sustained; we therefore have no way of knowing whether the patient died of old age or perhaps of long-term complications associated with the original injury.

272 The three case-studies are mentioned in Guglielmo da Saliceto, *Cyrurgia*, Book 2, chapter 5, and are quoted by Siraisi, 'How to write a Latin book on surgery', p. 103.

273 Galen, *In Hippocratis de articulis librum commentarii*, IV 5–6, cited in Hummel, *Das Kind und seine Krankheiten*, pp. 278–9.

274 Galen, *In Hippocratis de articulis librum commentarii*, IV 8, cited in Hummel, *Das Kind und seine Krankheiten*, pp. 278–9.

275 Galen, *De sanitate tuenda*, V 10, 40–44, cited in Hummel, *Das Kind und seine Krankheiten*, pp. 275–7.

276 Cameron, *Anglo-Saxon Medicine*, pp. 13–14.

277 *Leechdoms*, ed. Cockayne, 1, p. xxvi.

278 *Leechbook*, cited by Rubin, *Medieval English Medicine*, p. 131.
279 Cited in A. W. Beasley, 'Orthopaedic aspects of medieval medicine', *Journal of the Royal Society of Medicine*, 75, 1982, p. 972. Beasley described the illustrations accompanying the manuscript of *De balneis* as giving the impression of a 'community of resort hotels serving the bath houses themselves' (ibid.), which seems to demonstrate the popularity of such treatment methods.
280 *Laws of King Alfred*, 70, cited by W. Bonser, *The Medical Background of Anglo-Saxon England*, London: Wellcome Historical Medical Library, 1963, p. 105.
281 Rubin, *Medieval English Medicine*, p. 132.
282 Cf. F. M. Powicke (ed.), *Life of Ailred*, Edinburgh, 1964, p. 32, cited by Rubin, *Medieval English Medicine*, pp. 91–2.
283 Cf. E. A. Webb, *The Book of the Foundation of the Church of St Bartholomew*, London, Oxford: Oxford University Press, 1923, pp. 18–19, and V. C. Medvei and J. L. Thornton, *The Royal Hospital of St Bartholomew, 1123–1973*, London: Royal Hospital of Saint Bartholomew, 1974, p. 104.
284 Medvei and Thornton, *The Royal Hospital of St Bartholomew*, p. 101.
285 Cameron, *Anglo-Saxon Medicine*, pp. 13–14.
286 Rubin, *Medieval English Medicine*, p. 75.
287 Ingulf, *Croylandensis historia*, in: *Rerum anglicarum scriptorum veterum* tomus i, 1684, pp. 16–17, quoted by Bonser, *The Medical Background of Anglo-Saxon England*, p. 413–14.
288 Cited in Bonser, *The Medical Background of Anglo-Saxon England*, pp. 416–17.
289 See Cameron, *Anglo-Saxon Medicine*, p. 16.
290 Albertus Magnus, *De animalibus*, XXII, ii, 61; cf. Thorndike, *A History of Magic and Experimental Science*, 2, p. 560.
291 John of Gaddesden, *Rosa Anglica*, ed. Wulff, *Irish Texts Society*, 35, 1929, p. 267, cited in Rubin, *Medieval English Medicine*, p. 207.
292 Cameron, *Anglo-Saxon Medicine*, pp. 16–17, citing *Leechdoms*, ed. Cockayne, 2, p. 284:

> Soðlice seo adl cymð on monnan æfter feowertigum oððer fiftigum wintra; gif he bið cealdre gecyndo yonne cymð æfter feowertigum, elcor cymð æfter fiftigum wintra his gærgetales. Gif hit gingran men gelimpe þonne bið tæt eaðlæcnere 7 ne bið seo ylce adl þeah þe ungleawe læcas wenan þæt þæt seo ylce healfdeade adl si. Hu gelic adl on man becume on geogoðe on sumum lime swa swa seo healfdeade adl on yldo deð? Ne bið hit seo healfdeade adl, ac hwilc æthwega yfel wæte bið gegoten on þæt lim þe hit on gesit, ac bið eaðlæcnere. Ac seo soðe healfdeade adl cymð æfter fiftigum wintra.

293 Now London, British Library, Royal 15 E II, fol. 165.
294 Henri de Mondeville, *Chirurgie*, cited in Pouchelle, *The Body and Surgery in the Middle Ages*, p. 17.
295 Cf. Siraisi, *Medieval and Early Renaissance Medicine*, p. 154.
296 Albucasis was translated into Latin by Gerardus of Cremona (1187).
297 Albucasis, *On Surgery and Instruments*, Book 3, ch. 22, transl. and ed. M. S. Spink and G. L. Lewis, London: Wellcome Institute of the History of Medicine, 1973, p. 784. It is interesting to compare Albucasis's non-interventionist moderation with the insistence of modern medicine to better a patient's condition at all costs. For example, people paralysed due to polio ended up suffering from post-polio syndrome, that is, permanent muscle damage, because overly-enthusiastic medical professionals believed that vigorous physical exercise would build up a person's muscle and allow them to be more normal, whereas the muscles in people affected by polio behave differently to muscles in able-bodied people (cf. Deborah Marks, *Disability: Controversial Debates and Psychosocial Perspectives*, London and New York: Routledge, 1999, p. 65).
298 Hummel, *Das Kind und seine Krankheiten*, p. 276.
299 Beasley, 'Orthopedic aspects of medieval medicine', pp. 970–1, and Garrison, *History of Medicine*, p. 154.

300 Beasley, 'Orthopedic aspects of medieval medicine', pp. 970–1.

301 'Tant quan cel os es de novel aissi mogutz.' Cited in Paterson, 'Military surgery', p. 140. Various treatment methods for dislocations are described by Raimon, see Paterson, pp. 140–2.

302 Now London, British Library, MS Sloane 1977, fol. 6.

303 Cf. Talbot, *Medicine in Medieval England*, p. 79.

304 H. E. Handerson, *Gilbertus Anglicus: Medicine of the Thirteenth Century*, Cleveland: Cleveland Medical Library Association, 1918, pp. 68–9.

305 Ibid., p. 69.

306 Book II, ch. 20, *The Surgery of Theoderic* c. A. D. 1267, transl. E. Campbell and J. Colton, vol. I, New York: Appleton – Century – Crofts, 1955, p. 160. This modern edition is based on the printed edition of 1498, where Theoderic's text is bound together with works by Guy de Chauliac.

307 Book II, ch. 23, ibid., p. 177.

308 Book II, ch. 21, ibid., pp. 171–2.

309 Book II, ch. 21, ibid., p. 173.

310 Book II, ch. 42, ibid., p. 202.

311 Cited in Anderson and Carter, 'An archaeological example of medieval trauma', p. 149.

312 Book II, ch. 25, *The Surgery of Theoderic*, p. 180.

313 Book II, ch. 23, ibid., pp. 177–8.

314 Book II, ch. 23, ibid., p. 178. See also the citation from Albucasis, at note 297.

315 Book II, ch. 23, *The Surgery of Theoderic*, p. 178. One may wonder whether the re-breaking of incorrectly healed bones may in fact have led to greater impairment and/or disfigurement than had the initial fracture been left as it knitted together. Not all practitioners of surgery and bonesetting will have followed the advice of Albucasis or Theoderic, so perhaps some impairment was iatrogenic in origin.

316 Book II, ch. 28, ibid.

317 Book II, ch. 29, ibid., p. 185.

318 Book II, ch. 36, ibid., p. 194.

319 Cited in Anderson and Carter, 'An archaeological example of medieval trauma', p. 149.

320 Book II. ch. 48, *The Surgery of Theoderic*.

321 Book II, ch. 30, ibid.

322 De Moulin, *A History of Surgery with Emphasis on the Netherlands*, p. 43.

323 Ibid.

324 Ibid.

325 Book II, ch. 34, *The Surgery of Theoderic*, p. 192.

326 Book II, ch. 44, ibid.

327 Book II, ch. 45, ibid.

328 In a manuscript, at Florence, Biblioteca Laurenziana, MS Plut. 74.7, fol. 200.

329 Book II, ch. 45, *The Surgery of Theoderic*.

330 '…compownede dislocaciouns…ben harde and perylouse…Furyermore an olde dislocacioun (i. vnioyntynge) and harde is harde and as it were inpossible to be curede.' Book V, doctrine 2, ch. 1, *The Cyrurgie of Guy de Chauliac*, p. 351.

331 Book II, ch. 38, *The Surgery of Theoderic*, p. 197.

332 Book II, ch. 40, ibid.

333 Book II, ch. 41, ibid., p. 200.

334 Book II, ch. 54, ibid., p. 218.

335 Garrison, *History of Medicine*, p. 155. He recommended trephining (that is, a form of trepanation, cutting out a round hole from the skull) in cases of depressed bone fragments and irritation of the dura mater.

336 Cf. V. Zimmermann, 'Die mittelalterliche Frakturbehandlung im Werk von Lanfrank und Guy de Chauliac', *Würzburger Medizinhistorische Mitteilungen*, 6, 1988, pp. 21–34.

Lanfranc also wrote a *Libellus (opusculum) de chirurgia* in 1293/4, which was given the short title *Chirurgia parva* in the later Middle Ages. Concerning the omission of vertebral fractures, it might be possible that Lanfranc did not discuss this topic because vertebral fracture often leads to paralysis, which would have been incurable, and therefore not something that Lanfranc or any other medical professional could have treated.

337 De Moulin, *A History of Surgery with Emphasis on the Netherlands*, p. 49.

338 Quoted in Talbot, *Medicine in Medieval England*, p. 105.

339 The illumination shows King Edmund distributing alms; the crippled man holding his leg at the typical ninety-degree angle is just visible on the far right. Manuscript produced at Bury St Edmunds by Master Alexis and studio, of *Life and Miracles of Edmund King and Martyr*, now in New York, Pierpont Morgan Library, MS M.736, fol. 9.

340 Illumination of St Germain blessing the infirm, in a manuscript of the *Légende Dorée* (*Golden Legend*), now Mâcon, Bibliothèque municipale, ms 3, fol. 171.

341 De Moulin, *A History of Surgery with Emphasis on the Netherlands*, pp. 56–7.

342 Cited by Beasley, 'Orthopaedic aspects of medieval medicine', p. 972.

343 'Ausgehend von der Maxime, daß keine Ursache mehr zur Mißbildung eines gebrochenen Gliedes beitrage als der Schmerz, der durch einen allzu festen Verband oder durch eine ungünstige Lagerung entsteht...', Zimmermann, 'Die mittelalterliche Frakturbehandlung', p. 27.

344 See Pouchelle, *The Body and Surgery in the Middle Ages*, pp. 7–8.

345 Now Vienna, Graphische Sammlung Albertina.

346 See a narration of the anecdote in Johann Mach, *Von Aussätzigen und Heiligen. Die Medizin in der mittelalterlichen Kunst Norddeutschlands*, Rostock: Konrad Reich Verlag, 1995, p. 55.

347 Kühnel, *Alltag im Spätmittelalter*, p. 143, and p. 87 for the surgeons' names.

348 Cameron, *Anglo-Saxon Medicine*, p. 171.

349 Cited ibid., p. 170.

350 Cited ibid., pp. 170–1.

351 'Pur os depescé, esplenture e bevre', line 1234, *La Novele Cirurgerie* (Anglo-Norman Text Society 46), ed. C. B. Hieatt and R. B. Jones, London: Anglo-Norman Text Society, 1990, p. 41.

352 See *La Novele Cirurgerie*, p. xxii.

353 Volker Zimmermann, 'Zwischen empirie und magie: die mittelalterliche frakturbehandlung durch die laienpraktiker', *Gesnerus*, 45, 1988, p. 344. The manuscript at Salzburg (Cod. M. III,3, fol. 204va) mentions: 'Zv eym gebrochen beyne solt du ym daz bein ziehen also daz es glich stee.'

354 Cf. F. Koelsch, *Beiträge zur Geschichte der Arbeitsmedizin* (Schriften-reihe der Bayerischen Landesärztekammer Bd. 8), Munich: Bayerische Landesärztekammer, 1976. On the history of occupational diseases cf. also the article by L. J. Goldwater, 'From Hippocrates to Ramazzini: early history of industrial medicine', *Annals of Medical History*, 8, 1936, pp. 27–35, which, however, glosses over the medieval period, save for patronisingly commenting that even as important a medical figure as Avicenna 'made no significant contribution to the science of industrial medicine' (ibid., p. 30).

355 L. Teleky, *History of Factory and Mine Hygiene*, New York: Columbia University Press, 1948, p. 7; cf. Koelsch, *Beiträge zur Geschichte der Arbeitsmedizin*, p. 101.

356 Arnald of Villanova, *Speculum medicinae*, f. 26va (cap. 84), cited by McVaugh, *Medicine Before the Plague*, p. 141.

357 There seems to have been some truth in the uncomfortable writing positions, though, which could lead to physical complications, cf. G. M. Parassoglou, 'Some thoughts on the postures of the ancient Greeks and Romans when writing on papyrus rolls', *Scrittura e Civilita*, 3, 1979.

358 Cited in M. Drogin, *Anathema! Medieval Scribes and the History of Book Curses*, Totowa and Montclair: O. Allanheld, 1983, p. 21. Further examples include this *explicit* by the

scribe Florencio written in a manuscript dating from 945: 'He who knows not how to write thinks that writing is no labour, but be certain, and I assure you that it is true, it is a painful task. It extinguishes the light from the eyes, it bends the back, it crushes the viscera and the ribs, it brings forth pain to the kidneys, and weariness to the whole body': (ibid., pp. 17–18). And Prior Petrus of Santo Domingo de Silos wrote around 1091–1109 at his conclusion to the *Beatus Commentary on the Apocalypse* (British Library MS Add. 11695): 'A man who knows not how to write may think this is no great feat. But only try to do it yourself and you will learn how arduous is the writer's task. It dims your eyes, makes your back ache, and knits your chest and belly together – it is a terrible ordeal for the whole body' (ibid., p. 19). So similar is this complaint by Prior Petro to the earlier one by Florencio that it may well have been copied, or be a part of the same standard, formulaic expression.

359 As late as the early fifteenth century Thomas Hoccleve complained about the bad backs, stomach pains and blurred visions from which professional scribes suffered, cf. Rawcliffe, *Medicine and Society in Later Medieval England*, p. 184. Rawcliffe surmises that the 'demand for salves and washes to ease tired eyes' must have been enormous (ibid.).

360 Cf. Koelsch, *Beiträge zur Geschichte der Arbeitsmedizin*, p. 227. Another writer, Hartmann von der Aue in his *Iwein*, took up Chrétien's description, and alluded to the problems and complaints of the women who were spinning and weaving (ibid.).

361 Ibid., p. 227. There is an illustration of the warming room, which Koelsch calls a sauna, on p. 228.

362 C. L. Paul Trüb, *Heilige und Krankheit* (Geschichte und Gesellschaft. Bochumer Historische Studien, Bd. 19), Stuttgart: Klett – Cotta, 1978, pp. 282–3.

363 Ibid., p. 273.

364 Ibid., p. 285.

365 Cf. the article by G. Grupe, 'Metastasizing carcinoma in a medieval skeleton: differential diagnosis and etiology', *American Journal of Physical Anthropology*, 75, 1988, pp. 369–74.

366 George Rosen, *The History of Miners' Diseases*, New York: Schuman's, 1943.

367 Ibid., pp. 47–8.

368 Ibid., p. 39.

369 Ibid., pp. 54–5.

370 Ibid., p. 58.

371 Ibid., p. 59.

372 Ibid., pp. 60–1.

373 Ibid., pp. 62–3.

374 Ibid., p. 69.

375 Ibid., p. 70.

376 Ibid., pp. 42–4.

377 Ibid., p. 87.

378 Rawcliffe, *Medicine and Society in Later Medieval England*, p. 3, cites the case of the Provençal army, which in 1374 had about a quarter of all its recruits displaying signs of badly scarred hands or faces, plus the unspecified assertion that many English soldiers during the Hundred Years War returned home in a mutilated state.

379 Park, *Doctors and Medicine in Early Renaissance Florence*, pp. 87–8.

380 Cited by V. Nutton, 'Continuity or rediscovery? the city physician in classical antiquity and medieval Italy', in: A. W. Russell (ed.), *The Town and State Physician in Europe from the Middle Ages to the Enlightenment* (Wolfenbütteler Forschungen Bd. 17), Wolfenbüttel: Herzog August Bibliothek, 1981, pp. 26–7.

381 Ibid.

382 Ibid., p. 29.

383 Park, *Doctors and Medicine in Early Renaissance Florence*, p. 91.

384 Ibid., pp. 91–3.

385 Paterson, 'Military surgery', pp. 117–18.

386 Siraisi, *Medieval and Early Renaissance Medicine*, p. 182. Cf. G. E. Gask, 'The medical services of Henry the Fifth's campaign on the Somme in 1415', in: Gask (ed.), *Essays in the History of Medicine*, pp. 94–102. For some more fifteenth-century examples of surgeons and other medical staff accompanying campaigns, see Rawcliffe, *Medicine and Society in Later Medieval England*, p. 140.

387 Illumination in a manuscript of *History of the Romans* produced for Philip the Bold of Burgundy, dated 1465, now Florence, Biblioteca Laurenziana, MS Med. Palat. 156, 1, fol. 181v.

388 Gask, *Essays in the History of Medicine*, p. 63.

389 Susan Edgington, 'Medical knowledge in the crusading armies: the evidence of Albert of Aachen and others', in: Malcolm Barber (ed.), *The Military Orders: Fighting for the Faith and Caring for the Sick*, Aldershot: Ashgate, 1994, pp. 320–6. Interestingly, one crusade account, the *Historia* of Baudri of Dol, mentioned that the sick should be 'supported by a public dole until they have recovered' (cited ibid., p. 324). This seems to indicate that provision was made for the welfare of not just nobles, knights and officers, but of the ordinary soldiers as well.

390 'In obsidione castrorum necessarii sunt medici et maxima vulnera curare scientes.' Cited in Getz, *Medicine in the English Middle Ages*, p. 32 and p. 108 note 126.

391 Paterson, 'Military surgery', p. 125.

392 Ibid., p. 144. Cf. D. Jacquart, *Le Milieu médical en France du XIIIe au XVe siècle*, Paris: Champion, 1981, p. 118.

393 Paterson, 'Military surgery', pp. 144–5. The verses cited by Paterson refer to the presence of doctors at the siege of Beaucaire in 1216, and at the first (1217) and second (1218) sieges of Toulouse.

394 Siraisi, *Medieval and Early Renaissance Medicine*, p. 176.

395 *The Cyrurgie of Guy de Chauliac*, p. 10, which is a fifteenth-century Middle English translation of Guy's *Inventarium seu collectorium in parte cyrurgicali medicine*, originally written at Avignon in 1363. Cf. Siraisi, *Medieval and Early Renaissance Medicine*, p. 35.

396 Translation of phrase and discussion in Siraisi, *Medieval and Early Renaissance Medicine*, p. 176.

397 *Parzival*, 10. 506: 'er begreif der linden einen ast,/er sleiz ein luoft drab als ein rôr/ (er was zer wunden niht ein tôr):/ den schoup er zer tjost in den lîp./dô bat er sûgen daz wîp,/ unz daz bluot gein ir vlôz.' Wolfram von Eschenbach, *Parzival*, 2, pp. 128–31.

398 According to Schipperges, *Die Kranken im Mittelalter*, p. 159, Wolfram von Eschenbach was citing chapter 100 of the second book of Albucasis's *Surgery*, which Gerard of Cremona had translated into Latin in the late twelfth century; this section was entitled *De vulnere eius que est inter spatulas*. Cf. Bernhard D. Haage, 'Chirurgie nach Abu l'Qasim im <Parzifal> Wolframs von Eschenbach', *Clio Medica*, 19, 1984, pp. 193–205.

399 Parzival, 10. 516–17:

> si riten dannen beide,/ ûf eine liehte heide./ ein crût Gâwân dâ stênde sach,/ des würze er wunden helfe jach./ do erbeizte der werde/ nider zuo der erde:/ er gruop si, wider ûf er saz./ diu vrouwe ir rede ouch niht vergaz,/ si sprach 'kan der geselle mîn/ arzet unde ritter sîn,/ Er mac sich harte wol bejagen,/ gelernet er bühsen veile tragen'.

> (Wolfram von Eschenbach, *Parzival*, 2, pp. 146–7)

400 Heidelberg, Universitätsbibliothek, Cod. Pal. Germ. 848, fol. 158r.

401 Compare the dress of the man in the white cap here in the Manesse codex with the dress we know for certain to be a surgeon's in a French manuscript of Roger's *Chirurgia* (London, British Library, MS Sloane 1977, fol. 6): both the Manesse codex and the *Chirurgia* manuscript date from the early fourteenth century, so that we can make such comparisons relating to apparel.

402 For a discussion of the problematic term 'magical', and differences between modern and medieval concepts of 'magic', see the introductory remarks in my article 'Responses to physical impairment in Medieval Europe: between magic and medicine', *Medizin, Gesellschaft und Geschichte*, 18, 1999, pp. 9–35.

403 William Langland, *Piers the Ploughman*, transl. and intro. J. F. Goodridge, Harmondsworth: Penguin, first published 1959, revised edn, 1966, pp. 161–2

404 Cited in Finucane, *Miracles and Pilgrims*, p. 69. Cf. Lynn Thorndike, *Michael Scot*, London, 1965, p. 78. In the earlier middle ages, authorities were not so tolerant: Caesarius of Arles, in discussing the healing practices of women for their infirm children, defines the use of magic for such purposes as the complement of abortion, even as more cruel than abortion (sermo LII, *Sancti Caesarii Arelatensis sermones*, ed. G. Morin, Corpus Christianorum Series Latina 103, Turnhout: Brepols, 1963, pp. 230–3, especially p. 232:5–6).

405 I have discussed incidences of such transference rituals elsewhere (Metzler, 'Responses to physical impairment in medieval Europe: between magic and medicine', *Medizin, Gesellschaft und Geschichte*, 18, 1999.

406 Richard Kieckhefer, *Magic in the Middle Ages*, Cambridge: Cambridge University Press, 1989, p. 59.

407 Jean-Claude Schmitt, *The Holy Greyhound: Guinefort, Healer of Children Since the Thirteenth Century*, transl. M. Thom, Cambridge and Paris: Cambridge University Press, 1983.

408 Another aspect of the cult of St Guinefort revolved around changeling beliefs, whereby sick or impaired children were believed to be 'bogus' children, who had been substituted for a mother's 'real' child by supernatural beings, the 'real' child having been abducted by fawns, pixies, demons or such like. Besides the discussion of this topos in Schmitt, *The Holy Greyhound*, and my own contribution (Metzler, 'Responses to physical impairment in medieval Europe', pp. 24–5), the changeling belief is dealt with by Carl Haffter, 'The changeling: history and psychodynamics of attitudes to handicapped children in European folklore', *Journal of the History of the Behavioural Sciences*, 4, 1968, pp. 55–61, and L. Röhrich, 'Zwerge in Sage und Märchen', in: Alfred Enderle, Dietrich Meyerhöfer and Gerd Unverfehrt (eds), *Kleine Menschen – Große Kunst. Kleinwuchs aus künstlerischer und medizinischer Sicht*, Hamm: Artcolor Verlag, 1992, pp. 53–4. In southern Europe, especially in Greece, one encounters the legend of the *kalikandjarai* who exchange healthy babies for sickly and whineing infants. This exchange is possible because the infant has not yet been baptised, since the unbaptised baby is seen as 'still a piece of flesh' (Claudine Fabre-Vassas, *The Singular Beast: Jews, Christians, and the Pig*, transl. C. Volk, New York: Columbia University Press, 1997, p. 274).

409 The Old English text reads: 'Se wifman se hire cild afedan ne mæg. Gange to gewitenes mannes birgenne 7 stæppe Þonne Þriwa ofer Þa byrgenne 7 cweðe Þonne Þriwa Þas word: Þis me to bote Þære laÞan lætbyrde; Þis me to bote Þære swæran swærtbyrde; Þis me to bote Þære laðan lambyrde.' Cited in Grattan and Singer, *Anglo-Saxon Magic and Medicine*, pp. 188–90.

410 On the 'nocturnal visitors', see Bonser, *The Medical Background of Anglo-Saxon England*, p. 269. Anglo-Saxon reference can be found in *Leechbook* III, lxi: 'wið ælfcynne and nihtgengan and ðám mannum ðe deófol mid hæmð'. See also the discussion of 'nightwalkers' by Audrey L. Meaney, 'The Anglo-Saxon view of illness', in: Campbell, Hall and Klausner (eds), *Health, Disease and Healing in Medieval Culture*, p. 20. For a more detailed discussion of the influence of otherworldy, supernatural beings in Anglo-Saxon culture see Jolly, *Popular Religion in Late Saxon England*.

411 Salzburg, Cod. M. III, 3, fol. 396 rb, cf. Zimmermann, 'Zwischen Empirie und Magie', p. 349:

> Dem ein bein brichet es sy wie es wolle. Der neme eines hundes welpffen der eines dages alt ist vnd sol ym sin hut abe ziehen vnn sol sin hern dar jnne legen vnd sol daz legen uber daz gebrochen beine so heylet es gantz wider.

412 Salzburg, Cod. M. III, 3, fol. 396 rb, cf. Zimmermann, 'Zwischen Empirie und Magie', p. 345.
413 Getz, *Medicine in the English Middle Ages*, p. 90.

5 Medieval miracles and impairment

1 Raymond Van Dam, *Saints and their Miracles in Late Antique Gaul*, Princeton, NJ: Princeton University Press, 1993.
2 André Vauchez, *Sainthood in the Later Middle Ages*, transl. J. Birrell, Cambridge: Cambridge University Press, 1997.
3 Michael E. Goodich, *Violence and Miracle in the Fourteenth Century: Private Grief and Public Salvation*, Chicago, IL and London: University of Chicago Press, 1995.
4 Benedicta Ward, *Miracles and the Medieval Mind: Theory, Record and Event 1000–1215*, Aldershot: Wildwood House, first published 1982, revised edn, 1987.
5 Ronald C. Finucane, *Miracles and Pilgrims: Popular Beliefs in Medieval England*, Basingstoke: Macmillan, first published 1977, new edn, 1995, and Finucane, *The Rescue of the Innocents: Endangered Children in Medieval Miracles*, Basingstoke and London: Macmillan, 1997.
6 Eleanora C. Gordon, 'Child health in the middle ages as seen in the miracles of five English saints, A.D. 1150–1220', *Bulletin of the History of Medicine*, 60, 1986, pp. 502–22.
7 Finucane, *The Rescue of the Innocents*.
8 Finucane, *Miracles and Pilgrims*, p. 103.
9 Ibid., Finucane suggests these paralyses may be hemiplegia, but points out that medieval terminology employed 'paralysis' in a very loose sense.
10 Ibid., p. 104. The *contracta* refers to a miracle of St Thomas Cantilupe. Pierre-André Sigal, *L'homme et le miracle dans la France médiévale (XIe–XIIe siècle)*, Paris: Éditions du Cerf, 1985, p. 240, also discusses the terminology employed by medieval writers for the varieties of mobility impairments; he mentions *contractus, aridus, debilitatus, emortuus* (having a deadened limb), *mancus* (inability to move the upper limbs), and *claudus* (inability to move the lower limbs).
11 Ibid.
12 On this issue see also the discussion in Raymond Van Dam, *Leadership and Community in Late Antique Gaul*, Berkeley, Los Angeles, CA and London: University of California Press, 1985, pp. 258–60, who argues that modern scepticism toward miracles, the dismissal of medieval impairments as 'psychological illusions', and strict reliance upon a scientific, rationalistic viewpoint just serve to obscure our understanding of a past society 'by imposing on it our own misgivings' (p. 259).
13 Finucane, *Miracles and Pilgrims*, p. 103. In his introduction to the paperback edition of *Miracles and Pilgrims*, Finucane addressed the criticisms voiced by some reviews of his work, that on the one hand he had attempted to identify the ailments too specifically, while on the other hand he was faulted for not being more specific and mathematically detailed (ibid., p. 3).
14 Sigal, *L'homme et le miracle*, does attempt to categorise illnesses and impairments in medieval miracle stories according to modern medical criteria. His chapter on miracle healings (chapter 5 *L'homme et le miracle*) is arranged by modern type of illness, for example, blindness and eye disorders; deafness, speech and hearing disorders; mental illness; 'neurological' disorders, to which Sigal ascribes most mobility impairments; fevers and infectious diseases; tumours and ulcers; haemorrhages, traumas and wounds; St Anthony's fire ('mal des ardents'); a category Sigal termed 'diverse illnesses'; serious illnesses that have not been identified; and resurrections. One may observe the problem Sigal faced in trying to impose modern medical categories onto the medieval narrative. Sigal was to a degree aware of this. He believed the cause of an illness or impairment was rarely given in the sources because, on the one hand, the lack of medical knowledge in the medieval period, as he presumed, prevented

accurate diagnosis, and, on the other hand, diagnosis was of no particular interest to the hagiographers (Sigal, p. 228). The latter point is perfectly valid, but modern scholarly opinions on the standards achieved by medieval medicine have advanced somewhat since Sigal's statement.

15 See Ward, *Miracles and the Medieval Mind*, pp. 29–31.

16 Ronald C. Finucane, *The Rescue of the Innocents*, p. 3.

17 See also the description of the types of questions posed by a papal commission into the canonisation of Thomas Cantilupe in 1307, in Finucane, *Miracles and Pilgrims*, p. 53.

18 For a valuable source collection of hagiographical material in translation cf. Thomas Head (ed.), *Medieval Hagiography: An Anthology*, New York and London: Routledge, 2001.

19 Their status as twins may in itself be of interest: in many cultures, from medieval Christian Europe to modern West African tribal cultures, twins are believed to have special powers, or the birth of twins is believed to hold portents of good or evil. On twins in general, see John Lash, *Twins and the Double*, London: Thames & Hudson, 1993. For medieval concepts of twins, cf. J. M. Thijssen, 'Twins as monsters: Albertus Magnus's theory of the generation of twins and its philosophical context', *Bulletin of the History of Medicine*, 61, 1987, pp. 237–46.

20 For example in the painting by Fra Angelico, made 1439–42, on a predella for the altarpiece of San Marco, now at Florence, Museo di San Marco.

21 J. M. Riddle, 'Theory and practice in medieval medicine', *Viator*, 5, 1974, p. 166; cf. Anneliese Wittmann, *Kosmas und Damian. Kultausbreitung und Volksdevotion*, Berlin: E. Schmidt, 1967.

22 V. L. Bullough, 'The development of medical guilds at Paris', *Medievalia et humanistica*, 12, 1958, p. 36. Apparently St Louis founded the college at the instigation of his surgeon, Jean Pitard. Since the historic Jean Pitard died in 1327 or 1328, he is highly unlikely to have been the surgeon during Louis' crusade of 1248–54, as the story claims.

23 Emil F. Frey, 'Saints in medical history', *Clio Medica*, 14, 1979, pp. 35–70, provides a list with brief description of many saints and their associated patronage of specific diseases, as well as their depiction in art, together with a useful bibliography of hagiographical material.

24 S. v. 'Giles', in D. H. Farmer, *The Oxford Dictionary of Saints*, Oxford: Oxford University Press, 3rd edn, 1992.

25 There seems to have been an interplay between the saint's cult and the depiction of Giles as lame, mainly in thirteenth-century France. 'The process of translating the *vita* into pictorial form seems therefore to have collaborated with, if it did not inspire, the invention of the lame Giles and the cult's association with the crippled.' (Marcia Kupfer, *The Art of Healing: Painting for the Sick and the Sinner in a Medieval Town*, Pennsylvania: Pennsylvania State University Press, 2003, p. 95. With regard to the hagiographical image of Giles as lame, Kupfer cites Ethel Claire Jones, *St Gilles: Essai d'histoire littéraire*, Paris, 1914, who had argued that the tradition, making Giles lame had originated in England, seen for example in the dedication of a church to Giles in London's 'Cripplegate' during the last decade of the twelfth century.

26 S. v. 'Gilbert', in Farmer, *The Oxford Dictionary of Saints*. Farmer regrettably does not mention in what way Gilbert of Sempringham had been impaired. However, Shulamith Shahar, *Childhood in the Middle Ages*, London and New York: Routledge, 1992, p. 148, refers to Gilbert as 'an ugly and misshapen child' who had to eat with the family's servants, and who was intimidated by his father to such a degree that he became what we would now refer to as 'retarded', so that he 'was considered slow-witted' (cf. also *Acta Sanctorum*, Feb. 1, p. 572).

27 S. v. 'Osmund', in Farmer, *The Oxford Dictionary of Saints*.

28 Cf. C. L. Paul Trüb, *Heilige und Krankheit* (Bochumer Historische Studien 19), Stuttgart: Klett-Cotta, 1978.

29 D. Guthrie, *A History of Medicine*, London: Nelson, 1945, pp. 98–100.

30 Farmer, *The Oxford Dictionary of Saints*, s. v. 'Dunstan', 'Thomas', 'Raphael'.
31 Tobit became blinded after warm sparrow dung fell into his eyes, and his physicians failed to cure him (Tobit 2:10); after eight years he was cured when his son Tobias rubbed his eyes with the gall of a fish (Tobit 11:11–13), according to what Raphael had told Tobias to do.
32 Guthrie, *A History of Medicine*, pp. 98–100.
33 Trüb, *Heilige und Krankheit*, provides a comprehensive listing of saints and their area of patronage, covering patronage by saints of eye diseases and blindness (pp. 272–4), gout and rheumatic disorders (pp. 282–3), lameness and crippling disorders (pp. 284–5) and hearing disorders (p. 286).
34 Vauchez, *Sainthood in the Later Middle Ages*, p. 466.
35 Ibid., p. 468. Vauchez based his data on various processes of canonisation, for the period 1201–1300 on: St Gilbert of Sempringham (process 1201), St Hugh of Lincoln (1219), Hugh of Bonnevaux (*c.*1221), John Cacciafronte of Vicenza (1223–4), Ambrose of Massa (1240), Lawrence Loricatus (1240), Simon of Collazzone (1252), Philip of Bourges (1265–6); and for the period 1301–1417 on: St Peter of Morrone (1306), St Louis of Anjou (1307), St Nicholas of Tolentino (1323), St Yves (1330), Delphine of Puimichel (1363), Charles of Blois (1371), Urban V (1381), Peter of Luxembourg (1389–90), Dorothy of Montau (1404–6) and Nicholas of Linköping (1417).
36 Pierre-André Sigal, 'Maladie, pèlerinage et guérison au XIIe siècle. Les miracles de saint Gibrien à Reims', *Annales Économies, Sociétés, Civilisations*, 24(6), 1969, pp. 1522–39. St Gibrien appears to have been one of the insular missionaries active in Merovingian Gaul, dying there around 509. Shortly after the transportation of the saint's body to Reims cathedral in 1154 miracles at his shrine began to multiply, and it is during the period April to August 1154 that the 102 miracles were recorded by one of the monks at Reims.
37 'Presque tous cherchent à prouver que le saint qu'ils célèbrent est supérieur à tous les autres, et qu'il guérit ceux qui ont fait en vain d'autres pèlerinages.' Sigal, 'Maladie, pèlerinage et guérison au XIIe siècle', p. 1523.
38 Ibid. In his later book, *L'homme et le miracle*, Sigal again emphasises the healing function of medieval saints, in that healing miracles are almost to be seen as miracles *per se* in the eleventh and twelfth centuries. Medieval saints 'ressemblant en cela aux thaumaturges de presque toutes les époques' (*L'homme et le miracle*, p. 227).
39 Ibid., p. 1526.
40 Ibid., p. 1527 note 1.
41 Ibid., p. 1527. It is interesting to note that in the description of individual cases, the medieval writer has regarded it as sufficient that someone had lost the use of a limb, where the muscles had atrophied, for this to be termed a 'contracted' (*contractus*) or 'whithered' (*aridus*) limb. Sometimes the writer has mentioned an underlying cause, such as a badly reduced fracture or an infection, which led to the loss of use of a limb.
42 Ibid., pp. 1527–8.
43 Ibid., p. 1527.
44 Ibid.
45 For all further details regarding these texts, such as which editions used, location of original manuscript(s), and structure of the texts, I would kindly ask the reader to refer to the relevant introduction to each miracle collection given in the Appendix.
46 This figure includes miracles that are just listed by the writers without further details, for example, the short list in Appendix M prologue to second part, which provides a shorthand itemisation of pilgrims cured at Rocamadour.
47 See Appendix W VII.i.
48 I refer the reader to the relevant sections in the Appendix for a more detailed analysis of the individual breakdown into healing categories as far as the miracles by these three saints are concerned.

49 Finucane, *Miracles and Pilgrims*, p. 59.

50 Benedicta Ward, in her seminal study of medieval notions of miracles, seems to think that cures fall into patterns which were evidenced at shrines everywhere; she explains these patterns as being constituted by a mixture of medical diagnosis and literary example from the gospels (Ward, *Miracles and the Medieval Mind*, pp. 34–5).

51 Sigal, 'Maladie, pèlerinage et guérison au XIIe siècle', p. 1528: 'Pourquoi cette pré-dominance? Y avait-il réellement une très forte proportion de paralysés et d'aveugles dans la population souffrante du Moyen Age, ou bien y a-t-il là imitation d'un mod-èle évangélique auquel on ne peut s'empêcher de penser, les deux miraculés typiques du Nouveau Testament étant justement l'aveugle et le paralytique?'

52 Ibid., p. 1528 note 2, citing Evelyne Patlagean, 'Ancienne hagiographie byzantine et histoire sociale', *Annales Économies, Sociétés, Civilisations*, 1968, p. 119, who argued that it was evidently a mixture of both biblical imitation and reality.

53 Marcus Bull, *The Miracles of Our Lady at Rocamadour: Analysis and Translation*, Woodbridge, NJ: Boydell Press, 1999, p. 13.

54 Not to mention the healing of the insane or lunatics, as in the healing of the madman of Gerasa (Matthew 8:28–34, Mark 5:1–20, Luke 8:26–39), not discussed further since mental disability is not the concern of this book.

55 Matthew 9:1–8, Mark 2:1–12, Luke 5:17–26.

56 Matthew 12:9–14, Mark 3:1–6, Luke 6:6–11, also discussed by Jerome, *Commentary* on Matthew 12:13. According to a later tradition, this man had been a bricklayer who could no longer go about his trade due to his withered hand, and had to beg for a living, cf. H. Krauss and E. Uthemann, *Was Bilder erzählen. Die klassischen Geschichten aus Antike und Christentum in der abendländischen Malerei*, Munich: C. H. Beck, 1987, pp. 287–91.

57 Mark 10:46–52, Luke 18:35–43, though two beggars are mentioned at Matthew 20:29–34.

58 Mentioned only by John 5:1–18.

59 Mentioned only by John 9, but then concerns the entire chapter.

60 Cf. D. W. Amundsen and G. B. Ferngren, 'The Early Christian Tradition', in: R. L. Numbers and D. W. Amundsen (eds), *Caring and Curing: Health and Medicine in the Western Religious Traditions*, New York and London: Collier Macmillan, 1986, pp. 44–5.

61 Ibid., p. 45.

62 John 9:2–3.

63 John 5:14: the man just cured at the pool of Bethesda is told to go away and sin no more, lest something worse (i.e. worse than being lame) happen to him.

64 Eadmer, *Vita Anselmi*, Book II.liii, cf. *The Life of St Anselm Archbishop of Canterbury by Eadmer*, ed. and transl. R. W. Southern, London and Edinburgh: T. Nelson, 1962, p. 131: 'quidam homo pedes suos baculo regente'.

65 Ibid., 'Virtus crucis Christi illuminet oculos istos, et ab eis omnem infirmitatem depellat, integraeque sanitate restituat.'

66 Matthew 11:5.

67 Luke 7:22.

68 Isaiah 35:5 and 61:1.

69 Physicians are barely mentioned in the Bible, and where they are, their powers and skills are seen as quite inferior to divine healing, such as in the story of king Asa (2 Chronicles 16:12–13), who died aged 93 after seeking help unsuccessfully from his doctors and not from God.

70 John 11:37.

71 Matthew 15:31.

72 Mark 7:37.

73 Luke 11:14.

74 Appendix E MII 24.

75 John 9:17.

76 Appendix F 1.1.
77 Appendix F 1.2.
78 Appendix F 1.28.
79 Appendix F 1.29.
80 Appendix G 222: 'Sancto Godrico medicante'.
81 Appendix I V: 'manuque protensa quasi medici functus officio, oculos...tetigit'.
82 Appendix F 2.4.
83 Luke 13:11–13.
84 Appendix M III.10.
85 See also the discussion in Ward, *Miracles and the Medieval Mind*, pp. 3–8.
86 Acts 3:10.
87 William McCready, *Miracles and the Venerable Bede*, Toronto: Pontifical Institute of Medieval Studies, 1994, p. 56; cf. Bede, *In Abacuc, Corpus Christianorum Series latina* (hereafter CCSL.), Turnhout: Brepols, 1953, vol. 119B, p. 400, and *In Marc.*, CCSL., vol. 120, pp. 474–5 on the reactions of the scribes, as they deal with Christ's healing miracle of the paralytic in Mark 2:22. Bede further commented on the New Testament miracles, *In Marc.*, CCSL., vol. 120, p. 534, on healing as an allegory of spiritual cure, and in *Hom. Evan.*, CCSL., vol. 122, p. 220, on the healing of the deaf-mute man in Mark 7, and *In Marc.*, CCSL., vol. 120, p. 567, on the healing of the blind man in Mark 8.
88 McCready, *Miracles and the Venerable Bede*, p. 108.
89 Ælfric, *Homilies*, cited in: Karen Louise Jolly, *Popular Religion in Late Saxon England: Elf Charms in Context*, Chapel Hill, NC and London: University of North Carolina Press, 1996, p. 84. See also *The Homilies of Ælfric*, ed. Benjamin Thorpe, 2 vols, London: Ælfric Society, 1844 and 1846, vol. 1, p. 292, with further references to miracles on p. 304.
90 Cf. Jolly, *Popular Religion in Late Saxon England*, p. 69.
91 Thomas of Celano, *Vita Prima*, 121, cited by: Eamon Duffy, 'Finding St Francis: early images, early lives', in: Peter Biller and A. J. Minnis (eds), *Medieval Theology and the Natural Body* (York Studies in Medieval Theology 1), York: York Medieval Press, 1997, p. 213.
92 Reminiscent of the list of impairments cured by Christ given at Matthew 11:15 and Luke 7:22.
93 Painting depicting the miracles of St Francis: at top St Francis heals crippled people, below he heals a lame man, located in the church of San Francesco.
94 Appendix G cap.cxxii: 'In nomine Jesu Christi Nazareni, surge et ambula'.
95 For example, at Matthew 9:7, Mark 2:12 and John 5:9, where Christ told paralytic and lame people to 'rise and walk'.
96 Dan Michel, *Ayenbite of Inwyt*, ed. Richard Morris, *Early English Text Society*, o. s. 23, 1866, new edn, Pamela Gradon, reissue 1965, p. 56. The *Ayenbite* was written around 1340 by Dan Michel (Michel of Northgate) at Canterbury, who in his preface claims the text is all his own (p. 1). It is, however, a literal translation from the French into Middle English of *Le somme des Vices et de Virtues*, composed for Philip II of France in 1279 by the Dominican Laurentius Gallus. See also the discussion in G. R. Owst, *Literature and Pulpit in Medieval England: A Neglected Chapter in the History of English Letters and of the English People*, Oxford: Blackwell, 2nd edn, 1966, p. 438.
97 Cf. Matthew 20:30–34, Mark 10:46–52, Luke 18:35–43, where the man is called Bartimæus.
98 Lecture presented by Prof. Vivian Nutton, 'God, Galen and the depaganisation of ancient medicine', University of York, 21 May 1999.
99 Bull, *The Miracles of Our Lady of Rocamadour*, p. 13.
100 Ibid.
101 Ibid., It is interesting to note that Bull does not cite or list in his bibliography a single medieval medical text, or even a modern work on medical history, when making this statement.

102 Ibid., p. 14.
103 Miracle I.48, Bull, *The Miracles of Our Lady of Rocamadour*, p. 132.
104 Prologue, ibid., p. 98.
105 Miracle I.7, ibid., p. 107.
106 Miracle I.14, ibid., p. 112.
107 Miracle I.28, ibid., 1999.
108 Miracle I.43, ibid., p. 129.
109 Ibid.
110 Vauchez, *Sainthood in the Later Middle Ages*, p. 466.
111 Bede, *Life of Cuthbert*, ch. 45, in: *The Age of Bede*, transl. J. F. Webb, London: Penguin, 1983, pp. 99–100.
112 Ibid., p. 99.
113 Ibid.
114 McCready, *Miracles and the Venerable Bede*, p. 43. Bede relates more accounts of miraculous healings in his own time in *Historica ecclesiastica gentis Anglorum* (modern edition: *Ecclesiastical History of the English People*, transl. L. Sherley-Price, London: Penguin, 1990): sick people are healed and miracles frequently take place to this day at St Albans (1.7, p. 54); the church of Paulinus at Lincoln may be in ruins, but miracles of healing still take place there (II.16, p. 134); and at St Chad's tomb in Lichfield there is a shrine-like little house made of wood, with holes in the wall so that people can put their hands through to gather dust, which is then mixed with water and given to sick people and animals to drink (IV.3, p. 211). However, none of these miracles contemporary to Bede are further specified, they are just general healing miracles of 'sick' people.
115 Valerie J. Flint, 'The early medieval "medicus," the saint – and the enchanter', *Social History of Medicine*, 2, 1989, pp. 127–45.
116 Gregory of Tours, *The History of the Franks*, V.6, transl. Lewis Thorpe, London: Penguin, 1974, p. 263.
117 Flint, 'The early medieval "medicus" ', pp. 134–5 and note 27.
118 Gregory of Tours, *The History of the Franks*, V.6, pp. 263–4.
119 Flint, 'The early medieval "medicus" ', p. 135 ff.
120 When Gregory of Tours had a stomach ache he tried hot baths and poultices first – fairly typical medical treatment – but after enduring constant pain for six days, he turned to the relics of St Martin and was cured instantly (Gregory of Tours, *The Wonders of St Martin*, book iv, cf. Edward James, 'A sense of wonder: Gregory of Tours, medicine and science', in M. A. Meyers (ed.), *The Culture of Christendom: Essays in Medieval History in commemoration of Denis L. T. Bethell*, London and Rio Grande: Hambledon Press, 1993, p. 56). Gregory criticised physicians and other healers not because of what kind of treatment they offered, but because, in his view, they did not apparently 'recognize the subordination of themselves and their remedies to beliefs in the exclusive curative power of Christian relics and saints' (Van Dam, *Leadership and Community in Late Antique Gaul*, p. 262).
121 Appendix E MI 45. It is not made clear by the text whether the reference to 'others' refers to other forms of treatment, for example, by physicians, or to unsuccessful visits to other saints' shrines.
122 Appendix G 131.
123 Appendix G 115.
124 Appendix G 103: 'pedum et tibiarum tumorem incurabilem... quem nulla medicinalis industria mitigare vel curare'.
125 Appendix G 160.
126 Appendix E MI 104.
127 Appendix E MI 67.
128 Appendix E MI 94. Medicine was regarded as an 'art', as an addition to the seven liberal arts.

129 Appendix E MII 5.
130 Appendix J XVIII. Gilbert was blinded in punishment for a transgression, which may explain the inefficiency of secular medicine, since heavenly punishment was lifted by heavenly cure – a case of like needs to be cured with like, perhaps.
131 Appendix F L.5.
132 Appendix I II.
133 Appendix I VI: 'Aderant medici, arte et labore plurimo agentes, ut dolorem ei aut tollerent aut lenirent.'
134 Appendix W VI.xii: 'Medici frustra laborantes adhibentur.'
135 Appendix W III.vii: 'licet in illis multum expenderit, curari potuit medicos'.
136 Appendix M I.15.
137 Appendix M I.20.
138 Appendix M I.24. This is another case where the original impairment was caused by deliberate divine punishment for a transgression, so that the cure also had to be a divine one.
139 Appendix M I.35. The squire was also punished for transgression.
140 Appendix M III.3.
141 Appendix M III.21.
142 Appendix M II.15.
143 Appendix M II.18.
144 Appendix M II.24.
145 Appendix M II.41.
146 Appendix W IV.ix: 'mihi uouere uolo se nullam ulterius alteram preter huiusmodi meam suscepturum medicinam'; 'medicis persuadentibus tandem heu consensit, et fallacis medicine asylo se contulit'.
147 Finucane, *Miracles and Pilgrims*, p. 59.
148 On the 'hierarchy of resort' in anthropology see Arthur Kleinman, *Patients and Healers in the Context of Culture: Exploration of the Borderline Between Anthropology, Medicine, and Psychiatry*, Berkeley and Los Angeles, CA: University of California Press, 1980, and Allan Young, 'The Anthropologies of Illness and Sickness, *Annual Review of Anthropology*, 11, 1982, pp. 257–85; for this concept in the medieval period there is some discussion by Katherine Park, 'Medicine and society in medieval Europe, 500–1500', in: A. Wear (ed.), *Medicine and Society: Historical Essays*, Cambridge: Cambridge University Press, rpt. 1993, pp. 59–90, especially p. 73.
149 In a study of Southern Italian hagiographical texts of the ninth to eleventh centuries, Clare Pilsworth ('Medicine and Hagiography in Italy *c.*800–*c.*1000', *Social History of Medicine*, 13(2), 2000, p. 259) mentions several references to the failure of doctors to heal patients. It is a distinctive feature of Neapolitan hagiographical sources of that period that pilgrims, who had previously been unable to obtain a cure, are cured by the saint through incubation at the saint's tomb. The failure of physicians also features in Northern Italian hagiographies, but is not as prominent a topos as in the Southern hagiography of the same period.
150 Finucane, p. 64.
151 Bede, *Ecclesiastical History of the English People*, Book V ch. 6, pp. 272–4.
152 Ibid., p. 274.
153 William of Malmesbury, *De gestis reguum Anglorum*, ii.224, cited by Wilfred Bonser, *The Medical Background of Anglo-Saxon England*, London: Wellcome Historical Medical Library, 1963, pp. 182 and 273. On the same day as Wulfwin, a further three blind men and one monocular man were cured through the water touched by Edward the Confessor.
154 Helen Lubin and P. Barker (eds), *The Worcester Pilgrim*, Worcester: Worcester Cathedral Publications, 1990, p. 30, cf. Robert Nicholl, *St Oswald and St Wulfstan: Their Shrines and Miracles*, n.p., 1989.
155 Appendix V RO 11: 'pedem eius sese abscissurum esse'.

156 Ian McDougall, 'The third instrument of medicine: some accounts of surgery in medieval Iceland', in: Sheila Campbell, Bert Hall and David Klausner (eds), *Health, Disease and Healing in Medieval Culture*, Basingstoke and London: Macmillan, 1992, p. 60.

157 Appendix E MII 20. Of course, this story can also be read as a moralising tale, whereby heavenly (that is, saintly) medicine has to be presented as the superior medicine over mundane physic.

158 Appendix F 4.17.

159 Appendix M II.32.

160 Appendix F 1.1.

161 Appendix J XVIII.

162 Appendix W IV.ix. William the sacrist dies of his illness four days after breaking his vow. This is the only case among the sources I have studied in detail where the afflicted person is not given a chance to redeem themselves, and in repentance to obtain a cure.

163 Appendix G 220.

164 An analysis of the works of Gregory of Tours by Michael Sierck (*Festtag und Politik. Studien zur Tagewahl karolingischer Herrscher*, Cologne, 1995, cited by Arnold Angenendt, *Geschichte der Religiosität im Mittelalter*, Darmstadt: Wissenschaftliche Buchgesellschaft, 1997, p. 622) found 24 cases where the hands of workers dried up or shrivelled, five cases of blinding, one instance each of lameness in hands and feet, backwards twisting of the face and birth of a crippled child. Such punishments for disobeyance of particularly the special status of Sunday (*Sonntagsschändung*) carry with them in the majority of cases an action of drying up, related to heat in other words, or of fire and light (losing one's sight) – all punishments that can be connected with *Sun*day and can therefore be interpreted as mirroring punishments (*spiegelnde Strafen*). Such narratives of punishment then take on a moral and symbolic meaning, rather than reflecting a belief in the actual punishment of transgressions.

165 The story is related by Abbot Samson, *Opus de miraculis de S. Ædmundi*, I.viii, cited by Thomas Arnold (ed.), *Memorials of St Edmund's Abbey*, Rolls Series, 1890, vol. i, p. 134. Another source for the same story is Herman of Bury, *Miracles of St Edmund*, written *c.*1100, also in Arnold, *Memorials*, pp. 53–4. None other than Guibert of Nogent also related this episode, stating that soon after the sacrilege Leofstan 'wasted away with a permanent palsy of both hands' (*Self and Society in Medieval France*, III.20, John F. Benton (ed.), Toronto: University of Toronto Press, 1984, p. 225).

166 Cf. Denis Bethell, 'The miracles of St Ithamar', *Analecta Bollandiana*, 89, 1971, p. 424.

167 Appendix F 3.6.

168 Appendix F 1.2.

169 Appendix F 3.10. Similarly, another lord and fifty of his men were blinded when they tried to seize lands belonging to St Foy's abbey, and again they were healed after suitable repentance (F 3.14). And yet another lord and all his children either died miserably or were impaired in punishment for the lord's 'great hostility' to St Foy (F 3.17).

170 Appendix F 1.15.

171 Appendix F 1.15.

172 Appendix F 1.1.

173 Appendix F 1.1. There is a similar cycle of miracles related of St Benedict, where the paralytic peasant who was cured was also struck with his original affliction each time he sinned by fornicating (*The Book of Sainte Foy*, transl. with an intro. and notes Pamela Sheingorn, Philadelphia, PA: University of Pennsylvania Press, 1995, p. 290 note 18).

174 Appendix M I.4. Similarly, a knight who harassed a pilgrim was punished with ergotism in his foot (M I.24). And the thieves who attacked three pilgrims were struck blind and paralysed (M II.9).

175 Appendix M I.6.

176 Appendix M I.3.

177 Appendix M II.24.
178 Appendix M I.35.
179 Appendix M I.22. Interestingly, going to the local church of St Anthony did not help this woman, instead she had to make the far longer journey to Rocamadour to obtain a cure.
180 Appendix M II.26.
181 Appendix M III.11.
182 Finucane, *The Rescue of the Innocents*, p. 80, citing Reginald R. Darlington (ed.), *The Vita Wulfstani of William of Malmesbury... and the Miracles*, London: Camden Society Third Series, vol. 40, 1928, p. 140.
183 Van Dam, *Leadership and Community in Late Antique Gaul*, ch. 'Illness, Healing, and Relic Cults', pp. 256–76.
184 For example, in Gregory of Tour's *Life of St Julian*, a man who ploughed on a Sunday ended up with a paralysed hand, cf. Van Dam, *Leadership and Community in Late Antique Gaul*, p. 271.
185 On this topic see also my discussion in Chapter 3.1 of sin and illness in medieval thought.
186 Appendix G 222.
187 Appendix G 222: 'qui forte hoc non peccati sui meritis pertulit'.
188 Appendix G 222: 'fortassis nec ipse neque parentes ejus peccaverant'.
189 John 9:1–7.
190 Appendix E MII 20.
191 Appendix G 160.
192 Appendix W VI.viii.
193 Appendix E MI 92.
194 Appendix E MI 75.
195 Appendix E MI 25.
196 Appendix E MI 89.
197 Appendix E MII 24.
198 Appendix F 4.24. Hugh was cured instantaneously, and immediately carried on with his job of taking the load of rocks down to the church – a model workman.
199 Appendix G 46.
200 Finucane, *Miracles and Pilgrims*, p. 110. Children could be injured, impaired or killed in accidents involving drowning, smothering, burning, falling from trees, impaling themselves on implements and choking on a pilgrim badge from Thomas Becket's shrine. Adults could be dragged by horses, fall down wells, injured during wrestling matches, struck by lightning, fall through a floor onto the stone tomb in the room below, or simply trip over while running and sprain an ankle.
201 For an alternative view of miracle, sin and illness as punishment, one may look at the hagiographical writings of Gregory of Tours. His *Miracles* of St Martin and St Julian reflect a notion of illness as caused by sin, cf. Van Dam, *Saints and their Miracles in Late Antique Gaul*. However, Gregory was writing in the late sixth century, and the corpus of texts I studied range from the ninth to the thirteenth centuries.
202 Finucane, *Miracles and Pilgrims*, p. 72.
203 Jacques de Vitry [Jacobus Vitriacensis], *The Exempla or Illustrative Stories from the Sermones vulgares of Jacques de Vitry* (Publications of the Folk-lore Society 26), ed. Thomas F. Crane, London: Folk-lore Society, 1890, *exempla* no. 254.
204 Ibid.
205 Finucane, *Miracles and Pilgrims*, pp. 70–1, citing MS Vat. Lat. 4015, fol. 46r–47v, 86r.
206 Ibid., p. 70, citing MS Vat. Lat. 4015, fol. 46v.
207 Cf. J. Wortley, 'Three Not-So-Miraculous Miracles', in: Campbell, Hall and Klausner (eds), *Health, Disease and Healing in Medieval Culture*, Basingstoke: Macmillan, 1992, pp. 165–7.
208 'Silentio quoque praeterire placuit, innumeros homines tam per lavaturam manuum ejus, quam per reliquias ciborum ejus de ante illum clam eo subtractas a diversis languoribus

sed maxime febribus curatos.' Eadmer, *Vita Anselmi*, Book I.xxxv, ed. Southern, p. 61. Eadmer composed two versions of his *Vita*, a short version *c.*1112–4, and a long version *c.*1114–25, and it is on this final longer version that Southern has based his edition.

209 'et virum in hoc nichil quod miraculo posset ascribi velle facere', ibid., Book II.xl, p. 118.

210 'At ille nichil hoc ad se pertinere, sed ipsius fidei ac meritis beati martiris ad quem divertit ascribendum asserens.' Ibid., Book II.xli, p. 119.

211 'tam extraneum factum nulla sibi ratione temptandum', Ibid., Book II.xlii, p. 120.

212 Appendix E MI 66. A young woman with a twisted face is also said to appear as if her teeth were disfigured (E MI 57).

213 Appendix E MI 70.

214 Appendix E MI 82.

215 Appendix E MI 106. Another child is described as a 'monster' in one of the miracles Finucane refers to, where a baby girl, born prematurely after her mother had an accident, was so deformed she appeared 'a monstrous imitation' of a child: 'Her thighs were twisted and badly joined at the hips, there were horrendous concavities on her back, and her digestive powers were so weak that anything given for nourishment was vomited up.' The fact that she nevertheless survived for nine months in this condition is cited by Finucane as evidence for parental care and affection, when to historians examining abandonment and infanticide this baby would appear to have been a prime candidate (Finucane, *The Rescue of the Innocents*, p. 25, citing Paul Grosjean (ed.), *Henrici VI Angliae Regis Miracula Postuma*, Subsidia Hagiographica, 22, 1935, pp. 223–4).

216 Appendix E MI 14: 'Sie verletzte nämlich den Gesichts- und Geruchsinn der Menschen.'

217 Appendix E MI 44.

218 Appendix M II.15.

219 Appendix J III: 'nature defectu'.

220 Appendix J XIII: 'que ab ineunte etate diris indignationis sue legibus natura ita multaverat, ut contracto utroque poplite, spasmum pati putaretur'.

221 Appendix J XII: 'Hanc autem adolescentulam a nativitate sua ita natura dampnaverat.'

222 Appendix W VII.xvi: 'cui ex nature uitio pedum tali natibus adheserant'.

223 Appendix W VI.xi: 'debilitas dolenda'.

224 Appendix F 2.4.

225 Appendix F 2.4.

226 Appendix F. 4.13.

227 Appendix I XVI: 'nature vitio deformis'.

228 Numbers 22:28.

229 Appendix I XVI: 'et sciet quia Deo nichil est difficile, nichil contra naturam nature auctori factu impossibile'.

230 See my article 'Responses to Physical Impairment in Medieval Europe: Between Magic and Medicine', *Medizin, Gesellschaft und Geschichte*, 18, 1999.

231 Appendix F 2.7.

232 Appendix W III.xxvii: 'fere emortuum'.

233 Appendix M II.24.

234 Psalms 21:7.

235 Appendix M II.24.

236 Appendix M II.32.

237 Appendix M II.32.

238 Appendix M III.3.

239 Appendix G 111.

240 Appendix G 168.

241 Appendix G 191.

242 Finucane, *Miracles and Pilgrims*, p. 74. In his later book on children and miracles, Finucane cites the twelfth-century case of a girl of about 15 who was suffering for some four years from what the source refers to as 'cancer'. She was at one point also

described as seeming neither alive nor dead. However, this state lasted for only a few days, and appears to be indicative of the 'crisis' or turning point in her story, as it is then that her parents appeal to Thomas Becket, and she recovers within a day (Finucane, *The Rescue of the Innocents*, pp. 85–6).

243 Miracle I.49, Bull, *The Miracles of Our Lady of Rocamadour*, p. 133.
244 In discussing the work of Jean-Claude Schmitt on the cult of the Holy Greyhound, St Guinefort, Marcia Kupfer also speaks of the fate of the sickly in the thirteenth century, who call upon Guinefort, 'whose condition left them languishing painfully between life and death' (Kupfer, *The Art of Healing*, p. 30).
245 Sigal, *L'homme et le miracle*, p. 240, also pointed out that many of his samples of miracle narratives gave frequent descriptions of the effects of impairment, including the incapacity of moving one's limbs as well as the incapacity to work. He further described how the *miracula* mentioned cases of impairment: 'lorsque le mal est plus complexe ou plus étrange, les descriptions sont plus développées mais elles insistent plus sur les conséquences de l'infirmité que sur les caractères de cell-ci, d'où des phrases telles ≪un homme était tellement atteint qu'il ne pouvait plus porter ses mains à sa bouche≫ ou ≪…marcher sans l'aide de béquilles≫ ou ≪…s'occuper à aucun travail≫ etc.' (ibid., p. 228).
246 Appendix V V5.
247 Appendix F I.15.
248 Appendix F 2.4.
249 Appendix M II.41.
250 Appendix I III and I IV.
251 Appendix J XXIII.
252 Appendix J X.
253 Appendix W V.xxii.
254 Appendix W VII.ix.
255 Finucane, *The Rescue of the Innocents*, pp. 57–8.
256 Appendix G cap. clviii: 'vix de lectulo potuisset exsurgere'.
257 Appendix G cap. lxxxv: 'reclinabatur et efferebatur, manibus alienis'. The 'triple stick' is a particularly intriguing detail provided in this source, since perhaps it refers to the kind of mobility aid sometimes depicted in illuminated manuscripts. This contraption appears to be a modified form of those baby walkers often shown in the miniatures, and closely resembles a modern zimmer frame, sometimes on wheels, with three or four legs – see notes 414 and ff.
258 Appendix G 203. Another man, with contorted and contracted feet, had lost all movement of his shins and was incapable of walking (G 28). A man with gout was unable to walk for two years (G 57).
259 Appendix G 158.
260 Appendix G 92 and G 93. Also, a little girl with a contracted right hand and right foot could not move for half a year (G 37).
261 Appendix G 50. Another woman was paralysed in all her body so that she was unable to move (G 62).
262 Appendix G 91.
263 Appendix E MI 31. This was also the case for another girl whose right hand was swollen (E MII 23).
264 Appendix E MI 66.
265 Appendix E MI 22.
266 Appendix E MI 86.
267 Appendix E MI 62.
268 Appendix G 36.
269 Appendix G 26.
270 Appendix G 66. There was also a boy who was so weakened, he could not move without others' aid (G 120), while another youth could not move without a crutch due to a weakness of his knee (G 65).

271 Appendix G 205. There was also a paralysed woman who could not move to do any work (G 13).

272 Appendix G 187.

273 Appendix E MI 44. Another boy had a shaking arm which made his hand 'useless', and his head was inclined so that he could not upright himself, nor stand up unaided, nor could he use his left leg (E MII 19).

274 Appendix E MI 90.

275 Appendix E MI 98. Also, a youth was bedridden, unable to walk and had to be carried about by other people (E MI 51).

276 Appendix E MI 15. His cure is quite interesting in itself, since after his visit to the tomb of St Elisabeth, he was only healed of the trembling eyes, hands and arms, but to be mobile he had to use a crutch. Apparently this mobility aid was only necessary at first, and after returning home, his shins had a chance to develop enough for him to stand unsupported. He was then able to walk unaided on level ground, and only needed one crutch to manage with sloping terrain. The entire process sounds very much like a 'natural' healing process, as opposed to a sudden miracle cure, and could perhaps be explained as a form of cure reminiscent of modern physiotherapeutic practice.

277 Appendix E MI 19.

278 Appendix E MI 4.

279 Appendix E MI 101: 'wie ein Holz.'

280 Appendix E MI 56.

281 Appendix E MI 52. The woman described the physical effects of her condition to the protocol writers, saying that if hot coals were to fall on her feet, she would be unable to move or withdraw her feet of her own accord.

282 Appendix E MI 95.

283 Appendix E MI 82.

284 Appendix E MI 26.

285 Appendix F L.3.

286 Appendix W VII. xiv: 'Non se propriis ualebat uiribus eleuare, neque absque adiuuantis adminiculo a latere in latus quandoque conuertere. Neruis quoque in ceruicem contractis, ad augmentum incommodi, humero sinistro sinistra mala tam inseparabiliter adherebat, ut alteri alterum incastrari cerneres atque in nullas omnino partes inflexo humero ceruix flecti preualebat. Multiplex igitur incommodum, pedibus podagricis incessus, manibus contractis attactus, capitique humero cohercenti consuetudinarius uidendi, erigendi, conuertendi et comedendi negabatur usus. Quotiens enim manducandi perurgebat necessitas, cibo super terram uel asserem comminuto, humi procumbens, et ad instar pecudis oppetens, id solum poterat manducare quod lingua uel dentibus contingebat attingere. Toto igitur impos et imbecillis corpore alienis uertebatur, erigebatur, et circumferebatur manibus.'

287 Appendix W V.xv: 'et ea dolore partus atque angustia contractis membrorum neruis tantam corporis incurrit imbecillitatem, ut multis postea diebus neque se ipsam manibus pascere neque pedibus posset ambulare'.

288 Appendix W V.xv: 'Et factum est, que tristis et aliene opis aduenerat indigua, leta cum suis regreditur gressibus propriis confisa.'

289 Appendix W III.xxvii: 'Hi filium decennem toto corpore inbecillem attulerunt, quia gressu proprio illuc uenirenequaquam poterat, quoniam a multis idebus se mouere seu conuertere impotens erat.'

290 Appendix W III.xxii.

291 Appendix W III.xiv: 'nec sine baculo gressum figeret, nec omnino aliquid operis manibus efficere posset'.

292 Brian Kemp thinks this awkward passage may possibly stem from a corruption in the manuscript, fol. 174r. The Latin reads: 'Pes circumflexus pedis officium diffitens ita peruertebatur ut calcis crates cratis articuli articulorum locum clavellata usurparent.'

293 Appendix J XX: 'Haque puella sibi facta mutilata, aliisque miserabile a noverca sua plurimis lascessita iniuriis, variis affecta obprobriis.'
294 The stepmother at one point complains that the girl has still not been to a shrine for a successful cure, rejecting her as if she were 'damaged goods' sent back for returns: ' "Aha, you went away a cripple and, look, you have come back a cripple. Go away from me," she said, "and crawl where you will, for you shall certainly not stay under my roof" ' (Appendix J XX).
295 Appendix J XX.
296 It is interesting to note that Finucane, discussing one of the child healing miracles, refers to one of the protagonists, a 9-year-old girl who was immobile, therefore had to be carried everywhere by her mother, and needed help feeding herself, as being 'literally a burden', even though the citations from his source make no direct mention of the apparent 'burdensome' aspect (Finucane, *The Rescue of the Innocents*, p. 57).
297 Appendix F 2.7.
298 Appendix G 217: 'onerosior sibi et cunctis amicis suis apparuit'.
299 Appendix J XVIII.
300 Henry Mayr-Harting, 'Functions of a twelfth-century shrine: the miracles of St Frideswide', in: Henry Mayr-Harting and R. I Moore (eds), *Studies in Medieval History Presented to R. C. H. Davis*, London: Hambledon Press, 1985, p. 199. Cf. *Acta Sanctorum*, October viii, 45.
301 Appendix F L.5.
302 Appendix F 4.10.
303 Finucane, *Miracles and Pilgrims*, pp. 149–50. Finucane also argued that the nobility wished to disassociate themselves from the impairments, the 'blindness and lameness and contorted limbs' (ibid.), with which the common peasantry approached thaumaturgic shrines.
304 Ibid., p. 4.
305 Rudolf Hiestand, 'Kranker König-Kranker Bauer', in: Peter Wunderli (ed.), *Der kranke Mensch in Mittelalter und Renaissance* (Studia humaniora. Düsseldorfer Studien zu Mittelalter und Renaissance. Band 5), Düsseldorf: Droste Verlag, 1986, pp. 61–77.
306 Appendix II M II.24.
307 Appendix E MI 21.
308 Appendix M I.17.
309 Appendix W V.xxiii: 'obsurduerant aures adeoque inualuerat incommodum, ut nisi tuum illius auribus os applicares ab ipsa nequaquam audiri posses...Vnde et in publicum prodire uerebatur, et non nisi domesticorum utebatur alloquiis. Timebat enim ualde ne surdiciei sue obprobrium aliene quandoque noticie prodiret in risum'.
310 The theme of the old person, especially of the old woman, as a comic object, to be ridiculed and mocked, is already found in classical antiquity, where the *vetula* appears in drama, and in the visual arts, as a figure of fun. One may compare such antique notions with medieval depictions of old women, for example, a late fifteenth-century sculpture of an old woman (probably a *vanitas mundi* allegory) from the upper Rhine region, showing the physical deterioration of old age in graphic detail.
311 Appendix F 2.4.
312 Appendix F 2.4: 'This miracle caused great joy for all, and even for those who were mocking her. But these must have been ignorant and stupid schoolboys if they didn't know that Christ deigned to cure an old woman who had a curvature of the spine for eighteen years, [Luke 13:11–13] and an old man who lay paralyzed in the portico of a pool for 38 years, [John 5:2–9] both of whom had given up hope of a cure long before.'
313 Appendix F 2.4.
314 Appendix F 2.4.
315 Appendix F L.3.
316 Appendix F L.3.

317 Sigal, *L'homme et le miracle*, p. 240, regards this position of the affected limb as very characteristic of this type of mobility impairment: 'les deux jambs sont repliées en arrière si bien que les talons adhèrent aux fesses'.

318 Appendix G 221.

319 Appendix W VII.x: 'genibus innixus et manualibus gradiens scabellis.... Arefactis siquidem neruis, contracto poplite, ac desiccatis tibiis, usus illi negabatur gradiendi'. A contracted woman is mentioned, too, who is simply described as 'poor' without further detail (W VII.xii).

320 Appendix E MI 48: 'da er Bettler war, und nichts hatte, in der Kirche öffentlich von Gläubigen Almosen bettelte'.

321 Appendix V O 10.

322 Appendix I XVI: 'pauper quidem rebus, sed fide dives, etatis ut videbatur iuvenilis, sed nature vitio deformis'.

323 Appendix M I.39.

324 Appendix M I.39. Other instances where the supplicant has to make a non-verbal or silent vow, which the texts specifically emphasise as something extraordinary, can be found in M I.45 and W VII.i; and at M III.10, where a merchant who was robbed and badly wounded turned to the Virgin 'in his heart', imploring her help, 'even though he was unable to open his mouth because of the circumstances in which he found himself'.

325 Appendix F 3.23.

326 Finucane, *The Rescue of the Innocents*, pp. 81–2. John had begged from the ages of about nine to about sixteen, when, in 1287 or 1288, he travelled from his native Ludlow to the shrine of Cantilupe at Hereford. There he started to develop a stump where his tongue should have been, subsequently returning home to Ludlow, but it was not until a second visit to the shrine at Hereford that he was totally cured. Finucane points out that the sources frequently mention the suspicions of fraud contemporaries had, so that the boy John was often forced to open his mouth for inspection by local people who wanted to make sure the boy really was speech-impaired and not faking his affliction for the sake of more successful begging.

327 Appendix J XVIII: 'Raros enim amicos repperit adversitas, paucissimos paupertas, fere nullos medicantium cecitas.'

328 Appendix J XVIII.

329 Appendix W IV.ii: 'famis et mortalitatis diebus cum aliis in domo sua pauperibus cecum quendam ipse habuerat'.

330 Appendix E MI 3. Interestingly, it was her stepfather who took her to the shrine of St Elisabeth, which may indicate that her changed family circumstances could have had more to do with her impoverishment than her impairment.

331 Appendix F 4.3.

332 Appendix F 4.13.

333 Appendix M I.38.

334 Finucane, *Miracles and Pilgrims*, p. 47, citing narratives from the miracles or *vitae* of St Thomas Becket, St Hugh of Lincoln and St Osmund of Salisbury.

335 Ibid., Charity could also be 'compulsory', as in the case of the peasants of Arundel Castle, who were ordered by the lady of a nearby village to take in and look after her orthopaedically impaired washerwoman (ibid.).

336 Appendix F 2.4.

337 Appendix E MI 45: 'und er bettelte nicht mehr wie vorher, sondern ernährte sich von der Arbeit seiner Hände'.

338 Appendix F 4.12. The girl's presence outside the monastic church is compared in the text with that of the lame man healed by St Peter [Acts 3:2] who also 'once sought alms from those entering the Temple to pray there' (F 4.12).

339 Appendix E MI 76.

340 Appendix M I.21.

341 Appendix F 3.23.

342 Appendix E MI 89.

343 Appendix M II.15.

344 Appendix W VI.xi: 'Hanc Petrus presbiter de Langeham uilla episcopi per multum tempus elemosine gratia in domo sua tenuit, pauit, et uestiuit.'

345 Metalwork panel on the shrine of St Elisabeth, Marburg cathedral.

346 Appendix V W 8.

347 Finucane, *Miracles and Pilgrims*, p. 48. In his later book on child miracles, Finucane does make more mention of the mobility or immobility of his case studies (cf. Finucane, *The Rescue of the Innocents*, pp. 56–8, 122).

348 Appendix W VI.xi.

349 Appendix E MI 51.

350 For example, a woman with hands and arms contracted since birth was 'brought' to St Godric's shrine by others (Appendix G 182), and a man was 'taken' to the same shrine by his friends (G 187).

351 Appendix E MI 12. Also, one Goda, wife of Copman of Norwich, had herself carried to St William's shrine (W V.xxii).

352 Appendix E MI 72. Additionally, a 2-year-old boy was carried by his mother (E MI 55), and another girl was carried by her father on his back (E MII 8), while a boy who was blind, mute and deaf from birth was carried to St Foy's shrine by both of his parents (F 1.28). A severely impaired 8-year-old girl was carried to Norwich in her mother's arms (W VII.xiv).

353 Appendix F 1.15. An incurably injured warrior, whose friends and vassals had carried him home after he initially sustained the wounds, also had himself carried to Conques (F 2.7). During a procession at Conques, '[e]ach person who was sick or physically impaired was carried to the procession as it passed' (F L.3). Finucane also mentions the case of a crippled girl who was carried by her mother on her back to the tomb of St Louis at Marseille (Finucane, *The Rescue of the Innocents*, p. 56).

354 Appendix V G (S) II.37.

355 Appendix E MI 3.

356 Appendix E MII 12: 'weil sie nicht anders transportiert werden konnte'.

357 Appendix E MII 12: 'die die Träger verschiedener Güter benutzen'.

358 Appendix F 2.4.

359 Appendix F 4.12.

360 Appendix M I.38.

361 Finucane, *Miracles and Pilgrims*, p. 86, based on *The Life and Miracles of St Thomas Cantilupe, Bishop of Hereford, Acta Sanctorum*, I Oct., 1765, pp. 622–3.

362 Illumination from Jehan Henry's *Livre de Vie Active*, produced at Paris in 1482/3 for the sisters of the Hôtel Dieu.

363 Illumination in early fifteenth-century *Meditationes Vitae Christi*, London, British Library, MS Royal 20.B.IV, fol. 61v.

364 Appendix F L.3.

365 Appendix E MI 15.

366 Appendix W VI.xi: 'Quam si quandoque recuperande sanitatis gratia sacra uisitare loca concupisset, illus equo ad instar sacci pleni in transuersum deportare faciebat.'

367 Finucane, *Miracles and Pilgrims*, p. 86. Cf. J. O. Halliwell (ed.), *The Miracles of Simon de Montfort, Camden Society*, 15, 1840, pp. 82 and 108.

368 Appendix G 121. In other instances, a paralytic man was brought by his mother on horseback (G 135), and a woman who had lost the ability to walk was taken to the shrine on horseback by her husband (G205).

369 Appendix W V.xv.

370 Appendix E MI 19.

371 Appendix E MI 52.

372 Appendix E MI 59.

373 Appendix E MI 28. A young boy was also only partially cured at the shrine, where he was still lying in the vehicle he came in (E MI 70).

374 Appendix E MII 10/11. In St Godric's miracle narratives, a man bedridden with 'weakness' is also transported to the shrine in a cart (G 68).

375 Appendix V G (S) II.13.

376 Appendix V RO 13. This is an interesting mode of transport for the date of the miracle. Theoretically, this push-cart should not equated with what we would think of as a wheelbarrow. The wheelbarrow only appeared in western Europe in the twelfth or early thirteenth century, as an 'import' from China (cf. F. and J. Gies, *Cathedral, Forge, and Waterwheel: Technology and Invention in the Middle Ages*, New York: Harper Collins, 1994, p. 92).

377 Appendix W VI.xii. Since the St William text was composed in the 1170s, it is possible that this 'handbarrow' could actually be a proper wheelbarrow.

378 Finucane, *Miracles and Pilgrims*, p. 86. Finucane is apparently citing evidence from *The Life and Miracles of St Thomas Cantilupe, Bishop of Hereford, Acta Sanctorum*, I Oct., 1765, pp. 650 and 689. In his later book on child miracles, Finucane also cites the same miracle, this time in more detail. The protagonist of the cure was a 19-year-old girl, Alice, who had been crippled by accident some 10 years earlier. Together with her father, who sometimes carried her about on a day-to-day basis when she did not drag herself along the ground after her him, she lived by begging in London. In 1303 Alice's father decided to appeal to St Thomas Cantilupe, and began collecting and saving up enough alms to purchase a wheelbarrow, in which he then placed his daughter and wheeled her all the way from London to Hereford. Finucane quotes the notaries' report from the shrine, who described it as 'a little cart with one wheel which her father pushed in front of him with his hands' (*parvum currum unius rote quem pater ante se manibus pellebat*) (Finucane, *The Rescue of the Innocents*, p. 122 and p. 240 note 93).

379 This shows a crippled man being transported in a wheelbarrow who is given alms (London, British Library, MS Additional 42130, fol. 186v).

380 Appendix F 3.22.

381 Appendix G 139.

382 Appendix W VII.xvi: 'in uehiculo rotatili aduehitur, quod ciueriam appellant'.

383 Appendix W VII.xvi: 'itidem in ciueria aduehitur rotatili'.

384 Appendix J XXIII.

385 Appendix W VI.xi.

386 Appendix W VI.xi.

387 There are further dramatic descriptions of the conditions in which sufferers, this time mainly of non-impairing conditions, arrive at in church during the crisis point of their illness, cf. *Acta Sanctorum*, October viii, 35, 66, 67, 88, 89, 93, for the shrine of St Frideswide at Oxford, and Brian Kemp, 'The Miracles of the Hand of St James', *Berkshire Archaeological Journal*, 65, 1970, miracle nos. II, XX, XXIV.

388 Or servants who could take them to shrines, as in the case of a woman in the St Godric stories (Appendix G 142).

389 Finucane, *Miracles and Pilgrims*, p. 86. Finucane's irritating method of annotation in his earlier work does not allow the reader to follow up his sources with certainty: his example could come from a miracle of St Frideswide or of St Hedwig. In his book on child miracles, Finucane mentions a boy Ceptus in connection with a miracle by Clara of Montefalco, who used crutches because his 'feet were so twisted that he walked on the sides rather than the soles of his feet' (Finucane, *The Rescue of the Innocents*, p. 58).

390 Appendix W VII.xi: 'duobus quos uulgo potentias uocant baculis gressus utcumque dirigens, et imbecilles artus sustentans.'

391 Appendix F 4.13.

392 Appendix W III.xiv: 'nec sine baculo gressum figeret'.

393 Appendix W VI.xi: 'quod si quandoque de loco se ad locum transferre uoluisset, imbecillia baculo membra sustentans, uel gressus modicum proficeret uel nonnumquam nec in modico preualeret'.

394 Appendix G 16.

395 Appendix G 19.

396 Appendix G 46: 'duobus baculis sub alterutri lateris axe suffultus'.

397 Appendix G 117.

398 Appendix G 65.

399 Appendix G 16: 'sis sese protrahens quadrupes'.

400 Appendix E MI 5. A little boy who had been unable to walk all his life had used crutches before his miracle cure (E MI 65), and a 16-year-old boy could only walk with difficulty supported on crutches (E MI 95).

401 Appendix E MI 15. An 8-year-old girl began walking with crutches after her mother had visited the tomb, until one Sunday the girl was cured fully (E MI 87).

402 Appendix E MI 25. Another man was described by one of the witnesses as being able to move around supported on crutches, after lying ill for 20 weeks (E MI 29), while a man injured in an accident began to walk at first with the aid of crutches before his complete cure (E MI 75). A woman had been bedridden for weeks before she could walk with her lamed leg supported by crutches (E MI 89). A 9-year-old boy also gradually began to lose his lameness and rely less on his stick, until he finally no longer needed it at all (E MI 79).

403 Appendix E MII 9.

404 Appendix E MI 28. A 3-year-old boy was also the subject of a partial cure: after being initially unable to even crawl, he became able to right himself up with the aid of sticks, finally walking supported by a crutch (E MI 44). And a 16-year-old boy, who had to be carried everywhere by other people, began to start walking weakly and using crutches, then just using one crutch, until he was finally able to discard that one, too (E MI 51).

405 Appendix E MI 86.

406 Appendix E MI 62: 'auf zu diesem Zweck besonders hergestellten Stöcken'.

407 Finucane, in his brief passage dealing with the mobility issues of the impaired, also mentions hand-trestles, and additionally the use of wheeled platforms on which people pushed themselves about (Finucane, *Miracles and Pilgrims*, p. 86).

408 Metalwork panel on the mid-thirteenth century shrine of St Elisabeth in Marburg cathedral, showing the saint distributing alms to the needy who include cripples.

409 Appendix W V.xiv: 'hec manualibus gradiens scabellis'.

410 Appendix W VII.x: 'genibus innixus et manualibus gradiens scabellis'.

411 Appendix W VII.xvi: 'Quandoque tamen sed cum necessitas ingruebat, genibus innixus scabellis ibat manualibus.'

412 Appendix G 221.

413 Appendix G lxxxv.

414 The baby walker was known from the thirteenth century, cf. Shulamith Shahar, *Childhood in the Middle Ages*, London and New York: Routledge, 1992, p. 92.

415 Child using a three-wheeled walker depicted in an illumination from a fourteenth-century manuscript in Copenhagen, Kongelige Bibliotek, MS 3384, fol.104v.

416 Marginal illumination in the *Heures de François de Guise*, now Chantilly, Musée Condé, MS 64, fol. 191r.

417 The tapestry originally hung in the town hall of Regensburg, but is now in Museum der Stadt Regensburg.

418 Appendix W III.vii: 'Sicque factum est, ut que manibus alienis corpore inbecillis aduenerat, celesti operante medicina, nullius egens adminiculo incolumis rediret et sospes.'

419 Appendix W IV.xi.

420 Finucane, *The Rescue of the Innocents*, p. 56. The girl was cured in 1308 at the tomb of St Louis at Marseille.

421 Finucane, *The Rescue of the Innocents*, p. 57. This girl was cured after her family prayed to the recently deceased pope Urban V (d. 1370).

422 Appendix W VI.xii: 'cum ambulare proponeret, applicatis ad genua uel terre palmis, ipsa uel ipsam pro podio haberet'.

423 Appendix E MI 34.
424 Appendix E MI 48.
425 Appendix E MI 97.
426 Appendix E MI 82.
427 Marginal illumination in a fourteenth-century Book of Hours, now Baltimore, MD, Walters Art Gallery, MS 82, fol. 193v.
428 Appendix E MI 82: 'was er vorher auf keine Weise konnte'.
429 Appendix G 214: 'genibus pro pedibus super terram oportuit ipsam repere, si aliquando alicubi debuisset ire'.
430 Appendix G 218.
431 Appendix G 218.
432 Appendix F 4.3.
433 Appendix F 4.14.
434 Appendix F 4.15.
435 Appendix F 2.1.
436 Appendix F 3.6.
437 Appendix E MI 38.
438 Appendix E MI 50.
439 Appendix E MI 76.
440 Appendix E MI 78.
441 Appendix G 114.
442 Appendix G 222: 'aliis ducentibus'.
443 Appendix J XVIII.
444 Appendix M I.21.
445 Appendix W IV.xi.
446 Appendix W VI.viii.
447 Appendix V O 13.
448 Appendix I XIII.
449 Gregory of Tours, *Life of the Fathers*, transl. E. James, Liverpool: Liverpool University Press, 1991, p. 34. St Gallus proceeded to burn down the pagan temple, together with its wooden votives. Cf. V.I. Flint, *The Rise of Magic in Early Medieval Europe*, Oxford: Oxford University Press, 1991, pp. 72–3 and p. 210, where also other examples of the destruction of 'pagan' offerings and wonder-working imagery are detailed.
450 Ælfric, *Lives of the Saints*, ed. Skeat, *Early English Text Society*, orig. series 76, 82, 94, 114, 1881–1900, I, p. 451, § xxi, 11.149–55 and 11.431–4.
451 B. Nilson, *Cathedral Shrines of Medieval England*, Woodbridge, NJ: Boydell, 1998, p. 102; cf. E. M. Jancey, 'A Servant Speaks of His Master: Hugh le Barber's Evidence in 1307', in: M. Jancey (ed.), *St Thomas Cantilupe, Bishop of Hereford: Essays in his Honour*, Hereford: The Friends of Hereford Cathedral, 1982, pp. 200–1. It is interesting to note that Hugh appears to be a bit of a gambler (playing chess and dice), but that St Thomas Cantilupe, unlike some of the saints from my samples, does not take any punishing action for such immoral behaviour. St Foy, presumably, would have immediately struck Hugh blind again had she caught him examining the dots on dice.
452 Nilson, *Cathedral Shrines*, p. 102, cf. A. R. Malden (ed.), *The Canonisation of St Osmund*, Salisbury: no publisher, 1901, pp. 171–2.
453 Appendix G 16.
454 Appendix G 19.
455 Appendix G 65.
456 Appendix W VII.xi: 'ibique in signum sua podia dimisit'.
457 Appendix E MI 29.
458 Appendix E MI 76 and 100.
459 Appendix E MI 76.
460 A panel painting of *c*.1480, perhaps by Jan Pollak, in the parish church at Pipping, shows votive offerings lying in front of and adjacent to the shrine, and a wing of the

altarpiece, also *c*.1480, of St Wolfgang in Pipping depicts crutches, and models of limbs lying on the tomb of the saint.

461 This is an interesting reversal of the belief in the transference of illnesses: quasi-magical rituals, linked with the topos of the scapegoat, whereby an affliction is 'passed on' to an inanimate object, a plant, or an animal, cf. my discussion of these practices in medieval Europe, with particular reference to Anglo-Saxon England, in 'Responses to Physical Impairment in Medieval Europe', pp. 17–20, and also the discussion in Chapter 4.4. To me, the difference between beliefs in the transference of disease and beliefs in the transference of cures is only one of two sides of the same coin. If one has a belief in the transference of illness, then it is perhaps only logical to equally have a belief in the transference of healing powers.

462 B. Spencer, *Pilgrim Souvenirs and Secular Badges* (Medieval Finds from Excavations in London: 7), London: The Stationery Office, 1998, pp. 16–17.

463 Ibid., p. 18. Cf. also K. Köster, 'Mittelalterliche Pilgerzeichen', in: L. Kriss-Rettenbeck and G. Möhler (eds), *Wallfahrt kennt keine Grenzen*, Munich: Schnell & Steiner, 1984, pp. 203–23.

464 Appendix M I.23.

465 Appendix E MI 82.

466 Appendix W IV.v.

467 Appendix E MI 56.

468 Such as the cures at Appendix E MI 48, E MI 56 or E MII 12.

469 Appendix W VI.xi.

470 Appendix J XII.

471 Appendix E MI 12.

472 Appendix F L.5.

473 Appendix V RO 13.

474 Appendix M I.22.

475 Appendix M II.19. The Holy Sepulchre had no miracle-working relics on site, which may be one reason why the woman was not cured. Moreover, thaumaturgic shrines tended to cater for a local populace, if only for the purely pragmatic reason that impaired and sick people had difficulties travelling, as Benedicta Ward has pointed out: 'Healing shrines are of necessity local shrines' (Ward, *Miracles and the Medieval Mind*, p. 125).

476 Mayr-Harting, 'Functions of a Twelfth-Century Shrine', p. 195. Cf. for St Frideswide: *Acta Sanctorum*, October viii, 13, 31, 49, 66, and for the hand of St James: Kemp, 'The Miracles of the Hand of St James', miracle no. VIII. The hospital of St Mary Magdalen at Reading may well have had a function in connection with the shrine visitors. Mayr-Harting also cites the description in miracle accounts of 'mopping up' done by the custodians of the shrine after what appear to have been physically rather messy miraculous healings (Mayr-Harting, 'Functions', p. 195).

477 Finucane, *Miracles and Pilgrims*, p. 67.

478 Also called the fire of St Lawrence, or fire of St Silvanus, and having St Andrew associated with the disease, sometimes in France also associated with St Martial, see Kupfer, *The Art of Healing*, pp. 55–6.

479 Ibid.

480 The *Miracles* of St Silvanus (Paris, Bibliothèque Nationale, MS lat. 5317, fols. 3v–5v) recounts seven tales, three of which relate to cures of 'ergotism'. Silvanus seems to have specialised in curing people afflicted by the convulsive form of ergotism. Here they are a woman 'lying for many days in the *porticus* of this church (*per dies multos jacens in porticus hujus ecclesiae*)' who suffered from contractions in her arms and legs; a man 'with all his limbs shaking (*omnibus membris ejus trementibus*)' who was unable to raise his hand to his head; and another woman with spasms so severe her heels touched her buttocks ('*femina…quae contracta, calcaneis posterioribus adhaesis*'), these latter contortions being characteristic of convulsive ergotism, while her left hand was withered and shrivelled

(*perdita* and *arida*) implying variously anaesthesia and paralysis, or shrinkage, loss of sensation and mummification or drying out indicative of gangrene (which could be a consequence of ergotism). The severely affected woman was restored by her miracle cure so that she was able to extend her knees and stand up, and her hand revived (literally warmed up, *incaluit*). Medically, this might possibly be a case of the rare but known combination of the convulsive type of ergotism with the gangrenous variety. The miracles and possible medical explanations are cited in Kupfer, *The Art of Healing*, p. 52.

481 Ibid., p. 52 note 25, cf. Annie Saunier, *'Le pauvre malade' dans le cadre hospitalier médiéval: France du nord, vers 1300–1500*, Paris, 1993, p. 67.

482 A doctor Boucher writing in 1762 observed of the 1749 outbreak that the 'contractions of flexors were so violent in some subjects that they made the heels almost touch the buttocks', and then gangrene set in (cited by Kupfer, *The Art of Healing*, p. 52, and noted by George Barger, *Ergot and Ergotism*, London: Gurney and Jackson, 1931, p. 60). The last modern outbreak of ergotism is described in J. G. Fuller, *The Day of Saint Anthony's Fire*, London: Hutchinson, 1969, pp. 98–9.

483 James, 'A Sense of Wonder', p. 48.

484 'Sociosomatic' was the term preferred by V. Skultans, in an article 'Empathy and healing: aspects of spiritualist ritual', in: J. B. Loudon (ed.) *Social Anthropology and Medicine*, London and New York: Academic Press, 1976, pp. 190–222. Cf. Van Dam, *Leadership and Community in Late Antique Gaul*, p. 260.

485 During the twelfth century, most of the visitors to the shrine at Oxford (and the one at Reading) seem to have come from within a forty-mile radius of the site; they consisted mainly of knights, townsmen, and the upper peasantry. Mayr-Harting argues that just as people in the twelfth century began to have aspirations to enhanced legal and political status, so 'ordinary' people began to aspire to better health as well, and shrines provided a form of supplementary medical care to that offered by physicians, or shrines were used after a visit to a medical doctor had failed, or a combination of both was utilised (Mayr-Harting, 'Functions of a Twelfth-Century Shrine', pp. 196–7).

486 Ælfric, *Lives of the Saints*, I, p. 451, § xxi, 11.149–55 and 11.431–4.

487 Mayr-Harting, 'Functions of a twelfth-century shrine', p. 205, cf. *Acta Sanctorum*, October viii, 30.

488 I have argued this point regarding the contrast between public miracle and private medical healing more fully in my article 'Responses to Physical Impairment in Medieval Europe', pp. 32–3.

489 P. R. L. Brown, 'The rise and function of the holy man in antiquity', *Journal of Roman Studies*, 61, 1971, p. 96, cited by: Mayr-Harting, 'Functions of a Twelfth-Century Shrine', p. 205.

490 Mayr-Harting, 'Functions of a twelfth-century shrine', pp. 205–6. Mayr-Harting also assumes that sufferers of physical and mental illness 'were often the subjects of social repudiation in the twelfth century, as in other ages' (ibid.). A ritualistic cure could then also function as a means of reversing such repudiation.

491 Wortley, 'Three not-so-miraculous miracles', pp. 159–68. The miracle at the shrine of Sts Cosmas and Damian is the twenty-fourth in a collection dated to the seventh or eighth centuries; the second miracle refers to exemplum 254 of Jacques de Vitry, *Exempla* (see also note 203); and the third miracle story is from a Greek manuscript dated to after 1111.

492 P. W. Halligan, J. C. Marshall, G. R. Fink, D. T. Wade and R. S. J. Frackowiak, 'The functional anatomy of a hysterical paralysis', *Cognition*, 64(1), 1997, pp. B1–B8.

493 Finucane, *Miracles and Pilgrims*, p. 79.

494 Ibid. There is a serious problem with this inference: the jury is still out as to whether *rheumatoid* arthritis was actually present in medieval Europe – other forms of arthritis can be found in the palaeopathological record for the period, but the rheumatoid version appears to have been absent.

495 Ibid., p. 80.

496 Finucane, *Miracles and Pilgrims*, p. 91.
497 Ibid., p. 148.
498 Ibid.
499 There is a plethora of books and articles on the subject of the gendered construction of 'hysteria', amongst which worth pointing out are: Elaine Showalter, *The Female Malady: Women, Madness and English Culture*, New York: Penguin, 1985 and Jane Ussher, *Women's Madness: Misogyny or Mental Illness?*, London and New York: Harvester Wheatsheaf, 1991.
500 Finucane, *Miracles and Pilgrims*, p. 148.
501 Appendix M I.16. Two other miracles, this time from St Foy's narrative, also deal with the gradual regaining of sight by the visually impaired. One, concerning a boy who had his pupils pierced (F 4.3), is obviously not a realistically possible cure, but the analogy given in this miracle is interesting, in that it cites the biblical story (Matthew 8:24) of receiving gradual sightedness; the other story (F 4.14) is equally implausible, but again describes the gradual increase of vision the man in question gains: 'It seemed to him that he could make out human shapes as one does in the wavery light of dawn, but he couldn't really tell who they were.'
502 Appendix E MI 58.
503 Appendix E MI 86: 'sondern so, daß man ihn nach der Art der Kinder, die sprechen lernen, verstand'.
504 Appendix E MI 70.
505 Appendix E MI 44.
506 Appendix E MI 28: 'und jetzt geht er sehr gut'.
507 Appendix E MI 33.

6 Conclusion

  1 Charles T. Wood, 'The doctors' dilemma: sin, salvation, and the menstrual cycle in medieval thought', *Speculum*, 56, 1981.
  2 A recent publication (Emma Cave, *The Mother of All Crimes: Human Rights, Criminalization and the Child Born Alive*, Aldershot: Ashgate, 2004) considers precisely this topic: when 'bad' mothers are criminalised for their actions during pregnancy, and how pregnancy is becoming a crime zone in modern Britain and America.
  3 Umberto Eco in conversation with Christopher Frayling, cited in Frayling, *Strange Landscape: A Journey through the Middle Ages*, London: BBC Books, 1995, p. 13.
  4 Cf. Miri Rubin, *Corpus Christi: The Eucharist in Late Medieval Culture*, Cambridge: Cambridge University Press, 1991, p. 13.
  5 Cf. Caroline Walker Bynum, 'Warum das ganze Theater mit dem Körper? Die Sicht einer Mediävistin', *Historische Anthropologie*, IV 1, 1996, p. 14.
  6 Harald Kleinschmidt, *Understanding the Middle Ages: The Transformation of Ideas and Attitudes in the Medieval World*, Woodbridge, NJ: Boydell, 2000, p. 337.
  7 Ibid. This autodynamic perception of the body had an immediate impact on how action was regarded among the elites, but the larger part of the rural population retained their heterodynamic attitudes up until the fifteenth century, according to Kleinschmidt.

Appendix: medieval miracle narratives

  1 This is how Jessop and James translate *scabellarius*, meaning a person who moves about with hand-trestles; Latham's *Revised Medieval Latin Word-List* translates the word as 'person using a crutch'. Personally, I regard the hand-trestle user as the more correct meaning, especially since Thomas of Monmouth elsewhere refers to 'crutch' with a different word, *baculum*, or once, *potentia*, which the 'vulgar' commonly use to refer to crutches.

2 'Wens' is Jessop and James' translation of *gutturnosus*. I prefer the translation given in Latham, *Revised Medieval Latin Word-List*, as 'goitrous'.

3 She is also the subject of a miraculous cure for pain in her limbs (gout) in W III.xiv.

4 Latham's *Revised Medieval Latin Word-List* actually gives 'wheelbarrow' for *civeria rotatilis*, occuring in a text *c*.1172, which sounds far more plausible to me than the 'litter' euphemistically translated by Jessop and James, all the more so, since depictions of impaired people from later centuries, for example, the early fourteenth century Luttrell Psalter, still depict the disabled person in a wheelbarrow.

5 Alan Coates, *English Medieval Books: The Reading Abbey Collections from Foundation to Dispersal*, Oxford: Clarendon, 1999, p. 33.

6 Ibid., p. 35.

7 Brian Kemp thinks this awkward passage may possibly stem from a corruption in the manuscript, fol. 174r.

8 Cf. a Rhenisch panel painting of around 1500 by the Master of Holy Kinship, with St Elisabeth accompanied by a crippled beggar, who acts almost as her emblem, in the same way as St Gundula, who is shown alongside Elisabeth, carries a lantern as her emblem [Cologne, Wallraff Richartz Museum, inventory number WRM 165].

Select bibliography

Primary sources

Ælfric, *Lives of the Saints*, ed. Skeat, *Early English Text Society*, orig. series 76, 82, 94, 114, 1881–1900

Alberti, Leon Battista, *I libri della famiglia*, *The Family in Renaissance Florence*, transl. Renée Neu Watkins, Columbia, MO: University of South Carolina Press, 1969

Albucasis, *On Surgery and Instruments*, transl. and ed. M. S. Spink and G. L. Lewis, London: Wellcome Institute of the History of Medicine, 1973

Ancrene Wisse: Guide for Anchoresses, transl. and intro. Hugh White, London: Penguin Books, 1993

The Apocrypha According to the Authorised Version, London: Eyre and Spottiswoode, n.d.

Arnold, Thomas (ed.), *Memorials of St Edmund's Abbey*, Rolls Series, 1890

Augustine, *De vera religione*, XL, 75, *Corpus Christianorum. Series Latina*, Turnhout: Brepols, vol. 32, 1954

—— *The Confessions of Augustine*, ed. John Gibb and William Montgomery, New York: Arno Press, 1979

—— *Concerning the City of God against the Pagans*, transl. H. Bettenson, London, 1972, rpt. 1984

Bede, *In Marc.*, *Corpus Christianorum Series Latina*, Turnhout: Brepols, vol. 120, 1953

—— *Life of Cuthbert*, in: *The Age of Bede*, transl. J. F. Webb, London: Penguin, 1983

—— *Ecclesiastical History of the English People*, transl. Leo Sherley-Price, London: Penguin, first published 1955, rev. edn, 1990

Biblia Sacra iuxta Vulgatam Versionem, ed. B. Fischer, I. Gribomont, H. F. D. Sparks and W. Thiele, Stuttgart: Deutsche Bibelgesellschaft, 4th edn, 1994

The Book of Sainte Foy, transl. with an intro. and notes Pamela Sheingorn, Philadelphia, PA: University of Pennsylvania Press, 1995

Corpus Iuris Canonicis, ed. E. Friedberg, 2 vols, Leipzig: Tauchnitz, 1879

The Cyrurgie of Guy de Chauliac, ed. M. S. Ogden, *Early English Text Society*, no. 265, 1971

Dan Michel, *Ayenbite of Inwyt*, ed. Richard Morris, *Early English Text Society*, orig. series 23, 1866, new edn, Pamela Gradon, reissue 1965

De spermate, ed. Päivi Pahta *Medieval Embryology in the Vernacular: The Case of* De Spermate (Mémoires de la Société Néophilologique de Helsinki LIII), Helsinki: Société Néophilologique, 1998

Eadmer, *Vita Anselmi, The Life of St Anselm Archbishop of Canterbury by Eadmer*, ed. and transl. R. W. Southern, London and Edinburgh: T. Nelson

Everyman and Medieval Miracle Plays, ed. A. C. Cawley, London and Melbourne: Dent, first published 1956, new edn, and rpt. 1977

Gilbertus Anglicus, *Healing and Society in Medieval England: A Middle English Translation of the Pharmaceutical Writings of Gilbertus Anglicus*, ed. Faye M. Getz, Wisconsin: University of Wisconsin Press, 1991

Gregory of Tours, *The History of the Franks*, transl. Lewis Thorpe, London: Penguin, 1974
——*Life of the Fathers*, transl. E. James, Liverpool: Liverpool University Press, 1991

Gregory the Great, *Moralia in Iob*, Libri XI–XXII, *Corpus Christianorum Series Latina*, vol. CXLIII, Turnhout: Brepols, 1979

Hildegard of Bingen, *On Natural Philosophy and Medicine: Selections from Cause et Cure*, transl. and ed. Margret Berger, Cambridge, MA: D. S. Brewer, 1999
——*Heilwissen: Von den Ursachen und der Behandlung von Krankheiten*, transl. and ed. Manfred Pawlik, Freiburg, Basle and Vienna: Herder, 1994

Isidore of Seville, *Isidori Hispalensis Episcopi Etymologiarum sive Originum*, ed. W. M. Lindsay, 2 vols, Oxford: Clarendon, 1911

'Isidore of Seville: the medical writings', trans. with intro. and commentary William D. Sharpe, *Transactions of the American Philosophical Society*, new series 54 (2), 1964, pp. 3–75

Jacques de Vitry [Jacobus Vitriacensis], *The Exempla or Illustrative Stories from the Sermones vulgares of Jacques de Vitry* (Publications of the Folk-lore Society 26), ed. Thomas F. Crane, London: Folk-lore Society, 1890

John of Salisbury, *Policraticus: Of the Frivolities of Courtiers and the Footprints of Philosophers* (Cambridge Texts in the History of Political Thought), ed. and transl. Cary J. Nederman, Cambridge: Cambridge University Press, 1990

The Kalendar of Sheepehards (c.1585), facsimile ed. with intro. by S. K. Heninger, Jr, New York: Scholar's Facsimiles and Reprints, 1979

Konrad von Eichstätt, *Das Regimen Sanitatis Konrads von Eichstätt: Quellen – Texte – Wirkungsgeschichte* (Sudhoffs Archiv Beihefte 35), ed. Christa Hagenmeyer, Stuttgart: Franz Steiner, 1995

La Novele Cirurgerie (Anglo-Norman Text Society 46), ed. C. B. Hieatt and R. B. Jones, London: Anglo-Norman Text Society, 1990

La regola Salernitana, ed. A. Altamura, Naples: Società editrice napoletana, 1977

Langland, William, *Piers the Ploughman*, transl. and intro. J. F. Goodridge, Harmondsworth: Penguin, first published 1959, rev. edn, 1966

Leechdoms, Wortcunning and Starcraft of Early England, ed. T. O. Cockayne, 3 vols, *Rolls Series*, 1864–6

Libellus de Vita et Miraculis S. Godrici, Heremitæ de Finchale, auctore Reginaldo Monacho Dunelmensi, ed. J. Stevenson, *Surtees Society*, 20, 1845

The Life and Miracles of St William of Norwich by Thomas of Monmouth, ed. and transl. A. Jessop and M. R. James, Cambridge: Cambridge University Press, 1896

Marchant, Guy, *The Kalendar and Compost of Shepherds*, intro. G. C. Heseltine, London: P. Davies, 1931

Medizinische Kasuistik in den »Miracula Sancte Elyzabet«. Medizinhistorische Analyse und Übersetzung der Wunderprotokolle am Grab der Elisabeth von Thüringen (1207–1231), ed. Jürgen Jansen (Marburger Schriften zur Medizingeschichte Band 15), Frankfurt A. M., Bern and New York: Verlag Peter Lang, 1985

The Miracles of Our Lady of Rocamadour: Analysis and Translation, transl. Marcus Bull, Woodbridge, NJ: Boydell Press, 1999

'The miracles of St Ithamar', ed. and intro. Denis Bethell, *Analecta Bollandiana*, 89, 1971, pp. 421–37

'The miracles of the hand of St James', transl. and intro. Brian Kemp, *Berkshire Archaeological Journal*, 65, 1970, pp. 1–19

Orderic Vitalis, *The Ecclesiastical History of Orderic Vitalis*, ed. M. Chibnall, Oxford: Clarendon, 6 vols, 1969–80

Otto of Freising, *The Two Cities*, transl. and ed. C. C. Mierow A. P. Evans and C. Knapp, New York: Columbia University Press, 1966

Patrologia Latina, ed. J. P. Migne, 161 vols, Paris: Garnier, 1857–1939

Peter of Celle: Selected Works, ed. and transl. Hugh Feiss, Kalamazoo, MI: Cistercian Publications, 1987

The Prose Salernitan Questions: Edited from a Bodleian Manuscript (Auct. F. 3.10) (Auctores Britannici Medii Aevi V), ed. Brian Lawn, London: British Academy, 1979

The School of Salernum: Regimen Sanitatis Salernis, ed. John Harington, Salerno: Ente Provinciale per il Turismo, 1953

Soranus' Gynecology, transl. Owsei Temkin, Baltimore, MD and London: Johns Hopkins University Press, orig. pbl. 1956, rpt. 1991

Sources for the History of Medicine in Late Medieval England, transl. and ed. Carole Rawcliffe, Kalamazoo, MI: Medieval Institute Publications, 1995

The Surgery of Theoderic c.AD 1267, transl. E. Campbell and J. Colton, vol. I, New York: Appleton – Century – Crofts, 1955

William of Malmesbury, *De gestis regum Anglorum*, ed. W. Stubbs, *Rolls Series*, 90, 1887

Wolfram von Eschenbach, *Parzival*, transl. and ed. Wolfgang Spiewok, 2 vols, Stuttgart: Philipp Reclam, 1981

Secondary sources

Abberley, Paul, 'The concept of oppression and the development of a social theory of disability', *Disability, Handicap and Society*, 2 (1), 1987, pp. 5–19

Agrimini, Jole and Chiara Crisciani, 'Wohltätigkeit und Beistand in der mittelalterlichen christlichen Kultur', in: Mirko D. Grmek (ed.), *Die Geschichte des medizinischen Denkens. Antike und Mittelalter*, transl. C. Fiedler and S. Dietrich, Munich: C. H. Beck, 1996

Alexandre-Bidon, Danièle and Didier Lett, *Children in the Middle Ages: Fifth–Fifteenth Centuries*, transl. J. Gladding, Notre Dame: University of Notre Dame Press, 1999

Amundsen, Darrel W., *Medicine, Society, and Faith in the Ancient and Medieval Worlds*, Baltimore, MD and London: Johns Hopkins University Press, 1996

Amundsen, D. W. and G. B. Ferngren, 'The early Christian tradition', in: R. L. Numbers and D. W. Amundsen (eds), *Caring and Curing: Health and Medicine in the Western Religious Traditions*, New York and London: Collier Macmillan, 1986

Anderson, T. and A. R. Carter, 'An archaeological example of medieval trauma', *Journal of Palaeopathology*, 6, 1994

Angenendt, Arnold, ' "In meinem Fleisch werde ich Gott sehen." Bernward und die Reliquien', in exhibition catalogue: *Bernward von Hildesheim und das Zeitalter der Ottonen*, M. Brandt and A. Eggebrecht (eds), 1, Hildesheim and Mainz: Philipp von Zabern, 1993

——*Geschichte der Religiosität im Mittelalter*, Darmstadt: Wissenschaftliche Buchgesellschaft, 1997

Arano, L. C., *The Medieval Health Handbook: Tacuinum Sanitatis*, New York: George Braziller, 1976

Atkinson, Clarissa W., *The Oldest Vocation: Christian Motherhood in the Middle Ages*, Ithaca, NY and London: Cornell University Press, 1991

Auty, Robert (ed.), *Lexikon des Mittelalters*, 9 vols, Munich: Artemis Verlag, 1997–9

Baldwin, John H., *The Language of Sex: Five Voices from Northern France around 1200*, Chicago, IL and London: University of Chicago Press, 1994

Barber, Malcolm (ed.), *The Military Orders: Fighting for the Faith and Caring for the Sick*, Aldershot: Ashgate, 1994

Barnes, Colin, 'Theories of disability and the origins of the oppression of disabled people in western society', in: L. Barton (ed.), *Disability and Society: Emerging Issues and Insights*, London: Longman, 1996

Barnes, C. and G. Mercer (eds), *Exploring the Divide: Illness and Disability*, Leeds: Disability Press, 1996

Barnes, C., G. Mercer and T. Shakespeare, *Exploring Disability: A Sociological Introduction*, Cambridge, MA: Polity, 1999

Barton, L. (ed.), *Disability and Society: Emerging Issues and Insights*, London: Longman, 1996

Bassett, S. (ed.), *Death in Towns: Urban Responses to the Dying and the Dead, 100–1600*, Leicester: Leicester University Press, 1992

Beasley, A. W., 'Orthopaedic aspects of medieval medicine', *Journal of the Royal Society of Medicine*, 75, 1982, pp. 970–5

Benskin, M., 'For a wound in the head: a late medieval view of the brain', *Neuphilologische Mitteilungen*, 86 (2), 1985, pp. 199–215

Biller, Peter, 'Childbirth in the Middle Ages', *History Today*, 36 (8), 1986, pp. 42–9

—— 'Views of Jews from Paris around 1300: Christian or 'Scientific'?', in: D. Wood (ed.), *Christianity and Judaism* (Studies in Church History 29), Oxford: Blackwell, 1992

Biller, Peter and A. J. Minnis (eds), *Medieval Theology and the Natural Body* (York Studies in Medieval Theology 1), York: York Medieval Press, 1997

Biraben, Jean-Noël, 'Das medizinische Denken und die Krankheiten in Europa', in: Mirko D. Grmek (ed.), *Die Geschichte des medizinischen Denkens. Antike und Mittelalter*, transl. C. Fiedler and S. Dietrich, Munich: C. H. Beck, 1996

Bischoff, Bernard and Michael Lapidge, *Biblical Commentaries from the Canterbury School of Theodore and Hadrian* (Cambridge Studies in Anglo-Saxon England 10), Cambridge: Cambridge University Press, 1994

Bodine, Ann, 'Androcentrism in prescriptive grammar: singular "they," sex-indefinite "he," and "he or she" ', *Language in Society*, 4, 1975, rpt. in: D. Cameron (ed.), *The Feminist Critique of Language: A Reader*, London and New York: Routledge, 1990, pp. 166–86

Bonser, Wilfred, *The Medical Background of Anglo-Saxon England*, London: Wellcome Historical Medical Library, 1963

Boseley, Sarah, 'Cleft palates linked to pregnancy stress', *Guardian*, 8 September 2000

Boswell, D. M. and J. M. Wingrove (eds), *The Handicapped Person in the Community: A Reader and Sourcebook*, London: Tavistock Publications, 1974

Boswell, John, *The Kindness of Strangers: The Abandonment of Children in Western Europe from Late Antiquity to the Renaissance*, New York: Pantheon Books, 1988

Brandt, M. and A. Eggebrecht (eds), *Bernward von Hildesheim und das Zeitalter der Ottonen*, 2 vols, Hildesheim and Mainz, 1993

Bredberg, Elizabeth, 'Writing disability history: problems, perspectives and sources', *Disability and Society*, 14 (2), 1999, pp. 189–201

Brim, C. J., *Medicine in the Bible*, New York: Froben, 1936

Brindle, David, 'Study shows disabled prejudice', *Guardian*, 26 May 1998

Brody, S. N., *The Disease of the Soul: Leprosy in Medieval Literature*, Ithaca, NY: Cornell University Press, 1974

Brothwell, D. and A. T. Sandison (eds), *Diseases in Antiquity*, Springfield, MA: C. C. Thomas, 1967

Brown, Elizabeth A. R., 'The tyranny of a construct: feudalism and historians of Medieval Europe', in: Lester K. Little and Barbara H. Rosenwein (eds), *Debating the Middle Ages*, Malden and Oxford: Blackwell, 1998, pp. 148–69

Brown, Peter, *The Body and Society: Men, Women and Sexual Renunciation in Early Christianity*, London: Columbia University Press, 1989

Brundage, James A., *Law, Sex and Christian Society in Medieval Europe*, Chicago, IL: University of Chicago Press, 1987

Bull, Marcus, *The Miracles of Our Lady of Rocamadour: Analysis and Translation*, Woodbridge, NJ: Boydell Press, 1999

Bullough, Vern L., 'The development of medical guilds at Paris', *Medievalia et humanistica*, 12, 1958, pp. 34–40

——*Sexual Variance in Society and History*, New York, London, Sydney and Toronto: Wiley Interscience, 1976

Bullough, Vern L. and James A. Brundage, *Sexual Practices and the Medieval Church*, Buffalo, NY: Prometheus Books, 1982

Bunting, Madeleine, 'Wafer allergy bars priests', *Guardian*, 10 October 1995

Burnett, C. S. F., 'The Planets and the Development of the Embryo', in: Dunstan, G. R. (ed.), *The Human Embryo: Aristotle and the Arabic and European Traditions*, Exeter: University of Exeter Press, 1990, pp. 95–112

Bynum, Caroline Walker, *Holy Feast and Holy Fast: The Religious Significance of Food to Medieval Women*, Berkeley, Los Angeles, CA and London: University of California Press, 1987

——'The female body and religious practice in the later Middle Ages', in: Michel Feher (ed.), *Fragments for a History of the Human Body, Part One*, New York: Zone Books, 1989, pp. 161–219

——*Fragmentation and Redemption: Essays on Gender and the Human Body in Medieval Religion*, New York: Zone Books, 1992

——*The Resurrection of the Body in Western Christianity, 200–1336*, New York: Columbia University Press, 1995

—— 'Warum das ganze Theater mit dem Körper? Die Sicht einer Mediävistin', *Historische Anthropologie*, IV 1, 1996, pp. 1–33; published in English as 'Why all the fuss about the body? a medievalist's perspective', *Critical Inquiry*, 2, 1995, pp. 1–33

Cadden, Joan, *Meanings of Sex Difference in the Middle Ages: Medicine, Science, and Culture*, Cambridge: Cambridge University Press, 1993

Cameron, D. (ed.), *The Feminist Critique of Language: A Reader*, London and New York: Routledge, 1990

Cameron, M. L., *Anglo-Saxon Medicine*, Cambridge: Cambridge University Press, 1993

Campbell, Sheila, Bert Hall and David Klausner (eds), *Health, Disease and Healing in Medieval Culture*, Basingstoke and London: Macmillan, 1992

Centre Universitaire d'Etudes et de Recherches Médiévales d'Aix (eds), *Le beau et le laid au Moyen Âge* (Senefiance 43), Aix-en-Provence: CUER MA, 2000

Clarke, B., *Mental Disorder in Earlier Britain*, Cardiff: University of Wales Press, 1975

Coates, Alan, *English Medieval Books: The Reading Abbey Collections from Foundation to Dispersal*, Oxford: Clarendon, 1999

Cobban, Alan, *English University Life in the Middle Ages*, London: UCL Press, 1999

Cohen, Jeffrey Jerome, *Of Giants: Sex, Monsters, and the Middle Ages* (Medieval Cultures 17), Minneapolis, MN: University of Minnesota Press, 1999

——*Medieval Identity Machines* (Medieval Cultures 35), Minneapolis, MN: University of Minnesota Press, 2003

Daniels, Alison, 'Airline apology for bad form', *Guardian*, 30 July 1997

Davidson, F. (ed.), *The New Bible Commentary*, London: Intervarsity Fellowship, 2nd edn, 1954

De Mause, Lloyd (ed.), *The History of Childhood*, New York: Psychohistory Press, 1974

—— 'The Evolution of Childhood', in: Lloyd de Mause (ed.), *The History of Childhood*, New York: Psychohistory Press, 1974

De Moulin, D., *A History of Surgery with Emphasis on the Netherlands*, Dordrecht, Boston, MA and Lancaster: Nijhoff, 1988

Dinzelbacher, P., *Europa im Hochmittelalter 1050–1250. Eine Kultur- und Mentalitätsgeschichte*, Darmstadt: Primus Verlag, 2003

Dols, M. W., *Majnun: The Madman in Medieval Islamic Society*, Oxford: Oxford University Press, 1992

Douglas, Mary, *Purity and Danger: An Analysis of Concepts of Pollution and Taboo*, London: Routledge & Kegan Paul, 1966

Drogin, M., *Anathema! Medieval Scribes and the History of Book Curses*, Totowa and Montclair: O. Allanheld, 1983

Duffy, Eamon, 'Finding St Francis: early images, early lives', in: Peter Biller and A. J. Minnis (eds), *Medieval Theology and the Natural Body* (York Studies in Medieval Theology 1), York: York Medieval Press, 1997, pp. 193–236

Duft, J., *Notker der Arzt. Klostermedizin und Mönchsarzt im frühmittelalterlichen St. Gallen*, St. Gall: Fehr'sche Buchhandlung, 1972

Dunstan, G. R. (ed.), *The Human Embryo: Aristotle and the Arabic and European Traditions*, Exeter: University of Exeter Press, 1990

Eco, Umberto, 'Dreaming of the Middle Ages', in: Umberto (ed.), *Travels in Hyperreality*, transl. W. Weaver, London: Picador, 1987, pp. 61–72

—— *The Aesthetics of Thomas Aquinas*, London: Radius, 1988

—— *On Beauty*, transl. A. McEwen, London: Secker & Warburg, 2004

Edgington, Susan, 'Medical knowledge in the crusading armies: the evidence of Albert of Aachen and others', in: Malcolm Barber (ed.), *The Military Orders: Fighting for the Faith and Caring for the Sick*, Aldershot: Ashgate, 1994, pp. 320–6

—— 'Medical care in the hospital of St John in Jerusalem', in: H. Nicholson (ed.), *The Military Orders Volume 2: Welfare and Warfare*, Aldershot: Ashgate, 1998

Eldridge, M., *A History of the Treatment of Speech Disorders*, Edinburgh and London: E. & S. Livingstone, 1968

Elliott, Dyan, 'The physiology of rapture and female spirituality', in: Peter Biller and A. J. Minnis (eds), *Medieval Theology and the Natural Body* (York Studies in Medieval Theology 1), York: York Medieval Press, 1997

—— *Fallen Bodies: Pollution, Sexuality and Demonology in the Middle Ages*, Philadelphia, PA: University of Pennsylvania Press, 1999

Evans, M. L., 'Deaf and dumb in Ancient Greece', in: L. J. Davis (ed.), *The Disability Studies Reader*, New York and London: Routledge, 1997

Evans, R. J., *In Defence of History*, London: Granta, 1997

Fandrey, F., *Krüppel, Idioten, Irre. Zur Sozialgeschichte behinderter Menschen in Deutschland*, Stuttgart: Silberburg-Verlag, 1990

Farmer, D. H., *The Oxford Dictionary of Saints*, Oxford: Oxford University Press, 3rd edn, 1992

Farmer, Sharon, and Barbara H. Rosenwein (eds), *Monks and Nuns, Saints and Outcasts: Religion in Medieval Society*, Ithaca, NY and London: Cornell University Press, 2000

Feher, Michel (ed.), *Fragments for a History of the Human Body*, 3 parts, New York: Zone Books, 1989

Feldmann, H., *Die geschichtliche Entwicklung der Hörprüfungsmethoden*, Stuttgart: G. Thieme, 1960

Finkelstein, Vic, *Attitudes and Disabled People*, Geneva: World Health Organization, 1980

Finucane, Ronald C., *Miracles and Pilgrims: Popular Beliefs in Medieval England*, Basingstoke: Macmillan, first published 1977, new edn, 1995

——*The Rescue of the Innocents: Endangered Children in Medieval Miracles*, Basingstoke and London: Macmillan, 1997

Flint, Valerie I. J., 'The early medieval 'medicus', the saint – and the enchanter', *Social History of Medicine*, 2, 1989, pp. 127–45

——*The Rise of Magic in Early Medieval Europe*, Oxford: Oxford University Press, 1991

Frayling, C., *Strange Landscape: A Journey through the Middle Ages*, London: BBC Books, 1995

Frey, Emil F., 'Saints in medical history', *Clio Medica*, 14, 1979, pp. 35–70

Friedman, J. B., *The Monstrous Races in Medieval Art and Thought*, Cambridge, MA: Harvard University Press, 1981

Gans, Paul J., 'RE: Court Jester', mediev-l discussion group. Online posting of 18 February 1999. Available archives of discussion group at http: http://scholar.chem.nyu.edu/mediev-l/archives.html (accessed 12 April 2001)

García-Ballester, L., 'Introduction: practical medicine from Salerno to the Black Death', in: L. García-Ballester, R. French, J. Arrizabalaga and A. Cunningham (eds), *Practical Medicine from Salerno to the Black Death*, Cambridge: Cambridge University Press, 1994, pp. 1–29

García-Ballester, L., R. French, J. Arrizabalaga and A. Cunningham (eds), *Practical Medicine from Salerno to the Black Death*, Cambridge: Cambridge University Press, 1994

Garland, R., *The Eye of the Beholder*, London: Duckworth, 1995

Garrison, F. H., *History of Medicine*, Philadelphia, PA and London: W. B. Saunders, 2nd edn, 1929

Gask, G. E. (ed.), *Essays in the History of Medicine*, London: Butterworth & Co., 1950

Geller, Mark (University College London), 'Anatomy of Babylonian medicine', paper presented in the Department of Classics, University of Reading, February 1999

Getz, Faye, *Medicine in the English Middle Ages*, Princeton, NJ: Princeton University Press, 1998

Girard, René, *The Scapegoat*, transl. Y. Freccero, London: Athlone Press, 1986

Giuliani, L., 'Die seligen Krüppel. Zur Deutung von Mißgestalten in der hellenistischen Kleinkunst', *Archäologischer Anzeiger*, 1987, pp. 701–21

Gleeson, Brendan J., *Second Nature? The Socio-Spatial Production of Disability*, unpubl. PhD thesis, Melbourne, 1993

——'A geography for disabled people?', *Transactions of the Institute of British Geographers*, N.S. 21 (2), 1996, pp. 387–96

——'Disability studies: a historical materialist view', *Disability and Society*, 12 (2), 1997, pp. 179–202

Goffman, Erving, *Stigma: Notes on the Management of Spoiled Identity*, London: Penguin, 1968, rpt. 1990

Golledge, Reginald R., 'Geography and the disabled: a survey with special reference to the vision impaired and blind populations', *Transactions of the Institue of British Geographers*, N.S., 18, 1993, pp. 63–85

——'A response to Gleeson and Imrie', *Transactions of the Institute of British Geographers*, N.S., 21 (2), 1996, pp. 403–11

Goodich, Michael E., *From Birth to Old Age: The Human Life Cycle in Medieval Thought, 1250-1350*, Lanham, MD and London: University Press of America, 1989

—— *Violence and Miracle in the Fourteenth Century: Private Grief and Public Salvation*, Chicago, IL and London: University of Chicago Press, 1995

Goodrick, Edward W., and John R. Kohlenberger III, *The NIV Complete Concordance: The Complete Concordance to the New International Version*, London: Hodder and Stoughton, 1999

Gordon, Eleanora C., 'Child health in the Middle Ages as seen in the miracles of five English saints, AD 1150–1220', *Bulletin of the History of Medicine*, 60, 1986, pp. 502–22

Grattan, J. H. G. and C. Singer, *Anglo-Saxon Magic and Medicine Illustrated Specially from the Semi-Pagan Text 'Lacnunga'*, Oxford: Wellcome Historical Medical Museum, 1952

Gravitt, P., *Charity and Children in Renaissance Florence: The Ospedale degli Innocenti, 1410–1536*, Ann Arbor, MI: University of Michigan Press, 1990

Grmek, Mirko D. (ed.), *Die Geschichte des medizinischen Denkens. Antike und Mittelalter*, transl. C. Fiedler and S. Dietrich, Munich: C. H. Beck, 1996

Groebner, Valentin, *Defaced: The Visual Culture of Violence in the Late Middle Ages*, New York: Zone Books, 2004

Guthrie, D., *A History of Medicine*, London: Nelson, 1945

Hamilton, Bernard, 'The Cathars and Christian Perfection', in: Peter Biller and Barrie Dobson (eds), *The Medieval Church: Universities, Heresy, and the Religious Life. Essays in Honour of Gordon Leff*, Woodbridge: Boydell Press, 1999, pp. 5–23

Hand, Wayland D., 'Deformity, disease and physical ailment as divine retribution', in: Edith Ennen and Günter Wiegelmann (eds), *Festschrift Matthias Zender. Studien zu Volkskultur, Sprache und Landesgeschichte*, 1, Bonn: Ludwig Röhrscheid Verlag, 1972, pp. 519–25

—— *Magical Medicine: The Folkloric Component of Medicine in the Folk Belief, Custom, and Ritual of the Peoples of Europe and North America*, Berkeley, Los Angeles, CA and London: University of California Press, 1980

Handerson, H. E., *Gilbertus Anglicus: Medicine of the Thirteenth Century*, Cleveland, OH: Cleveland Medical Library Association, 1918

Harper-Bill, C. and R. Harvey (eds), *The Ideals and Practice of Medieval Knighthood II: Papers from the third Strawberry Hill conference 1986*, Woodbridge, NJ: Boydell Press, 1988

Hastings, James (ed.), *A Dictionary of the Bible*, 2 vols, Edinburgh: T. & T. Clark, 1900

Hauck, Karl, 'Gott als Arzt. Eine exemplarische Skizze mit Text- und Bildzeugnissen aus drei verschiedenen Religionen zu Phänomenen und Gebärden der Heilung', in: C. Meier and U. Ruberg (eds), *Text und Bild. Aspekte des Zusammenwirkens zweier Künste in Mittelalter und früher Neuzeit*, Wiesbaden: L. Reichert Verlag, 1980

Henderson, J., 'The Black Death in Florence: medical and communal responses', in: S. Bassett (ed.), *Death in Towns: Urban Responses to the Dying and the Dead, 100–1600*, Leicester: Leicester University Press, 1992, pp. 136–50

Herrmann, H., *Die Stellung unehelicher Kinder nach kanonischem Recht*, Amsterdam: Grüner, 1971

Herzlich, C. and J. Pierret, *Illness and Self in Society*, transl. E. Forster, Baltimore, MD: Johns Hopkins University Press, 1987

Hewson, M. Anthony, *Giles of Rome and the Medieval Theory of Conception: A Study of the De formatione corporis humani in utero*, London: Athlone Press, 1975

Hiestand, Rudolf, 'Kranker König – Kranker Bauer', in: Peter Wunderli (ed.), *Der kranke Mensch in Mittelalter und Renaissance* (Studia humaniora. Düsseldorfer Studien zu Mittelalter und Renaissance. Band 5), Düsseldorf: Droste Verlag, 1986, pp. 61–77

Holdsworth, C. and T. P. Wiseman (eds), *The Inheritance of Historiography 350–900*, Exeter: University of Exeter Press, 1986

Hölter, A., *Die Invaliden. Die vergessene Geschichte der Kriegskrüppel in der europäischen Literatur bis zum 19. Jahrhundert*, Stuttgart and Weimar: Metzler, 1995

Honecker, Martin, 'Christus medicus', in: Peter Wunderli (ed.), *Der kranke Mensch in Mittelalter und Renaissance* (Studia humaniora. Düsseldorfer Studien zu Mittelalter und Renaissance. Band 5), Düsseldorf: Droste Verlag, 1986, pp. 27–43

Howe, G. Melvyn, *People, Environment, Disease and Death: A Medical Geography of Britain through the Ages*, Cardiff: University of Wales Press, 1997

Huard, P. and M. D. Grmek, *Mille ans de chirurgie en occident: V^e–XVe siècles*, Paris: Dacosta, 1966

Huet, Marie-Hélène, *Monstrous Imagination*, Cambridge, MA and London: Harvard University Press, 1993

Hughes, Robert, *Heaven and Hell in Western Art*, London: Weidenfeld & Nicolson, 1968

Hughes, W. and K. Paterson, 'The social model of disability and the disappearing body: towards a sociology of impairment', *Disability and Society*, 12 (3), 1997, pp. 325–40

Huizinga, J., *The Waning of the Middle Ages*, transl. F. Hopman, Harmondsworth: Penguin, 1976

Hummel, Christine, *Das Kind und seine Krankheiten in der griechischen Medizin. Von Aretaios bis Johannes Aktuarios (1. bis 14. Jahrhundert)*, Frankfurt: Peter Lang, 1999

Husband, T (ed.), *The Wild Man: Medieval Myth and Symbolism*, New York: Metropolitan Museum of Art, 1980

Illich, Ivan, *Limits to Medicine. Medical Nemesis: The Expropriation of Health*, Harmondsworth: Penguin, 1977

Imrie, Rob, 'Ableist geographies, disablist spaces: towards a reconstruction of Golledge's "Geography and the disabled" ', *Transactions of the Institute of British Geographers*, N. S., 21 (2), 1996, pp. 397–403

Ingstad, Benedicte and Susan Reynolds Whyte (eds), *Disability and Culture*, Berkeley, Los Angeles, CA and London: University of California Press, 1995

Jacquart, Danielle and Claude Thomasset, *Sexuality and Medicine in the Middle Ages*, transl. M. Adamson, Cambridge: Polity, 1988

Jaeger, W., *Die Heilung des Blinden in der Kunst*, 2nd edn, Sigmaringen: Jan Thorbeke Verlag, 1976

James, Edward, 'A sense of wonder: Gregory of Tours, medicine and science', in: M. A. Meyers (ed.), *The Culture of Christendom: Essays in Medieval History in Commemoration of Denis L. T. Bethell*, London and Rio Grande: Hambledon Press, 1993, pp. 45–60

Jolly, Karen Louise, *Popular Religion in Late Saxon England: Elf Charms in Context*, Chapel Hill, NC and London: University of North Carolina Press, 1996

Kapani, Lakshmi, 'Notes on the Garbha-Upanishad', in: Feher, Michel (ed.), *Fragments for a History of the Human Body*, part three, New York: Zone Books, 1989

Kay, Sarah and Miri Rubin, *Framing Medieval Bodies*, Manchester and New York: Manchester University Press, 1994

Kealey, E. J., *Medieval Medicus: A Social History of Anglo-Norman Medicine*, Baltimore, MD: Johns Hopkins University Press, 1981

Kenny, Anthony, *Aquinas on Mind*, London: Routledge, 1994

Ketsch, P. and A. Kuhn (eds), *Frauen im Mittelalter: Band 1. Frauenarbeit im Mittelalter. Quellen und Materialien*, Düsseldorf: Schwann, 1983

Kieckhefer, Richard, *Magic in the Middle Ages*, Cambridge: Cambridge University Press, 1989

King, Helen, 'Making a man: becoming human in early Greek medicine', in: Dunstan, G. R. (ed.), *The Human Embryo: Aristotle and the Arabic and European Traditions*, Exeter: University of Exeter Press, 1990, pp. 10–19

Kleinschmidt, Harald, *Understanding the Middle Ages: The Transformation of Ideas and Attitudes in the Medieval World*, Woodbridge, NJ: Boydell, 2000

Knape, Joachim (Tübingen University), 'Historia: a medieval concept of knowledge?', paper presented at Leeds, International Medieval Congress, July 1998

Koelsch, F., *Beiträge zur Geschichte der Arbeitsmedizin* (Schriftenreihe der Bayerischen Landesärztekammer Bd. 8), Munich: Bayerische Landesärztekammer, 1967

Kotzur, H. J. (ed.), *Hildegard von Bingen 1098–1179*, Mainz: Philipp von Zabern, 1998

Koven, Seth, 'Remembering and dismemberment: crippled children, wounded soldiers, and the Great War in Great Britain', *American Historical Review*, 99 (4), 1994, pp. 1167–202

Krauss, H. and E. Uthemann, *Was Bilder erzählen. Die klassischen Geschichten aus Antike und Christentum in der abendländischen Malerei*, Munich: C. H. Beck, 1987

Kühnel, Harry (ed.), *Alltag im Spätmittelalter*, Graz, Vienna and Cologne: Edition Kaleidoskop, 1984

Kupfer, Marcia, *The Art of Healing: Painting for the Sick and the Sinner in a Medieval Town*, Pennsylvania, PA: Pennsylvania State University Press, 2003

Kurath, Hans (ed.) and Sherman M. Kuhn (associate ed.), *Middle English Dictionary*, Ann Arbor, MI: University of Michigan Press, 1954

Latham, R. E., *Revised Medieval Latin Word-List from British and Irish Sources*, London, 1965

Le Goff, Jacques, 'The framework of time and space', in: Jacques Le Goff (ed.) *Medieval Civilization*, Oxford: Blackwell, 1988, pp. 131–94

——*The Medieval Imagination*, transl. A. Goldhammer, Chicago, IL and London: University of Chicago Press, 1988

Le Vay, David, *The History of Orthopaedics: An Account of the Study and Practice of Orthopaedics from the Earliest Times to the Modern Era*, Cornforth and Park Ridge: Parthenon, 1990

Lecouteux, Claude, *Les nains et les elfes au moyen age*, Paris: Imago, 1988

Lemay, Helen Rodnite, 'Some thirteenth and fourteenth century lectures on female sexuality', *International Journal of Women's Studies*, 1 (4), 1978, pp. 391–400

——'Human sexuality in twelfth-through fifteenth-century scientific writings', in: Vern. L. Bullough and James Brundage (eds), *Sexual Practices and the Medieval Church*, Buffalo, NY: Prometheus Books, 1982, pp. 187–205

Lennon, Peter, '100 years of solitude', *Guardian*, 26 May 1999

Little, Lester K., and Barbara H. Rosenwein (eds), *Debating the Middle Ages*, Malden and Oxford: Blackwell, 1998

Longmore, P. K., 'Uncovering the hidden history of people with disabilities', *Reviews in American History*, 15, 1987, pp. 355–64

McCracken, Peggy, *The Curse of Eve, The Wound of the Hero: Blood, Gender, and Medieval Literature*, Philadelphia, PA: University of Pennsylvania Press, 2003

McCready, William D., *Miracles and the Venerable Bede*, Toronto: Pontifical Institute of Medieval Studies, 1994

McDougall, Ian, 'The third instrument of medicine: some accounts of surgery in medieval Iceland', in: Sheila Campbell, Bert Hall and David Klausner (eds), *Health, Disease and Healing in Medieval Culture*, Basingstoke and London: Macmillan, 1992

Mach, Johann, *Von Aussätzigen und Heiligen. Die Medizin in der mittelalterlichen Kunst Norddeutschlands*, Rostock: Konrad Reich Verlag, 1995

Mackelprang, R. W. and R. O. Salsgiver, 'People with disabilities and social work: historical and contemporary issues', *Social Work: Journal of the National Association of Social Workers*, 41 (1), 1996, pp. 7–14

McLaughlin, Mary M., 'Survivors and surrogates: children and parents from the ninth to the thirteenth centuries', in: De Mause, Lloyd (ed.), *The History of Childhood*, New York: Psychohistory Press, 1974, pp. 101–82

MacLehose, William F., 'Nurturing danger: high Medieval Medicine and the problem(s) of the child', in: John Carmi Parsons and Bonnie Wheeler (eds), *Medieval Mothering*, New York and London: Garland, 1996, pp. 3–24

McVaugh, M. R., *Medicine Before the Plague: Practitioners and Their Patients in the Crown of Aragon 1285–1345*, Cambridge: Cambridge University Press, 1993

Magdalino, P. (ed.), *The Perception of the Past in Twelfth-Century Europe*, London and Rio Grande: Hamledon Press, 1992

Maher, W. B. and B. Maher, 'The ship of fools: *Stultifera Navis* or *Ignis Fatuus?*', *American Psychologist*, 37 (7), 1982, pp. 756–61

Marks, Deborah, *Disability: Controversial Debates and Psychosocial Perspectives*, London and New York: Routledge, 1999

Mayr-Harting, Henry, 'Functions of a twelfth-century shrine: the miracles of St Frideswide', in: Henry Mayr-Harting and R. I. Moore (eds), *Studies in Medieval History Presented to R. C. H. Davis*, London: Hambledon Press, 1985

Mayr-Harting, Henry, and R. I. Moore (eds), *Studies in Medieval History Presented to R. C. H. Davis*, London: Hambledon Press, 1985

Meaney, Audrey L., 'The Anglo-Saxon view of illness', in: Sheila Campbell, Bert Hall and David Klausner (eds), *Health, Disease and Healing in Medieval Culture*, Basingstoke and London: Macmillan, 1992

Medvei, V. C. and J. L. Thornton, *The Royal Hospital of St Bartholomew, 1123–1973*, London: Royal Hospital of Saint Bartholomew, 1974

Meier, C. and U. Ruberg (eds), *Text und Bild. Aspekte des Zusammenwirkens zweier Künste in Mittelalter und früher Neuzeit*, Wiesbaden: L. Reichert Verlag, 1980

Mellinkoff, Ruth, *Outcasts: Signs of Otherness in Northern European Art of the Late Middle Ages*, 2 vols, Berkeley, Los Angeles, CA and Oxford: University of California Press, 1993

Merriam-Webster, *Merriam-Webster's Collegiate Dictionary*, Springfield, MA, 2004. Online. Available http://www.m-w.com (accessed 30 September 2004)

Metzler, Irina, 'Responses to physical impairment in Medieval Europe: between magic and medicine', *Medizin, Gesellschaft und Geschichte*, 18, 1999, pp. 9–35

Meyer, Heinz, 'Metaphern des Psaltertextes in den Illustrationen des Stuttgarter Bilderpsalters', in: C. Meier and U. Ruberg (eds), *Text und Bild. Aspekte des Zusammenwirkens zweier Künste in Mittelalter und früher Neuzeit*, Wiesbaden: L. Reichert Verlag, 1980

Michel, P., *Formosa deformitas. Bewältigungsformen des Hässlichen in mittelalterlicher Literatur*, Bonn: Bouvier, 1976

Michler, M., 'Die Krüppelleiden in 'De morbo sacro' und 'De articulis'', *Sudhoffs Archiv*, 45, 1961, pp. 303–28

Miles, M., 'Disability in an eastern religious context: historical perspectives', *Disability and Society*, 10 (1), 1995, pp. 49–69

Minois, Georges, *History of Old Age: From Antiquity to the Renaissance*, transl. S. H. Tenison, Cambridge and Oxford: Polity, 1989

Montserrat, Dominic (ed.), *Changing Bodies, Changing Meanings: Studies on the Human Body in Antiquity*, London and New York: Routledge, 1997

Müller, K. E., *Der Krüppel. Ethnologia passionis humanae*, Munich: C. H. Beck, 1996

Murphy, Robert, *The Body Silent*, London: Phoenix House, 1987

Neubert, Dieter and Günther Cloerkes, *Behinderung und Behinderte in verschiedenen Kulturen. Eine vergleichende Analyse ethnologischer Studien*, 2nd edn, Heidelberg: Edition Schindele, 1994

Nicholson, H. (ed.), *The Military Orders Volume 2: Welfare and Warfare*, Aldershot: Ashgate, 1998

Nilson, B., *Cathedral Shrines of Medieval England*, Woodbridge, NJ: Boydell Press, 1998

Noonan, J. T., *Contraception: A History of Its Treatment by the Catholic Theologians and Canonists*, Cambridge, MA: Harvard University Press, 1966

Norden, Martin F., *The Cinema of Isolation: A History of Physical Disability in the Movies*, New Brunswick, NJ: Rutgers University Press, 1994

Norri, J. *Names of Sickness in English, 1400–1550: An Exploration of the Lexical Field*, Helsinki: Academia Scientiarium Fennica, 1992

Nutton, V., 'Continuity or rediscovery? the city physician in Classical antiquity and medieval Italy', in: A. W. Russell (ed.), *The Town and State Physician in Europe from the Middle Ages to the Enlightenment* (Wolfenbütteler Forschungen Bd. 17), Wolfenbüttel: Herzog August Bibliothek, 1981, pp. 9–46

Ohry, A. and E. Dolev, 'Disabilities and handicapped people in the Bible', *Koroth*, 8 (5–6), 1982, pp. 63–7

Oliver, Mike, *The Politics of Disablement*, Basingstoke: Macmillan, 1990

——*Understanding Disability: From Theory to Practice*, Basingstoke: Macmillan, 1995

O'Neill, Ynez Violé, *Speech and Speech Disorders in Western Thought Before 1600* (Contributions in Medical History, Number 3), Westport, CT and London: Greenwood Press, 1980

Orchard, Bernard, Edmund F Sutcliffe, Reginald C. Fuller and Ralph Russell (eds), *A Catholic Commentary on Holy Scripture*, London: Nelson, 1953

Owst, G. R., *Literature and Pulpit in Medieval England: A Neglected Chapter in the History of English Letters and of the English People*, Oxford: Blackwell, 2nd edn, 1966

Park, K., *Doctors and Medicine in Early Renaissance Florence*, Princeton, NJ: Princeton University Press, 1985

Parsons, John Carmi and Bonnie Wheeler (eds), *Medieval Mothering*, New York and London: Garland, 1996

Paterson, Linda M., 'Military surgery: knights, sergeants and Raimon of Avignon's version of the *Chirurgia* of Roger of Salerno (1180–1209)', in: C. Harper-Bill and R. Harvey (eds), *The Ideals and Practice of Medieval Knighthood II: Papers from the third Strawberry Hill conference 1986*, Woodbridge, NJ: Boydell Press, 1988, pp. 117–46

Paton, Maureen, 'Hear me out', *Guardian*, 18 August 1998

Paxton, Frederick S., *Christianizing Death: The Creation of a Ritual Process in Early Medieval Europe*, Ithaca, NY and London: Cornell University Press, 1990

Payne, J. F., *English Medicine in Anglo-Saxon Times*, Oxford: Clarendon, 1904

Phillips, Anthony, *The Cambridge Bible Commentary: Deuteronomy*, Cambridge: Cambridge University Press, 1973

Pilsworth, Clare, 'Medicine, hagiography and manuscripts in Italy, *c.*800–*c.*1000', *Social History of Medicine*, 13 (2), 2000, pp. 253–64

Politzer, A., *A History of Otology*, transl. S. Milstein, C. Portnoff and A. Coleman from orig. German edition of 1907, I, Phoenix, AZ: Columella Press, 1981

Pool, Hannah, 'Zoo barred disabled "to spare the animals," ' *Guardian*, 6 July 1996

Porter, J. R., *The Cambridge Bible Commentary: Leviticus*, Cambridge: Cambridge University Press, 1976

Pouchelle, Marie-Christine, *The Body and Surgery in the Middle Ages*, transl. R. Morris, Cambridge: Polity, 1990

Price, B. B., 'The physical astronomy and astrology of Albertus Magnus', in: J. A. Weisheipl (ed.), *Albertus Magnus and the Sciences*, Toronto: Pontifical Institute of Medieval Studies, 1980

Prinz, Wolfram, 'Die Physiognomie', in: Wolfram Princy and Iris Marzik, *Die Storia oder die Kunst des Erzählens in der italienischen Malerei und Plastik des späten Mittelalters und der Frührenaissance 1260–1460*, Mainz: Philipp von Zabern, I, 2000

Rawcliffe, Carole, *Medicine and Society in Later Medieval England*, Stroud: Alan Sutton, 1995

Renger, J., 'Kranke, Krüppel, Debile – eine Randgruppe im Alten Orient?', in: Volker and Haas (eds), *Außenseiter und Randgruppen. Beiträge zu einer Sozialgeschichte des Alten Orients* (Xenia. Konstanzer althistorische Vorträge und Forschungen, Heft 32), Konstanz: Universitätsverlag, 1992, pp. 113–26

Richards, Peter, *The Medieval Leper and his Northern Heirs*, Cambridge: D. S. Brewer, 1977

Riddle, J. M., 'Theory and practice in Medieval medicine', *Viator*, 5, 1974, pp. 157–84

——'Ancient and Medieval chemotherapy for cancer', *Isis*, 76, 1985, pp. 319–30

Riley, J. C., 'Sickness in an early modern workplace', *Continuity and Change*, 2 (3), 1987, pp. 363–85

Roberts, Charlotte and Keith Manchester, *The Archaeology of Disease*, Stroud: Alan Sutton, 2nd edn, 1995

Rosen, G., *The History of Miners' Diseases*, New York: Schuman's, 1943

——*Madness in Society*, Chicago, IL and London: University of Chicago Press, 1968

Rosenthal, Joel T., *Old Age in Late Medieval England*, Philadelphia, PA: University of Pennsylvania Press, 1996

Roth, C., 'The qualification of Jewish physicians in the middle ages', *Speculum*, 28, 1953, pp. 834–43

Rubin, Miri, *Corpus Christi: The Eucharist in Late Medieval Culture*, Cambridge: Cambridge University Press, 1991

——'Medieval bodies: why now, and how?', in: Miri Rubin (ed.), *The Work of Jacques Le Goff and the Challenges of Medieval History*, Woodbridge, NJ: Boydell Press, 1997, pp. 209–17

Rubin, S., *Medieval English Medicine*, New York: Barnes and Noble, 1974

Russell, A. W. (ed.), *The Town and State Physician in Europe from the Middle Ages to the Enlightenment* (Wolfenbütteler Forschungen Bd. 17), Wolfenbüttel: Herzog August Bibliothek, 1981

Russell, Jeffrey Burton, *A History of Heaven: The Singing Silence*, Princeton, NJ: Princeton University Press, 1997

Russell, J. C., 'How many of the population were aged?' in: Michael M. Sheehan (ed.), *Aging and the Aged in Medieval Europe* (Papers in Medieval Studies 11), Toronto: Pontifical Institute of Medieval Studies, 1990, pp. 119–27

Schipperges, Heinrich, *Der Garten der Gesundheit. Medizin im Mittelalter*, Munich and Zurich: Artemis Verlag, 1985

——*Homo patiens. Zur Geschichte des kranken Menschen*, Munich and Zurich: Piper, 1985

——*Die Kranken im Mittelalter*, Munich: C. H. Beck, 3rd edn, 1993

Schlegel, K. F. (ed.), *Der Körperbehinderte in Mythologie und Kunst*, Stuttgart and New York: Thieme, 1983

Schmitt, Jean-Claude, *The Holy Greyhound: Guinefort, Healer of Children Since the Thirteenth Century*, transl. M. Thom, Cambridge and Paris: Cambridge University Press, 1983

Schreiner, Klaus and Norbert Schnitzler (eds), *Gepeinigt, begehrt vergessen: Symbolik und Sozialbezug des Körpers im späteten Mittelalter und in der frühen Neuzeit*, Munich: Wilhelm Fink Verlag, 1992

Scott, R. A., 'The construction of conceptions of stigma by professional experts', in: D. M. Boswell and J. M. Wingrove (eds), *The Handicapped Person in the Community: A Reader and Sourcebook*, London: Tavistock Publications, 1974

Seidler, Eduard, 'Historische Elemente des Umgangs mit Behinderung', in: U. Koch, G. Lucius-Hoene and R. Stegie (eds), *Handbuch der Rehabilitationspsychologie*, Berlin, Heidelberg, New York and London: Springer, 1988, pp. 3–20

Shahar, Shulamith, *Childhood in the Middle Ages*, transl. C. Galai, London and New York: Routledge, 1992

——*Growing Old in the Middle Ages: 'Winter Clothes Us in Shadow and Pain'*, London and New York: Routledge, 1997

Shearer, Ann, *Disability: Whose Handicap?*, Oxford: Blackwell, 1981

Sheehan, Michael M. (ed.), *Aging and the Aged in Medieval Europe* (Papers in Medieval Studies 11), Toronto: Pontifical Institute of Medieval Studies, 1990

Sheer, Jessica and Nora Groce, 'Impairment as a human constant: cross-cultural and historical perspectives on variation', *Journal of Social Studies*, 44 (1), 1988, pp. 23–37

Siebenthal, W. von, *Krankheit als Folge von Sünde. Eine medizinhistorische Untersuchung*, Hannover: Schmorl und von Seefeld, 1950

Sigal, Pierre-André, 'Maladie, pèlerinage et guérison au XIIe siècle. Les miracles de saint Gibrien à Reims', *Annales Économies, Sociétés, Civilisations*, 24 (6), 1969, pp. 1522–39

——*L'homme et le miracle dans la France médiévale (Xie–XIIe siècle)*, Paris: Éditions du Cerf, 1985

Siraisi, Nancy G., *Taddeo Alderotti and His Pupils: Two Generations of Italian Medical Learning*, Princeton, NJ: Princeton University Press, 1981

——*Medieval and Early Renaissance Medicine: An Introduction to Knowledge and Practice*, Chicago, IL and London: University of Chicago Press, 1990

——'How to write a Latin book on surgery: organizing principles and authorial devices in Guglielmo da Saliceto and Dino del Garbo' in: García-Ballester, L., R. French, J. Arrizabalaga and A. Cunningham, *Practical Medicine from Salerno to the Black Death*, Cambridge: Cambridge University Press, 1994, pp. 88–109

Skinner, Patricia, *Health and Medicine in Early Medieval Southern Italy*, Leiden, New York and Cologne: Brill, 1997

Solis-Cohen, Rosebud T., 'The exclusion of aliens from the United States for physical defects', *Bulletin of the History of Medicine*, 21, 1947, pp. 33–50

Spencer, B., *Pilgrim Souvenirs and Secular Badges* (Medieval Finds from Excavations in London: 7), London: The Stationery Office, 1998

Spencer, H. L., *English Preaching in the Late Middle Ages*, Oxford: Clarendon, 1993

Staff reporter, 'Cosmetic surgery for Down's children', *Guardian*, 5 June 1997

Stenek, N. H., 'Albert on the psychology of sense perception', in: J. A. Weisheipl (ed.), *Albertus Magnus and the Sciences*, Toronto: Pontifical Institute of Medieval Studies, 1980

Stiker, Henri-Jacques, *A History of Disability*, transl W. Sayers, Ann Arbor, MI: University of Michigan Press, 1999

Stone, Sharon Dale, 'The myth of bodily perfection', *Disability and Society*, 10 (4), 1995, pp. 413–24

Talbot, C. H. *Medicine in Medieval England*, London: Oldbourne, 1967

Talbot, C. H. and E. A. Hammond, *The Medical Practitioners in Medieval England: A Biographical Register*, London: Wellcome Historical Medical Library, 1965

Teleky, L., *History of Factory and Mine Hygiene*, New York: Columbia University Press, 1948

Temkin, Owsei, *The Falling Sickness: A History of Epilepsy from the Greeks to the Beginnings of Modern Neurology*, Baltimore, MD and London: Johns Hopkins University Press, 2nd rev. edn, 1971

Thorndike, Lynn, *A History of Magic and Experimental Science*, 8 vols, New York and London: Columbia University Press, 1923–58

Thurer, Shari, 'Disability and monstrosity: a look at literary distortions of handicapping conditions', *Rehabilitation Literature*, 41, 1980, pp. 12–15

Trüb, C. L. Paul, *Heilige und Krankheit* (Geschichte und Gesellschaft. Bochumer Historische Studien, Bd. 19), Stuttgart: Klett-Cotta, 1978

Tucker, M. J., 'The child as beginning and end: fifteenth and sixteenth century English childhood', in: Lloyd De Mause (ed.), *The History of Childhood*, New York: Psychohistory Press, 1974

University of Reading, Postgraduate Registration Form, Notes for Guidance, 1994

Van Dam, Raymond, *Leadership and Community in Late Antique Gaul*, Berkeley, Los Angeles, CA and London: University of California Press, 1985

——*Saints and their Miracles in Late Antique Gaul*, Princeton, NJ: Princeton University Press, 1993

Vauchez, André, *Sainthood in the Later Middle Ages*, transl. J. Birrell, Cambridge: Cambridge University Press, 1997

Vlahogiannis, N., 'Disabling bodies', in: Dominic Montserrat (ed.), *Changing Bodies, Changing Meanings: Studies on the Human Body in Antiquity*, London and New York: Routledge, 1997, pp. 13–36

Ward, Benedicta, *Miracles and the Medieval Mind: Theory, Record and Event 1000–1215*, Aldershot: Wildwood House, first published 1982, rev. edn, 1987

Watson, Frederick, *Civilization and the Cripple*, London: [s.n.] no publisher, 1930

Webb, E. A., *The Book of the Foundation of the Church of St Bartholomew, London*, Oxford: Oxford University Press, 1923

Weisheipl, J. A. (ed.), *Albertus Magnus and the Sciences*, Toronto: Pontifical Institute of Medieval Studies, 1980

Wells, Calvin, *Bones, Bodies and Disease*, London: Thames and Hudson, 1964

Werner, H., *Geschichte des Taubstummenproblems bis ins 17. Jahrhundert*, Jena: Gustav Fischer, 1932

Wilhelmy, W., 'Hildegards natur- und heilkundliches Schrifttum' in: H. J. Kotzur (ed.), *Hildegard von Bingen 1098–1179*, Mainz: Philipp von Zabern, 1998, pp. 284–303

——'Sexualität, Schwangerschaft und Geburt in den Schriften Hildegards von Bingen' in: H. J. Kotzur (ed.), *Hildegard von Bingen 1098–1179*, Mainz: Philipp von Zabern, 1998, pp. 334–41

Williams, David, *Deformed Discourse: The Function of the Monster in Mediaeval Thought and Literature*, Exeter: University of Exeter Press, 1996

Williams, G., 'Representing disability: some questions of phenomenology and politics', in: C. Barnes and G. Mercer (eds), *Exploring the Divide: Illness and Disability*, Leeds: Disability Press, 1996

Wisbey, Roy A., 'Die Darstellung des Häßlichen im Hoch- und Spätmittelalter', in: Wolfgang Harms and L. Peter Johnson (eds), *Deutsche Literatur des späten Mittelalters: Hamburger Colloquium 1973* (simultaneously published as *Publications of the Institute of Germanic Studies University of London*, vol. 22), Berlin: E. Schmidt, 1975, pp. 9–34

Wood, Charles T., 'The doctors' dilemma: sin, salvation, and the menstrual cycle in Medieval thought', *Speculum*, 56, 1981, pp. 710–27

Wortley, John, 'Three not-so-miraculous miracles', in: S. Campbell, B. Hall and D. Klausner (eds), *Health, Disease and Healing in Medieval Culture*, Basingstoke: Macmillan, 1992, pp. 159–68

Wunderli, Peter (ed.), *Der kranke Mensch in Mittelalter und Renaissance* (Studia humaniora. Düsseldorfer Studien zu Mittelalter und Renaissance. Band 5), Düsseldorf: Droste Verlag, 1986

Würtz, Hans, *Zerbrecht die Krücken. Krüppel-Probleme der Menschheit. Schicksalsstiefkinder aller Zeiten und Völker in Wort und Bild*, Leipzig: Leopold Voss, 1932

Young, Robert, *Analytical Concordance to the Bible*, London: Lutterworth Press, 6th edn, n.d. (after 1879)

Zimmermann, Volker, 'Die mittelalterliche Frakturbehandlung im Werk von Lanfrank und Guy de Chauliac', *Würzburger Medizinhistorische Mitteilungen*, 6, 1988, pp. 21–34

——'Zwischen Empirie und Magie: Die mittelalterliche Frakturbehandlung durch die Laienpraktiker', *Gesnerus*, 45, 1988, pp. 343–52

Ziolkowski, Jan, 'Avatars of ugliness in medieval literature', *The Modern Language Review*, 79, 1984, pp. 1–20

Index

Abberley, Paul 23
abbot 17, 141, 145, 147–8, 195, 213, 256
Achler, Elsbeth 48
Ada (in miracle) 210
Adwyn (carpenter) 106
Ælfric (abbot of Eynsham) 84, 137, 176, 180
aetiology 5–6, 32, 70–2, 74–5, 79, 93–4, 98, 123–4, 126, 140, 187–8
Agnes (in miracle) 214
Agricola 116, 117
ahistoricity of disability theories 9, 11, 21, 28, 36–7
Ailred of Rievaulx, Saint 47, 106
Alan of Lille 53
Alberti, Leon Battista 83
Albertus Magnus 54, 62, 66, 78, 80, 85, 87–8, 107, 188
Albucasis 103, 109–10, 113
Alderotti, Taddeo 77
Alditha (in miracle) 164, 208, 211
Alexander of Hales 50
Alexander of Tralles 74, 102
Alfred (king of England) 105
Alice of Essex (in miracle) 225
Alice of Schaerbeke 47
Alice of Stocking 95
Alpais of Cudot 48, 275 n.87
Ambrose of Milan, Saint 46
Amédée V (count of Savoy) 119
amputation 5, 55, 95, 114, 146, 154
Andrew, Saint 116, 228
Angenendt, Arnold 60
animals 3, 51, 53, 56, 78, 84, 88, 91–2, 107, 121, 128, 149, 170, 194, 201, 227
Anselm, Saint 56, 134–5, 152–3
Ansfrida (in miracle) 208
Anthony, Saint 148, 178, 217–18
anthropology 1–2, 17, 20, 23, 27–31, 35–6, 66, 108, 144, 153, 155, 157, 188

Apollonia, Saint 129
Apollonius of Citium 112
apoplexy 69, 74, 76, 79, 99
Archimataeus 75
Aretaios 73, 74
Aristotelianism 59, 80
Aristotle 78, 87
Arnald of Villanova 115
arthritis 47–8, 75, 77, 99, 108, 127, 181, 193, 208
Asa (biblical figure) 39
Asclepius 67
astrology 54, 83–5, 92, 95, 98, 123, 187
Augsburg 115
Augustine (bishop of Hippo), Saint 49–51, 56–8, 90, 136
Aurelianus, Saint 129
Avertin, Saint 129
Avicenna 80–1, 92, 101–2, 112

Balaam (biblical figure) 155, 206
Bald (physician) 103, 114
Baldwin (count of Flanders) 101
Baldwin (physician) 147
Bamberg 56
baptism 90
Baptista Trovamala de Salis 94
Barnes, Colin 35
Bartholomew (biblical figure) 138;
    see also Bartimaeus
Bartimaeus (biblical figure) 42, 272 n.40
Bartolomaeus Anglicus 66, 75, 93–4
beauty 48–54, 56–7, 63, 82, 91, 248
Bede: on miracles 45–6, 137, 141–2, 145
beggars 14, 18, 42, 113, 134, 145, 160, 165–7, 175, 193, 203, 245, 249; begging 151, 238
Benedict of Aniane, Saint 45
Benedict of Nursia, Saint 195
Bernard de Gordon 113

Bernard of Angers 132, 155, 194–6, 199
Bernarda (in miracle) 141
Bernardine, Saint 129
Berthold von Regensburg 88
Bertholdus (count) 77
Bethesda 42, 134
birth defects 80–1, 88–9, 94, 98, 198
bishop 40, 44, 104, 119, 127, 143, 145, 177, 196, 205
Blaise (Blasius), Saint 129
blind(ness) 4–5, 12, 17, 27, 29, 32, 38–46 *passim*, 53, 55–6, 62, 71, 78, 81, 87, 96–7, 101–2, 116, 129–30, 132–9, 142–5, 147–52, 155, 162, 167–8, 170–1, 175–8, 182, 192–3, 195–200, 202, 205, 208–13, 215–18, 220–2, 226–35 *passim*, 237–9, 241–2, 244–5, 250–8
Bologna 96, 118
Bonaventura Berlinghieri 138
Bonaventure of Bagnoregio, Saint 49, 58
Boniface, Saint 86
Bonser, Wilfred 122
Botilda (in miracle) 209
Bradwardyn, William (surgeon) 95
Brancus (in miracle) 224
Bredberg, Elizabeth 28
Bridget (Brigid, Bride), Saint 129
Brown, John (surgeon) 96
Brown, Peter 180
Bruges 108
Bull, Marcus 130, 134, 139–40
Bury St Edmunds 147, 210
Butler, Samuel 8
Bynum, Caroline Walker 18, 48, 58, 60, 62
Byzantium 14, 128

Caelius Aurelianus 74
Caesarius (bishop of Arles) 44–5
Cameron, M. L. 114
canon law 40–1, 45–7, 63, 67, 179
Canterbury 86, 107, 168, 177
Cantilupe, Thomas, Saint 152, 171, 177
Catharism 62, 64
Catherine of Siena 48
Celsus 97
Ceolnoth (archbishop of Canterbury) 107
charity 16–17, 26, 55, 118, 124, 153, 162, 165, 167–9, 185, 212, 235; charitable acts 106, 125, 168–9
Charlemagne 42
Chrétien de Troyes 53, 116

Christ 42, 45, 51, 55, 63, 67, 123, 133–9 *passim*, 150, 163, 170, 183, 187, 189, 198, 220, 228; *see also* Jesus
Cimabue 42
Claricia (in miracle) 143, 208
cleft palate 9
Cloerkes, Günther 5, 29, 31–3
clubfoot 5, 73, 105
Cohen, Beth 15
Cohen, Deborah 12
Colobern (in miracle) 208
Cologne 41, 80, 176
Combe, John 177
Compostela 129, 162, 177
conception 79, 81–2, 84–92, 98, 123
congenital impairment 1, 4, 15, 69, 71–2, 77–81, 84, 89–90, 92–3, 98, 102–3, 108, 123–4, 149–50, 154–5, 165–6, 172–3, 175, 178, 187–8, 234, 236, 238; *see also* birth defects
Conques 132, 148, 162, 167, 172, 194–205 *passim*
Constance 116, 191
Constantinus Africanus 83–4
Corneille, Saint 179
corporeality 60–2
Cosmas and Damian, Saints 128, 181
Creschas de Torre of Gerona 96
cripple 3–5, 7, 9, 12–14, 16–17, 21, 23, 29, 32, 42, 53–4, 82, 84, 88–9, 93, 106, 113, 125–6, 129–30, 136, 138, 143, 146, 148–9, 151, 156, 158, 161, 165–6, 168, 170–1, 173–4, 176, 180–1, 192, 194, 196, 210, 214, 217, 219, 222–4, 226, 237, 239, 245, 248–9, 257, 259
crutches 8, 13, 105, 150, 158–9, 169–70, 172–7, 182, 202, 214, 228, 230–1, 234, 236, 240–2, 244, 246, 248, 250, 252–3, 257
cultural concepts 1–10, 14–15, 17–19, 23–4, 26–30, 33, 35–8, 48, 55, 66, 80, 91, 128, 134, 153, 182–3, 185–9
Cuthbert, Saint 141–2
Cyprian, Saint 129

Dalton, John (barber) 95
Dan Michel 87
Dasen, V. 14
David (biblical figure) 39
De Beauvoir, Simone 21
deaf(ness) 4–5, 27, 32, 38–40, 42, 53, 74, 78, 87–8, 96–7, 102, 108, 123, 129–35 *passim*, 137–9, 155, 164, 166, 171,

176–7, 192–3, 196–8, 206, 208, 211,
   213, 218–19, 223, 227–34 *passim*, 237
deformity 13–15, 23, 40–1, 51, 55–8,
   93–4, 105–6, 199, 234, 255
Delumeau, Jean 16
Deschamps, Eustache 54
Devil 9, 48–9, 55, 138
disability studies 3, 11, 13, 16, 20, 22–4,
   27–8, 30, 32, 36–7, 43, 122, 140, 157,
   182–3, 186
disease 1, 4, 8, 13–14, 32, 41, 43–4, 46,
   48, 55, 57–8, 65, 67–9, 70–2, 74–6, 82,
   86, 89, 94–5, 98–9, 101–2, 106–8,
   115–17, 121, 126, 129, 130–1, 140,
   152, 163–4, 179–81, 183–4, 200, 213,
   216; *see also* illness; sickness
doctors 68, 70, 83, 94, 111, 117–19, 124,
   136, 140–1, 143–6 *passim*, 155, 157,
   197, 205–6, 209, 213, 216–17, 220–1,
   224, 232; *see also* physicians
Dolev, E. 39
Dorothy of Montau 47
Douglas, Mary 26
Downs, Laura Lee 27
dumb(ness) 3, 38–9, 74, 87, 104, 134–5,
   137–8, 143, 147–8, 166, 208, 210–11,
   213, 218–19, 224; *see also* mute(ness)
Dunstan, Saint 129
Dunwich (Suffolk) 106
dwarfism 14–15, 40–1, 57, 80–1
Dymphna, Saint 129

Eadmer 134, 152
Eco, Umberto 49, 188
Edmund (king of England)147
Edward I (king of England) 119
Edward the Confessor, Saint 147
Edwards, M. L. 15
elderly 27, 107, 143, 163, 174, 179, 232
Eli (biblical figure) 39
Elisabeth of Hungary, Saint 128, 132,
   136, 143, 147, 150, 153–4, 157–9, 163,
   166, 168–70, 173–5, 177–8, 182–3,
   235–59 *passim*
embryology 73, 81, 83–4
emic approach 9, 10, 34–5, 127, 186, 188
Ephraim 57
epilepsy 6, 69, 74, 79, 89, 99, 129–30,
   132–3, 144, 148, 156, 163, 215, 221,
   227–8, 238, 256; epileptic 4, 32, 82–3,
   224, 232–3, 237, 241, 243–4, 246,
   250–1, 255–6
Erasmus, Saint 129
ergotism 71, 179, 218

Ermarth, Elizabeth Deeds 19
etic approach 9, 10, 33, 34–5, 127,
   186, 188
Evesham 171

Faber, Felix 177
Farfa (Latium, Italy) 115
Fiacre, Saint 129
Finchale 177, 227–8, 233
Finkelstein, Vic 24
Finucane, Ronald 70, 126–7, 132, 145,
   149, 151–2, 157–8, 163, 166, 168–72
   passim, 174, 179, 181–2
Flint, Valerie 142
Flordon (England) 210
Florence 42, 97, 117–18
foetus 73, 80, 82–4, 86, 91–2, 124
food 92, 98, 123, 152, 160, 166–9, 182,
   196, 198, 204, 212, 214, 219–20, 232
Foucault, Michel 18, 24, 28
Fourth Lateran Council (1215) 46, 63, 67
Foy (Faith), Saint 131–2, 136, 146–8,
   150–1, 155–6, 158, 162–4, 166–8,
   170–1, 175, 178, 194–205 *passim*
fractures 33, 69, 96, 98, 100, 105–6,
   108–15, 117–18, 122, 124, 130–1,
   187, 238
Francis of Assisi, Saint 137, 138
François de Guise 174
Frankfurt 166, 245
Frederick II (emperor) 121
Frederick III (emperor) 114
Frideswide, Saint 162, 179–80

Galen 72, 74–5, 78, 104–5, 138
Gallus, Saint 131, 176, 191
Gallus of Clermont, Saint 176
Garland, Robert 15
Geert Grote 101
Gentile da Foligno 99
Gerald (in miracle) 156, 195, 223
Gerard of Cremona 101
Gerbert (in miracle) 147, 175, 195, 197
Gerbert of Creysse (in miracle) 167,
   170, 219
Gerona (Spain) 96
Gertrude of Helfta 47
Getz, Faye 124
giant 39; gargantuan 78
Gibrien, Saint 130, 131
Gilbert (in miracle) 143, 147, 162,
   167, 226
Gilbert of Sempringham 129
Gilbertus Anglicus 76, 79, 102, 109, 124

Giles, Saint 129
Giles of Rome 80, 91–2
Gilliva (in miracle) 176, 212
Girard, Réné 23
Giuliani, Luca 14
Gleeson, Brendan 24–6, 36, 157
God 9, 32, 40–1, 46–50 *passim*, 52–3,
    56–7, 62, 85, 87, 89–90, 92, 102, 120,
    134, 136–8 *passim*, 146, 155, 164, 166,
    188–9, 191, 196, 198, 207, 217, 221,
    223, 235, 245
Goda (in miracle) 211
Godfrey (in miracle) 144
Godfrey (son of count Hartman, in
    miracle) 158, 222
Godiva (in miracle) 209
Godric, Saint 132, 136, 138, 143, 147,
    150–1, 157–9, 165, 171, 173–7 *passim*,
    227–35 *passim*
Godric of Wortham (in miracle) 213
Goffman, Erving 22–3, 36–7
Goldeburga (in miracle) 209
Golledge, Reginald 24
Goodich, Michael 126
Gordon, Eleanora 126
Goslar 116–17
Göttingen 93
gout 69–70, 75–6, 81, 87, 105, 116, 137,
    160, 161, 208, 209, 214, 228–9
Gozbert (deacon) 191
Gozmar (in miracle) 166, 201
Gratian 86
Greer, Phil 8
Gregory IX (pope) 40, 46
Gregory of Tours 89, 126, 131, 142,
    147, 149, 176
Gregory the Great (pope) 57
Grenoble 224
Groce, Nora 27
Gudmundr Arason of Hólar (bishop)
    145–6
Guibert (in miracle) 146, 148, 195, 196
Guillelma (in miracle) 143, 224
Guillem Guerau (surgeon) 96
Guimerra, Saint 116
Guinefort, Saint 121
Gurevich, Aaron 28
Gurwan (in miracle) 167, 209
Guthlac, Saint 107
Guy de Chauliac 70, 75–6, 81, 100, 102,
    112–14, 119, 124

Haggard, H. W. 12
Haj, Fareed 15

Halligan, Peter 181
Haly Abbas 92
Hans Seyff of Göppingen 114
Harding, Snowy 7
harelip 5, 103–4
Harvey de Cornubia 119
Harwe, John (surgeon) 95
Hathewis (in miracle) 215
Hathvidis (in miracle) 217
hearing impairment 155, 166
Heinrich von Pfolspeundt 102
hemiplegia 107, 131
Henri de Mondeville 52, 72, 98, 107,
    114, 188
Henri de Saalma 179
Henry II (king of England) 219
Henry V (king of England) 95, 118
Hereford 170, 171, 177
Heribald (abbot of Tynemouth) 145
Herman of Reun 58
Herzlich, C. 7
Hiestand, Rudolf 163
Hilarius of Passau 114
Hilary of Poitiers 103
Hildegard of Bingen 59, 76, 78, 81,
    85, 102
Hippocrates 70, 105
historiography 9, 11–13, 18–20, 36, 186
Hoddle, Glen 8
hospital 2, 5, 93, 97, 101, 106, 167,
    178–9, 221, 232, 246, 249, 256
Howe, G. Melvyn 14
Huelina of Rochesburch (in miracle)
    154, 215
Huga (in miracle) 218
Hugh (master mason, in miracle) 150, 203
Hugh le Barber 177
Hugh of St Victor 52, 58
Hughes, W. 21
Humbert (in miracle) 155, 167,
    172, 202
humoral theories 69, 74–8, 81–2, 84, 91,
    96, 100, 108, 123, 187, 224
hunchback 5, 73, 75, 237, 251; hump
    (back) 154, 171, 174, 180, 208, 213,
    231, 241–3, 249–51, 253, 255–6
hydrocephalus 73, 93, 100–1

iatrogenic disorders 70, 94–7, 124
Ida (in miracle) 208
Idensen (Lower Saxony) 42
identity 7, 22, 26–7, 30, 35–6, 48, 59–62,
    63–4, 187
Illich, Ivan 32

illness 1, 6–7, 13–14, 17, 19, 30–1, 36, 39,
    42–8, 61, 63, 65, 67–8, 71, 77, 90, 106,
    108, 117, 121, 126–7, 129, 130, 134,
    140, 144–7, 149, 151, 156–8, 161, 163,
    181–3, 187, 194, 199, 200, 205–6, 208,
    213, 221–2, 224, 227, 231–4, 239,
    241–2, 247–8, 251; chronic 5–6, 65,
    129, 157; *see also* disease; sickness
imagination 12, 78, 127, 54; maternal
    90–3, 124, 187
incurability 41, 69–70, 79, 81, 94–5,
    102, 107, 123, 135–7, 139–40,
    143–5, 155–6, 159, 162, 164, 183,
    187, 194, 198, 219, 222, 226, 231,
    233, 249, 255
Ingstad, Benedicte 30
Ingulf 106–7
Innocent III (Lothario dei Segni, pope) 86
insanity 51, 83, 129, 132–3, 138, 227,
    229–33, 240, 255
institutions for disabled 1, 7, 12–13, 24,
    28, 31, 41, 167; institutionalisation of
    disabled 7, 12, 18, 66
Isidore of Seville 19, 69, 76, 79
Iso of St Gall 191
Ithamar, Saint 132, 136, 147, 155, 166,
    176, 205–7 *passim*

Jacob (biblical figure) 91–2
Jacques de Vitry 151–2, 181
James (apostle), Saint 132, 143, 147, 154,
    161–2, 167, 171, 175, 179, 200, 205,
    224–227 *passim*
Jeroboam (biblical figure) 39
Jerome, Saint 86
Jerusalem 5, 39, 158, 178, 221, 223
Jesus 38, 41–4, 134; *see also* Christ
Jews 17, 40, 58, 62, 142, 207
Job (biblical figure) 46
John (apostle), Saint 137
John (clerk, in miracle) 154, 224
John Duns Scotus 87
John Gori of San Gimignano 93
John of Beverley (bishop of Hexham),
    Saint 104, 145
John of Cornhill (surgeon) 95
John of Gaddesden 75, 107
John of Rupescissa 99
John of Salisbury 51–2
John of Trevisa 94
John Scotus Erigena 50, 58
John the Baptist 221
Julian of Norwich 47
Juliana (in miracle) 166, 219

Keach, Stacy 9
Kingesbyry (England) 107
Klapisch, Christiane 89
Kleinschmidt, Harald 189
Konrad von Eichstätt 79
Koven, Seth 12

Laban (biblical figure) 91–2
lame(ness) 5, 39–40, 42, 46, 56–7, 71, 74,
    76–7, 81, 83, 87–8, 109, 116, 121, 126,
    129, 131, 133–5, 137–8, 143, 151, 154,
    158–9, 162, 166, 168, 170–1, 173–6,
    178, 193–4, 196–7, 202–4, 208, 213,
    225, 228, 232, 234, 237, 239, 240,
    244–53 *passim*, 257
Lanfranc of Milan 100, 102, 112, 114
Lawrence, Saint 129
Lazarus (biblical figure) 135
Le Goff, Jacques 25, 35
Leofstan (abbot of Bury) 147
Leonides 73, 100
leprosy 1, 5, 14, 17, 70, 89, 151, 179, 232,
    261 n.16; leper 137; leprous 48, 83,
    87–8, 137, 233
Leunast of Burges (archdeacon) 142
Lille 179
Limburg 246
liminality 1, 31–2, 35, 37, 68, 108, 153,
    155–7, 163, 184, 188
limp 110, 112; limp limbs 111
Lindisfarne 141–2
Linz (Austria) 114
London 7, 96, 106, 171
Longmore, P. K. 43
Lot (biblical figure) 38
Lothario dei Segni (Innocent III, pope) 86
Louis IX (king of France), Saint
    128, 158
Louvain 41
Lucia (Lucy), Saint 129
Luther, Martin 55

Mackelprang, R. W. 43
macrocosm 51–2, 63; *see also* microcosm
McVaugh, Michael 66, 68
mad(ness) 18, 23, 86, 130–1, 137–8, 140,
    143, 148, 197, 208, 216, 218, 225, 228,
    232; *see also* mental illness
Marburg 177, 182, 235
Marchant, Guy 54
Margaret of Ypres 47
Marie de France 90
Mark, Deborah 13
Martin, Saint 89, 131, 142, 249

martyrs 46, 56–8, 61, 63, 153, 194, 204, 208, 219
Marx, Karl Friedrich Heinrich 93
Mary (Virgin, Our Lady) 132, 134, 141, 143, 146–8, 151, 163, 168, 178, 215–24 *passim*
Mary Magdalen, Saint 138
Masaccio 42
Masolino 42
Mathilda (in miracle) 162
Matilda (in miracle) 154, 169–72, 178, 212
Matteuccia Fransisci of Todi 121
Matthew of Vendôme 53
Maurus (in miracle) 192
Mayr-Harting, Henry 180
Meletius 74
Melinkoff, Ruth 55
Melksham 145
menstruation 11, 86–90, 98, 123
mental illness 6, 13, 242, 261 n.17; *see also* mad(ness)
mental impairment 3, 12, 16, 27, 71
mentality 16–17, 67, 72
Mephibosheth (biblical figure) 39
Meriadocus, Saint 129
Meschede 42
Mesue (John Damascene) 102
Michael Psellos 109
Michael Scot 121
Michler, M. 15
microcosm 51–2, 63; *see also* macrocosm
Milan 46, 224
Miles, M. 16
mobility of the impaired 4, 22, 55, 71, 110–11, 124, 127, 132–3, 140, 153, 158–9, 161, 165, 169–78 *passim*, 182–5, 188, 227, 256
monks 58, 74, 78, 106, 141, 147–8, 158, 164, 170, 191, 194–5, 200–1, 205, 207, 209, 221, 223, 225, 228, 230, 232, 255
monster 5, 15–16, 49–50, 53, 57, 80, 92, 122, 154, 175, 220, 251, 255, 270 n.143, 276 n.103, 280 n.168
Montpellier 82, 146, 222
Morestede, Thomas (surgeon) 118
Moses (biblical figure) 38, 40
Murphy, Robert 31
muscular dystrophy 7
mute(ness) 3–4, 42, 76, 78, 84, 97–8, 102, 130–3, 135, 137, 155, 162, 166, 168, 176, 192–4, 196–8, 201, 206–7, 210–11, 215–16, 218–20, 227, 230–1, 233–5, 237–8, 241, 248, 253; *see also* dumb(ness)

Neubert, Dieter 5, 29–33
Niccolò d'Este of Ferrara 77
Nicholas of Bari, Saint 116, 178, 239
Nider, Johannes 54
Ninove (Belgium) 179
Norwich 25, 92, 132, 147, 154, 165, 169, 171–4, 176–8, 207–15 *passim*

occupational disorders 115–17, 120, 124, 238
Ogden, Daniel 15
Ohry, A. 39
old age 6, 15–16, 39, 53, 56, 76, 84, 99, 108, 125, 136, 158, 160, 164, 168, 170, 174, 177, 197, 198, 203–4, 227, 236, 238, 257, 261 n.20
Oliver, Mike 23, 25–6
Øm (Denmark) 101
Orderic Vitalis 101
Oribasius 73, 100
Orléans 171, 194
orthopaedic impairment 5, 12–13, 15, 42, 84, 104, 108, 124, 154, 165–6, 169, 172–4, 176, 183, 235–8
Osmund (bishop of Salisbury), Saint 129, 177
Osyth, Saint 147
Otmar, Saint 131, 145, 191, 194
Otto of Freising 19, 57–8
Oxford 41, 152, 162, 171, 179–80, 227

palsy 4, 42, 75–6, 96, 107, 213
Paracelsus 116, 117
paralysed limbs 48, 76, 104, 106–7, 126, 145, 148–9, 152–4, 161, 163, 167–8, 170, 174, 181, 198, 200–2, 216, 220–1, 223, 226, 228–30, 243–4, 252
paralysis 5, 7, 69, 73–7 *passim*, 79, 82, 99, 106–7, 110, 123, 127, 129–31 *passim*, 133, 141, 143–4, 146–7, 156, 159, 163, 181, 207, 215, 222, 224, 236–7
Paris 128, 170
Paschors of Romans (in miracle) 218
Paterson, Linda 118–19
Patterson, K. 21
Paul (apostle), Saint 42, 134, 203
Paul of Aegina 73–4, 100, 115
Paulinus 46
Pavia 45, 219
Paxton, Frederick S. 45
Périgueux 166
Pescia 138
Peter (apostle), Saint 42, 56, 137, 203, 239
Peter (priest of Langham) 169, 212

Peter Lombard 58
Peter of Celle 47
Peter of Eboli 105
Peter of Luxemborg (cardinal) 131
Philip (apostle), Saint 42
physicians 35, 39, 47–8, 67–70, 74,
    79–80, 87, 93–5, 97, 99–102 *passim*,
    107, 109–10, 115, 118–21, 123, 135–6,
    138–47, 162, 167, 179–80, 183, 203–4,
    206, 208, 218, 221–3, 226, 235, 249,
    256–8; *see also* doctors
physiognomy 53–5, 63, 70, 278 n.140
Pierret, J. 7
pilgrimage 127, 141, 143–6, 149, 169–73
    passim, 177–8, 194–5, 216–17, 221–3
pilgrims 74, 113, 126, 129, 131, 139,
    142–3, 148, 151–4, 158, 162–3,
    165, 167–8, 176, 180–2, 185, 187,
    200, 216, 218–20, 236–8; pilgrim
    souvenirs 177
Pilsworthy, Clare 46
Pipping (Bavaria) 177
plague 1, 14, 39, 129
planets 83–5, 90, 123
plants 86, 92–3, 109, 120–1
Pliny 107
Poitou 131
Polilia (in miracle) 166, 219
postmodernism 18–19, 24
poverty 6, 11, 16–17, 19–20, 36, 39, 58,
    82, 99, 117–18, 153, 160, 162, 164–70,
    173, 196, 203, 206, 209–11, 213, 219,
    220, 226, 235
pregnancy 8, 12, 83, 88, 91–3, 98,
    122, 188
priest 35, 40–1, 43, 57, 67–8, 96, 136–7,
    145, 151–2, 169, 172, 178, 206–7, 212,
    215, 230, 233, 247, 274 n.77; priestly
    63, 189
progressionist view 11–12, 28, 36
psychogenic 181
psychosomatic 59–60, 180–1, 185

Raimon of Avignon 100, 101, 109, 119
Ralph (bishop of Chichester) 119
Raphael (archangel) 129
Ravenilda (in miracle) 176, 210
Raymond (in miracle) 162, 198, 223
Raymond of Penyafort 87
Reading 132, 154, 158, 161–2, 171,
    178–9, 224–7
Reginald of Durham 227
Reimbert (in miracle) 213
Reinfroi (lord, in miracle) 200

relics 107, 129, 141–5, 147, 151–2, 158,
    177–9, 181, 189–90, 194, 196–7,
    203–4, 225, 235
Renald Belloz (in miracle) 222
Renger, Johannes 16
resurrection 56–64, 232, 240
Revesby (England) 106
Rhabanus Maurus 50
Rhazes 92
Ricardus Anglicus (Ricardus Salernus)
    69, 70
Richard III (king of England) 55
Richard de Belmeis (bishop of
    London) 147
Richard of St Victor 58
Rigaud (in miracle) 163, 201
Riley, J. C. 21
Robert (count of Meulan) 143, 216
Robert (in miracle) 200, 217
Robert (lord, in miracle) 147
Robert of Flamborough 88
Rocamadour 134, 139, 140–1, 144,
    148–9, 151, 154, 156, 163, 166–70,
    177–8, 182, 215–24 *passim*
Roch, Saint 129
Rochester 132, 205
Rodez 196
Roesslin, Eucharius 94
Roger (in miracle) 209
Roger of Salerno (Ruggiero Frugardi)
    100, 101, 109, 119
Rolf, Simon (barber) 95
Rome 171, 178, 194, 199
Rosen, George 116–17
Rubin, Miri 35
Rubin, S. 106
Rufinus 86

Saint-Gilles (Provence, France) 129
Saint-Wandrille (France) 131
Salisbury 25, 177
Salsgiver, R. O. 43
Salzburg 115, 122
Samson of Old Sarum 168
San Baudelio de Berlanga (Soria, Spain) 41
Sankt Gallen (St Gall) 46, 131, 145, 171,
    178, 191–4 *passim*
Schett (in miracle) 213
Schmitt, Jean-Claude 122
Scholasticism 2, 66, 71, 87
Sebastian, Saint 129
Senorez (knight, in miracle) 223
senses 79, 81, 99, 103, 138, 154, 197,
    219–20, 240

Serafina of San Gimignano 7
Shahar, Shulamith 45
Shakespeare, Tom 23, 26
Shakespeare, William 55, 90
Shearer, Ann 22, 29
Sheer, Jessica 27
shrines 70, 74, 127–9, 131, 133, 139,
    142–5, 147, 149, 151, 153, 161–3, 165,
    167, 171–2, 175–81, 184–5, 187, 202,
    205, 212, 223, 225–6
sickness 5, 8, 23, 35, 39, 44–5, 47–9, 65,
    67, 70, 75, 81, 87, 102, 126, 192, 221,
    224, 236; *see also* disease; illness
Siena 117
Sigal, Pierre-André: on miracles 130–3
Siger (in miracle) 157, 200
Silvanus of Levroux, Saint 179
sin 1, 8, 13, 26, 32, 38–9, 41–7, 48–9, 55,
    62–3, 67–8, 87–90, 94, 123, 134–5,
    146, 150–1, 165, 184, 187–8, 195, 198,
    217, 235
Siraisi, Nancy 119
Siwate (in miracle) 174, 210
Skinner, Patricia 89
sociology 1–2, 20, 27, 65
Soranus 91
soul 14, 19, 38–9, 47, 49, 51–4, 57–61,
    62–4, 76, 80, 84, 91, 93, 103, 137, 146
spectacular healing 127, 161, 180, 199
speech impairment 15, 52, 97, 104, 152,
    154, 166, 168, 181–2
Stephana (in miracle) 144, 154, 169, 220
Stephen (in miracle) 197
Stephen of Bourbon 122
stereotype 3, 6, 9, 12–13, 15, 18, 26, 43,
    53–5, 130, 133, 182–3, 198
stigma 22–3, 37
Stiker, Henri-Jacques 16, 31
surgeons 69, 72, 94–8 *passim*, 101–
    108–12 *passim*, 114, 118–20, 123
    139, 141, 145, 180, 183, 188
surgery 6, 66, 68, 70, 96–7, 99–100
    102–4, 108–9, 112, 114–15, 118, 1...,
    123, 128, 145
swaddling: of infants 73, 94, 124
Swithun, Saint 176, 180

Talizat 170
Tanavelle 203
terminology 3–4, 20, 76, 131, 139,
    179, 224
Tertullian 57
Theoderic (Theoderico Borgognoni): on
    surgery 110–12, 124

Theodore of Tarsus 86
Theophilus 55
therapeutic: measures 1, 70–1, 74, 97–9,
    104–5, 107; miracles 125, 129–30, 135,
    183–5, 187
therapies 66, 78, 94, 96, 102, 104–6, 112,
    114, 121–2, 124–5, 145, 180, 183, 187;
    alternative 65, 121
Thomas (apostle), Saint 129
Thomas Aquinas, Saint 50, 51, 59, 61,
    62, 87
Thomas Becket, Saint 152, 168
Thomas of Cantimpré 66, 107
Thomas of Celano 137
Thomas of Froidmont 52, 277 n.119
Thomas of Monmouth 132, 207, 211–12
Thomas of York, in miracle 172, 214
Thurer, Shari 43
Thurstan 147
Tobit (biblical figure) 129
Tommaso del Garbo 71
tongue string: cutting of 97–8, 123
transcendence: of nature 35, 127,
    135–6, 183
transference: of illness 121–2, 177,
    328 n.461
Triduana, Saint 129
Tynemouth 145

ugliness 15, 48–55, 57, 63, 82, 92,
    95, 164
Ugo of Lucca 118
Ugo of Siena 77–8
Ulrich Ellenbog 115
Ulrich Engelberti of Strasbourg 51,
    276 n...
unive... 65–6, 68, 71
...nd 126, 149
...126, 141; on miracles
...iana de' Botti 47
Vincent of Beauvais 66, 91–2
visual impairment 35, 79, 102, 160, 163,
    172, 174–6
Vlahogiannis, Nicholas 15
Voerda, Nicasius 41
votive offering 49, 153, 176–7, 185,
    223, 250
Vulfran, Saint 131

Walahfrid Strabo 191
Walstan, Saint 116